PRACTICING PREVENTION FOR THE ELDERLY

RISA LAVIZZO-MOUREY
SUSAN C. DAY
DEBORAH DISERENS
JEANE ANN GRISSO

HANLEY & BELFUS, INC. / Philadelphia
The C.V. Mosby Company / St. Louis • Toronto • London

Publisher: HANLEY & BELFUS, INC.
                  210 South 13th Street
                  Philadelphia, PA 19107

North American and worldwide sales and distribution:
                  THE C.V. MOSBY COMPANY
                  11830 Westline Industrial Drive
                  St. Louis, MO 63146

In Canada: THE C.V. MOSBY COMPANY
                  5240 Finch Avenue East
                  Unit 1
                  Scarborough, Ontario M1S 4P2

PRACTICING PREVENTION FOR THE ELDERLY   ISBN 0-932883-17-6

Last digit is the print number: 9 8 7 6 5 4 3 2 1

DEDICATION

For our families,
Bob, Rel, Max, Wigs, William, Morgan,
Mark, Jesse, Seth and Jim,
who keep us healthy.

Contents

Foreword xi
   Anne R. Somers

Chapter 1

Preventive Care for the Elderly 1
   Risa Lavizzo-Mourey and Deborah Diserens

Chapter 2

Principles of Screening 11
   Susan C. Day

Chapter 3

Screening for Cancer in the Elderly 23
   Susan C. Day

Chapter 4

Immunization in the Elderly 37
   Richard V. Sims

Chapter 5

Preventing Adverse Drug Reactions in the Elderly 47
   Risa Lavizzo-Mourey

Chapter 6

Reducing Cardiovascular Risk in the Elderly 63
   Thomas H. Lee

Chapter 7

Exercise 75
   Jeane Ann Grisso

Chapter 8

Nutrition, Alcohol and Tobacco in Late Life 89
   Mary Ann Forciea

Chapter 9

Prevention of Osteoporotic Fractures **107**
Jeane Ann Grisso and Maurice Attie

Chapter 10

Preventing Dependence and Injury: An Approach to Sensory Changes ... **125**
Jeane Ann Grisso and Mathy D. Mezey

Chapter 11

Functional Status: An Approach to Tertiary Prevention **141**
Jerry C. Johnson and Mathy D. Mezey

Chapter 12

Optimizing Mental Function of the Elderly **153**
Gary L. Gottlieb

Chapter 13

Preventing Elder Abuse and Neglect **167**
Elizabeth Capezuti

Chapter 14

Urinary Incontinence **183**
Laurence H. Beck

Chapter 15

The Economics of Prevention in the Elderly **197**
John M. Eisenberg

Chapter 16

The Home Team **209**
Risa Lavizzo-Mourey

Appendix A

Assessment and Screening Instruments **215**

Appendix B

Prevention Flowsheet and Checklist **240**
Susan C. Day and Todd Goldberg

Index **247**

Contributors

Maurice Attie, M.D.
Assistant Professor of Medicine, University of Pennsylvania School of Medicine; Director, University of Pennsylvania Osteoporosis Center; Philadelphia, Pennsylvania

Laurence H. Beck, M.D.
Sylvan Eisman Professor of Medicine, University of Pennsylvania School of Medicine; Director, Program in Geriatric Medicine, University of Pennsylvania; Philadelphia, Pennsylvania

Elizabeth Capezuti, R.N., M.S.N.
Clinical Lecturer in Nursing and Gerontological Nurse Practitioner, School of Nursing, University of Pennsylvania, Philadelphia, Pennsylvania

Susan C. Day, M.D., M.P.H.
Assistant Professor of Medicine, University of Pennsylvania School of Medicine; Director of Evaluation for General Internal Medicine, American Board of Internal Medicine; Philadelphia, Pennsylvania

Deborah F. Diserens, M.Phil.
Research Associate, University of Pennsylvania School of Medicine, Philadelphia, Pennsylvania

John M. Eisenberg, M.D., M.B.A.
Sol Katz Professor of General Internal Medicine, University of Pennsylvania School of Medicine; Chief, Section of General Medicine; Senior Fellow, Leonard Davis Institute of Health Economics, University of Pennsylvania; Philadelphia, Pennsylvania

Mary Ann Forciea, M.D.
Assistant Professor of Medicine, University of Pennsylvania School of Medicine; Director, Geriatrics Evaluation Program, University of Pennsylvania; Philadelphia, Pennsylvania

Todd Goldberg, M.D.
Geriatrics Fellow, University of Pennsylvania School of Medicine, Philadelphia, Pennsylvania

Gary L. Gottlieb, M.D., M.B.A.
Assistant Professor of Psychiatry, University of Pennsylvania School of Medicine; Director, Section of Geriatric Psychiatry, Hospital of the University of Pennsylvania; Philadelphia, Pennsylvania

Jeane Ann Grisso, M.D., M.Sc.
Assistant Professor of Medicine, University of Pennsylvania School of Medicine, Philadelphia, Pennsylvania

Jerry C. Johnson, M.D.
Associate Professor of Medicine, University of Pennsylvania School of Medicine; Director, Geriatric Fellowship Program and Chief, Geriatrics Program, Philadelphia Veterans Administration Medicine Center; Philadelphia, Pennsylvania

Risa J. Lavizzo-Mourey, M.D., M.B.A.
Assistant Professor of Medicine, University of Pennsylvania School of Medicine; Assistant Professor of Health Care Systems, The Wharton School, University of Pennsylvania; Medical Director, Elmira Jeffries Memorial Home; Senior Fellow, Leonard Davis Institute of Health Economics, University of Pennsylvania; Philadelphia, Pennsylvania

Thomas H. Lee, M.D., M.Sc.
Assistant Professor of Medicine, Harvard University Medical School; Associate Physician, Brigham and Women's Hospital; Boston, Massachusetts

Mathy D. Mezey, Ed.D., R.N.
Professor of Gerontological Nursing, School of Nursing, University of Pennsylvania, Philadelphia, Pennsylvania

Richard V. Sims, M.D.
Assistant Professor of Medicine, University of Pennsylvania School of Medicine, Philadelphia, Pennsylvania

Anne R. Somers, Sc.D. (hon)
Adjunct Professor, Department of Environmental and Community Medicine, University of Medicine and Dentistry of New Jersey—Robert Wood Johnson Medical School, Piscataway, New Jersey

Preface

It is now a well-known fact that the elderly population is growing and that as much as 50 or 60 percent of a clinician's practice in the next 20 years will be 65 or older. Many of these patients can expect to live another 10 to 20 years. What is not as well-known is how clinicians can make important contributions to maintaining a high-quality, independent lifestyle for their older patients.

The importance of preventive care for the elderly is just beginning to be recognized. However, the heterogeneity of the elderly population and diversity of possible preventive measures, combined with the time and fiscal contraints on today's practitioners, make providing effective preventive care a challenge. To date there has been very little information available describing practical clinical interventions that will help clinicians meet this challenge within the context of a busy practice. This book is a unique resource, for both students and practitioners, that combines summaries of available research with specific recommendations and pragmatic strategies for *practicing* prevention for the elderly.

Risa Lavizzo-Mourey, M.D., M.B.A.
Susan C. Day, M.D., M.P.H.
Deborah Diserens, M.Phil.
Jeane Ann Grisso, M.D., M.Sc.

Acknowledgments

Creating a book is a process that brings into sharp focus the interdependence of human activities. We are grateful to those on whom we have depended.

We would like to thank the ARCO Foundation for recognizing the need to provide clinicians with information about preventive care for the elderly and for providing us with the financial support to do so.

We are also indebted to our colleagues both here at the University of Pennsylvania and across the country. This book would probably not have gotten beyond the stage of a good idea had we not been working in a Section of General Medicine where there is a climate of commitment to addressing the needs of the elderly and a belief in the promise of prevention. The book would not have even been an idea without the direction and research provided by those who have pioneered the effort to bring together the fields of Geriatrics and Prevention, one of whom, Anne Somers, we would like to thank in particular for her willing support and contribution of the Foreword.

We are especially grateful to those who have directly contributed to bringing words to the page. To those who have written individual chapters, we would like to express our appreciation for their willingness to contribute their expertise and for their patience with our requests for more. To those who have decoded handwriting and weathered with good nature what probably seemed like an interminable process of typing and retyping we offer heartfelt thanks, especially to Marie Kaufmann and Joanne Walter for initially handling the whole job, to Dianne Greer for her counsel in guiding us through the incompatibility of different word processing systems, to Ginnie Crouthamel for her sense of humor about the number of revisions, to Jacki Brown for the late hours and that special touch she has with the computer, and to Mary Ann Thrasher particularly for her assistance in designing the layout of the Prevention Flowsheet. Jody Goodrich's innumerable trips to the library and encouraging words kept the process moving.

We are grateful to Jack Hanley for his encouragement, support, able guidance, and patience. And, finally, we would like to thank John Eisenberg who, by proposing the project to begin with, gave us the opportunity to work together.

Risa Lavizzo-Mourey, M.D., M.B.A.
Susan C. Day, M.D., M.P.H.
Deborah Diserens, M.Phil.
Jeane Ann Grisso, M.D., M.Sc.

FOREWORD

Anne R. Somers, ScD (hon.)

The very concept of "health promotion and preventive care for the elderly" may appear to some as incongruent, even contradictory. Once an individual is 65 and has a suspicious cough or elevated blood pressure, isn't it "too late to lock the barn door?"

Far from accepting this pessimistic view, many leading gerontologists and geriatricians now believe that prevention is actually the key to effective health care for the elderly. The phrase "preventive gerontology" is increasingly used to encapsulate this new approach. Support comes from both public and professional sources.

On the public side, recent surveys have shown that elders are more prevention-minded than younger people. It is also well known that the elderly spend a disproportionate amount of their generally small incomes on health care and health-related products—frequently not wisely, but often the best they can do, given inadequate information and inadequate professional assistance.

Meanwhile, scientists have been documenting the fact that advancing age does not automatically bring disease and disability. On the contrary, it is increasingly asserted that chronological age is only one factor—and not the most important—in determination of health and functional status. For most of the major chronic diseases associated with advancing years—most cardiovascular disease, many cancers, osteoporosis, emphysema, cirrhosis of the liver, and others—it is now known that lifestyle, environmental factors, and genetic risk factors play a far more decisive role than age alone. Lifestyle and behavioral factors are particularly important. The U.S. Surgeon-General has said they may account for as much as half of all U.S. mortality today (U.S. Dept. of HEW, 1979). They are also generally subject to professional intervention and individual control. Even in the case of environmental and genetic factors, professional assistance and individual knowledge can often lead to corrective or at least ameliorative action.

The extent to which this new marriage of prevention and gerontology has progressed is indicated in the following statement by Drs. E.L. Bierman and William Hazzard (author of the concept of "preventive gerontology"), associate editors of one of the major new textbooks of geriatric medicine:

> Prevention or attenuation of the chronic diseases of aging should be the ultimate goal of geriatric practice. (Bierman and Hazzard, 1985)

Examples of this new professional interest abound:

• "Productive aging" is the phrase coined by Dr. Robert Butler, former Director, National Institute on Aging, and now Chairman, Department of

Geriatrics and Adult Development, Mount Sinai School of Medicine, New York City, to address "mobilization of the productive potential of the elders of society" (Butler and Gleason, 1985).

• "Successful aging" is the name given to a multi-million dollar research project funded by the MacArthur Foundation and directed by Dr. John Rowe. The study involves a long-term effort to identify the causes and "predictors" of "successful aging" and the investigators hope to produce a "risk profile" to facilitate early positive intervention in the aging process (MacArthur, 1985).

• The "extension of the adult prime" is a concept and goal articulated by the Aging Society Project of the Carnegie Corporation of New York (Pifer and Bronte, 1986).

• "Old Age Is Not What It Used To Be" is the title of a popular *New York Times* article summarizing recent neurological and psychological studies showing the malleability of the aging human brain and psyche and the continued opportunity for positive professional assistance (Tavris, 1987).

There are, of course, major distinctions between these and related concepts, programs, and statements. (One is a basic science research project; one is addressed primarily to practicing physicians; one to older people themselves; another addresses public policy.) What they have in common is a conviction based on accumulating evidence, albeit still incomplete, that the mechanisms of disease can be understood and, within certain limits, controlled, resulting in a positive, rather than a negative, approach to aging.

The challenge now facing those of us who share this conviction is threefold: (1) to strengthen the science base linking specific risk factors to specific disease outcomes, and linking specific modifications in these risk factors to modified outcomes; (2) to translate these basic scientific findings into practical guidelines that can be used by the public, physicians, and other caregivers to prevent or postpone individual disease and disability; and (3) to devise organizational, financial, and other socioeconomic modalities and policies to permit the incorporation of the new science base and prevention technologies into routine health care for the American people.

While this volume addresses all three of these challenges, the emphasis is clearly on the second, especially the development of preventive strategies for physicians, nurses, and other clinicians to use in their regular patient care, and modifications in medical education to better prepare future practitioners for this responsibility.

The need for such emphasis on implementation is tremendous. Despite the progress just noted at the conceptual and research levels, there is a serious lag in implementation, especially the integration of scientific findings into regular clinical practices. There is even some evidence of retrogression in this respect. For example, a 1986 Harris public opinion poll found that only 30 percent of adults had received "unsolicited advice about health habits" from a doctor, down from 36 percent in 1983 (Prevention Index, 1987). The 30 percent contrasted with 50 percent who said that some "health book or magazine caused reconsideration of habits."

There is no question but that physicians are still far from fulfilling their potential in terms of prevention for the elderly. Too few women are being screened for breast cancer. Even in such traditional medical areas as vaccination, performance is disappointing. To the frustration of flu experts, only about 20 percent of Americans in high-risk groups, including the elderly, are vaccinated each fall (LaForce, 1987) despite the evidence from controlled studies that flu vaccine is 70 to 80 percent effective. In the words of one influenza authority,

"Physicians have not been trained to think of the routine immunization needs of their adult patients; it's not part of their everyday sphere of thinking."

This is probably the key to the problem. Despite all the new developments, prevention still plays an insignificant role in the education of most physicians. For example, a survey of 90 medical schools found little attention to hypertension at either undergraduate or residency levels (Moser et al., 1985). Students received an average of only 18 hours of instruction in hypertension management over the course of four years despite the fact that high blood pressure is the most common chronic disease in America. A 1983–84 survey by the Association of American Medical Colleges reports that the proportion of medical schools with a clearly-defined nutrition course was only 17 percent, even less than in 1958 (National Academy of Sciences, 1985). Reviewing the obstacles to greater acceptance of prevention in regular medical practice, Dr. Robert Levy, former Director, National Heart Institute and now Professor of Medicine, Columbia University, said, "The key to acceptance of prevention/health promotion lies with the gatekeepers to the practice of medicine, the medical schools" (American Council on Life Insurance, 1985).

The best response to all such shortcomings—inadequate attention to prevention by clinicians and professional schools and overreliance by patients on non-professional sources of information—is not "to curse the darkness but to light a few candles." That is exactly what this handbook for practitioners attempts to do.

The authors, a talented group of young physician-educators at the University of Pennsylvania School of Medicine, have made a major contribution both to medical education and to patient care for the growing legions of America's elderly, so many of whom are seeking professional guidance on these issues. I commend it to all who are seriously interested in furthering the goal of a healthy, active and productive life for older Americans and an affordable health care system for the nation as a whole.

REFERENCES

American Council on Life Insurance and Health Insurance Association of America, Advisory Council on Education for Health: Minutes of a meeting, Washington, D.C., June 13, 1985, p 8.

Bierman EL, Hazzard WR: Middle age: Strategies for the prevention or attenuation of the chronic diseases of aging. In Andres R, Bierman EL, Hazzard WR (eds): Principles of Geriatric Medicine. New York, McGraw-Hill, 1985, pp 862–866.

Butler RN, Gleason HP (eds): Productive Aging: Enhancing Vitality in Later Life. New York, Springer Publishing Company, 1985.

LaForce FM: Immunizations, immunoprophylaxis, and chemoprophylaxis to prevent selected infections. JAMA 1987; 257:2467–2470.

J.D. and C.T. MacArthur Foundation: Successful aging: The focus of MacArthur Foundation study. Press release, Chicago, September 1985.

Moser M, Rowden DW, et al: Medical school education in hypertension management: A national survey. Am J Prev Med 1985; 1:12–17.

National Academy of Sciences, National Research Council, Committee on Nutrition in Medical Education: Nutrition Education in U.S. Medical Schools. Washington, D.C., National Academy Press, 1985, pp 63, 12.

Pifer A, Bronte DL (eds): Our Aging Society: Paradox and Promise. New York, Norton, 1986.

Prevention Index '87: A Report Card on the Nation's Health. Summary Report. Consumers' survey by Louis Harris & Associates, November 1986. Emmaus, PA, Rodale Press, 1987.

Tavris C: Old age is not what it used to be. New York Times, Good Health Magazine, September 27, 1987.

U.S. Department of Health, Education, and Welfare, Public Health Service. Healthy People: The Surgeon General's Report on Health Promotion and Disease Prevention, 1979.

1
PREVENTIVE CARE FOR THE ELDERLY

Risa Lavizzo-Mourey, MD, MBA
Deborah Diserens, MPhil

A CONCEPT WHOSE AGE HAS COME

Almost 400 years ago, in "As You Like It," Shakespeare described the world as a stage on which we, the actors, start out "mewling and puking," crest in activity in the middle of life and, thereafter, physically and mentally decline to a second childhood "sans eyes, sans teeth, sans everything." In recent years a shift has been occurring in this long-accepted script for aging. To borrow from Gershwin, "It ain't necessarily so."

The change in the conceptualization of aging is represented by those, such as Fries,[1] who contend that, while the length of the human life span is fixed, chronic disease can be postponed by changes in lifestyle, modifying the common physiological indicators of aging so that the average period of disability may be reduced and postponed until shortly before death. This "compression of morbidity" theory suggests that, although chronic disease may not be eliminated, its onset may be delayed, thereby changing notions of aging from a process of gradual decline in function to a sustained period of activity until a rapid onset of disease and curtailed period of disability before death. The preventive efforts of clinicians in encouraging strategies for modifying the aging process are of obvious importance.

While prevention has received a great deal of attention in the medical community in the last 15 to 20 years, little of this research or clinical activity has been addressed directly to the elderly population. Today, with the increasing emphasis on geriatric care, there is a rising awareness that clinicians' preventive efforts on behalf of the elderly can yield important benefits not only for individuals, by improving their quality of life, but also for society through potential cost savings. In addition, there is evidence that the elderly population may be more receptive to health-promoting information and activities than has been previously believed. Preventive care for the elderly is a concept whose age has come. The issue facing clinicians is that this awareness has not yet been fully realized in medical practice

EFFICACY OF PREVENTION FOR THE ELDERLY

Despite, or possibly because of, the fact that very little is yet known about the efficacy of many treatments in the elderly population, studies suggest that the elderly receive less screening than younger persons. Some controlled trial studies

1

have found no difference in mortality between those in the population who were screened and unscreened elderly control groups; however, as sensitivity to the particular needs of the elderly improves, it is likely that mortality will increasingly be considered only one measure of outcome in a group where prevention of disability, maintenance of function, and quality of life may be more important considerations. It is worthy of note that in the 1979 Department of Health and Human Services publication *Healthy People,*[2] the goal for older people is phrased in terms of reduction of days of restricted activity rather than death rates, as had previously been the case. (The stated goal is to reduce the average number of days of restricted activity to fewer than 30 days per year for people 65 and over by 1990. The average was 38.4 days in 1975 and 39.2 days in 1980.[3,4])

If primary prevention, the identification and reversal or elimination of risk factors, was universally implemented and effective, most of us would live disease- and accident-free into old age, with death occurring according to the schedule of our genetic limits. This would result in a rectangular survival curve for the population and sustained physical and mental function from birth to death for each person. While this ideal may describe our potential, a large percentage of the elderly population has already experienced some degree of decline in function. If a reduction in early mortality is the goal of preventive efforts, then most would agree that the elderly are an inappropriate target for encouraging the lifestyle changes implied by primary prevention. The pervasiveness of this attitude and of using mortality rates as the criterion of success for preventive efforts is reflected in what, up until recently, has been a virtual void of discussion of preventive care for the elderly. If the goal is shifted, however, from reduced mortality rates to sustained independence, avoidance of unnecessary disability, and restoration or maintenance of function, then secondary prevention, the detection of asymptomatic disease, and most especially tertiary prevention, the detection of symptomatic but unreported disease or impairment, are as important for the elderly as for younger populations. Perhaps more so. From this broader view of the aims of prevention, encouraging lifestyle changes in elderly patients is still important, not only for the purpose of avoiding disease but also as a way to reverse the effects of disease and restore function, where possible, or to minimize further decline. The underlying purpose of this book is to reinforce clinicians' efforts to strive for "preventive success" that includes outcomes measured not only by length of life but also by its sustained breadth.

Unfortunately, scientific research on the efficacy of various prevention strategies and interventions for the elderly is little past its infancy. Relatively few studies have been done, and those that have been done often yield conflicting results due to, among other factors, variability of the samples studied, the methods used, and the definition of outcomes. However, amidst what may initially appear a discouraging array of quasi-scientific opinions about "what to do," there has evolved fairly widespread agreement in the identification of those health problems of the elderly where preventive efforts of clinicians have the greatest potential to make a difference.

Mobility and Function. Mobility and function are the major factors used by older people to assess whether they are in relative good or poor health, and fully 50% of the elderly have some limitation in function that prevents them from being fully independent.[5,6] Yet, few clinicians systematically assess the functional status of their elderly patients, and even fewer have developed a network of other professionals who can assist in restoring function or developing compensatory strategies that may prevent further decline.

Sensory Loss. Five percent of persons over 65 have severe visual impairments, with the percentage who have some trouble seeing reaching as high as 50% in nursing homes, yet it is estimated that only a few percent receive adequate attention for their problems.[7] The prevalence of hearing impairment is 25% of those over 65, rising to 50% of those over 85.[8,9,10] Studies suggest that physicians may underestimate the prevalance of hearing impairment by 50% or more.[11] Detection of sensory loss and subsequent restoration of sensory function may eradicate, among other things, many psychiatric symptoms, including confusion, anxiety, fearfulness and depression, without the need for psychiatric intervention.[11]

Injuries. Injuries are the fifth leading cause of death in persons older than 65,[12] and each year almost 5 million elderly persons sustain non-fatal injuries, about 75% of them in the home.[13] The estimated costs per year due to hip fractures alone in those over 65 is 6.1 billion dollars.[14] Physician intervention, such as early detection of sensory loss and counseling patients in a timely fashion to make appropriate adjustments in the home environment, may prevent many injuries.

Exercise. The elderly tend to become unnecessarily sedentary. For example, in 1975 only 36% of adults over 65 reported taking regular walks,[15] yet there is increasing evidence that through exercise programs fitness can be regained,[16,17,18] with improvements in aerobic capacity, muscle strength, flexibility, range of motion and coordination. To the degree that elderly individuals' loss of function may be related to deconditioning, even small improvements in fitness may increase their independence and ability to care for themselves.

Adverse Drug Reactions. Nearly one-third of elderly patients report adverse reactions to medications,[19,20] with as many as 65% of these being avoidable. Adverse drug reactions account for as many as 10% of hospitalizations among the elderly.[19,21] Improved understanding of physiologic changes related to aging, increased awareness of potential drug interactions, and more frequent and careful review of medications are all important for the physician who wishes to minimize patients' adverse reactions to drugs.

Depression. It is estimated that 13–18% of persons over 65 have clinically significant depression.[22,23] Yet as many as 75% of elderly suffering from depression are unknown to the primary care physician,[24] which is unfortunate since studies suggest that from 55–80% of depressed elderly patients will respond to treatment.[25,26,27] The importance of detection and an increased awareness of the subtlety of presentations and causes of depression in the elderly is underscored by the fact that a large percentage of older patients show a preference for using medical providers to care for psychiatric problems.[28]

Immunizations. While influenza vaccine is probably 60–70% effective in reducing mortality and admission to the hospital in elderly patients when it is adequately matched to the epidemic virus of a season, physicians are currently providing immunizations for only half of their elderly patients who have chronic disease and only a third of their otherwise healthy elderly patients.[11] The situation is similar with pneumococcal vaccination. Assuming vaccination rates of only 22%, the U.S. Office of Technology Assessment estimated that immunization of elderly patients saved about 6.6 million dollars in medical costs associated with epidemic influenza in 1971.[29]

Nutrition. It is estimated that 30% of community-dwelling elderly individuals have diets deficient in at least one major nutrient,[30] and at the same time one study suggests that physicians may fail to recognize up to 50% of cases of malnutrition.[31] Dietary therapies, currently popular among the elderly, may lead to toxicity syndromes or interact with other medications. Improved awareness of proper nutritional guidelines is needed on the part of both clinicians and their elderly patients.

Alcoholism. The average estimate of the prevalence of alcoholism in the elderly is about 10%, yet "a disproportionately small number of the elderly with alcoholism receive therapy for it despite the fact that treatment may be as much as twice as effective as in younger persons."[11] All elderly should be educated about the accentuation of alcohol's immediate effects with aging and warned of potential alcohol-drug interactions.

Smoking. Smoking is still prevalent among those over 65: 17% for men and 12% for women.[32] Elderly smokers who stop can still expect moderate increases in life expectancy, and just 60–120 seconds of verbal advice from the physician has been associated with a significant increase in the quit rate.[33]

Cardiovascular Disease. For the last 20 years, mortality from ischemic heart disease in the U.S. has been steadily declining. Coronary artery disease nevertheless remains the leading cause of death among individuals over 65.[34] It has been projected that if risk factors and the efficacy of medical care remain constant, there will be a 40% increase in the incidence, mortality, and costs associated with coronary artery disease by the year 2010.[35] Making informed management decisions for elderly patients involves a careful weighing of the limited data available on risk factor control in the elderly and an individualized plan for diet, exercise and smoking cessation.

Hypertension. About 15% of whites and 30% of blacks 65 and older have diastolic hypertension, and 10 to 15% of all elderly have isolated systolic hypertension.[11] Among those over 75, the prevalence of systolic hypertension is 25% and is even higher for diastolic hypertension. This results in an increased risk for cardiovascular complications of approximately 30% for every 10 mmHg increment in systolic blood pressure.[36] One study suggested that among the hypertensive elderly, treatment results in a reduction in cardiovascular mortality by 27% and in cerebrovascular events by 52%.[37] Clearly, early detection and treatment of hypertension is very important in the elderly.

Cancer. The risk of developing cancer between 65 and 85 is 20%, with 50% of all cancers and 60% of all cancer deaths occurring in the 11% of the population that is over 65.[11] Recommended screening frequencies for the elderly have varied considerably in various published recommendations. Consideration of several screening criteria and a careful assessment of patient status and preferences should be used to develop an individualized screening plan for each elderly patient.

Osteoporosis. At least 50% of women are likely to develop a fracture in later life due to osteoporosis.[38] Fractures of the hip are associated with more deaths, disability and medical costs than all other osteoporotic fractures combined,[39] and almost 50% of all hip fractures occur in those over 80.[40] Individualized assessment and recommendations for estrogen replacement therapy, adequate calcium consumption and exercise, as well as appropriate measures to prevent falls, are all components of a preventive program designed to reduce the risk of osteoporotic fractures in the elderly.

Urinary Incontinence. The prevalence of urinary incontinence in community-dwelling elderly is estimated at from 5–15%.[41] It is a problem that often goes undetected due to both patient reluctance to discuss it and physician failure to ask. It can lead unnecessarily to anger, depression, self-imposed isolation and a subsequent, more global decline in function. Yet, if detected, management strategies are available.

Elder Abuse. It is estimated that 4% of elderly Americans, or about 1.1 million persons, are victims of elder abuse each year.[42] For many of these individuals, the physician may be the only contact outside the home who has the opportunity to detect abuse or neglect and initiate intervention.

This book offers specific practice recommendations about these and other areas to which clinicians can be additionally attentive in their assessment and care of elderly patients. These areas, in which elderly show a high incidence of disability or impairment, are currently under-assessed or too infrequently prevented or treated.

HEALTH BEHAVIOR OF THE ELDERLY

Clinicians, discouraged by what they perceive to be patient unwillingness to respond to advice about changes in behavior and health practices, may be heartened to find that they have a receptive audience in the elderly. If once considered an unlikely or uninterested group, the elderly, as indicated by a growing number of reports, may now be regarded as the segment of the population most likely to engage in healthy behaviors.

National surveys, reported in 1979 by the National Center for Health Statistics,[43,44] showed that the prevalence of favorable health practices increases with age. This conclusion has been reported in several other studies as well,[45,46,47,48] studies that showed that elderly smoke and drink alcohol and coffee less often, sleep 7 to 8 hours, eat breakfast, and maintain proper weight more often than other age segments of the population. A nationwide study in 1986 commissioned by the Rodale Press and conducted by Louis Harris and Associates[49] found that those over 65 had the best overall prevention index score on 21 health-seeking behaviors, despite the fact that they had lower income and lower education levels, factors usually predictive of lower preventive orientations. The Rodale/Harris report also indicated that many of the elderly are interested in more guidance in health promotion, with over 40% reporting that they felt there should be more emphasis on prevention in their health-care location. Two studies reported by Prohaska, Leventhal and others in 1985[50] and 1986[51] once again confirmed that elderly respondents report higher frequencies of health-promoting actions. In addition, these studies extended the range of activities considered, showing that the elderly are also more likely to engage in health practices aimed at reinterpreting stress and controlling emotions, factors shown to be important in coping with stressors and chronic illness.

The Prohaska and Leventhal studies also demonstrated, however, that while the elderly are more likely to act to promote their own health, at the same time they may underreport or not respond to ambiguous symptoms, because they attribute symptoms such as tiredness, weakness, or aching to simply being older. Other studies have reported just the opposite, that the elderly tend to overuse medical care due to hypervigilance to symptoms that may be benign.[52] What becomes apparent is that the elderly, due to their growing sense of vulnerability, tend to move to one extreme or the other in their response to symptoms. Thus, it becomes increasingly important for the clinician interested in preventive care for elderly patients to explore how each individual interprets his or her symptoms.

In sum, clinicians can expect that as their patients age they will be increasingly receptive to information about how to promote and maintain their health, but, at the same time, in order to insure a timely and appropriate preventive response to physical changes, the clinician needs to become increasingly attentive to how each individual assigns meaning to changing bodily sensations.

EDUCATIONAL AND PRACTICAL NEEDS OF CLINICIANS

As the scientific community and society-at-large experience a shift in world view about what it means to grow old, health researchers have identified those areas in which preventive care of the elderly is most in need of improvement, and the elderly themselves are showing a desire to maintain function and promote health through their actions. At the same time, however, there is still very little curricular time devoted to either Prevention or Geriatrics in medical schools and almost none devoted to the intersection of these two areas. Simon and Wilson[53] found in a recent survey of medical schools 484 courses with prevention content, 143 courses with some content on aging, but only 20 courses with both prevention and aging content. If the educational time devoted to preventive care for the elderly is currently minimal, it was all but non-existent in the education of most of the physicians now in practice. Simply put, physicians have not been provided with the information they need to promote health in the group that will comprise as much as 50% of the patient population they will see in the next 20 years, and they may find it difficult to get this information.

Until recently, there has been very little research describing what physicians actually believe and do with respect to prevention. In 1986 Valente and others published a report on a survey of 1,040 primary care physicians concerning their health promotion beliefs, attitudes and practices with patients of all ages.[54] Ninety-seven percent of the physicians believed they should engage in health-promoting practices with patients. Yet only 3 to 18% reported being very successful in helping patients achieve desired changes in various areas. Ninety percent of the physicians said that they were the person most responsible for health education in their office and, when asked about their potential success in achieving behavioral change, they reported that they believed they could be much more successful if given appropriate information and support. The type of health promotion assistance most frequently rated as valuable was information about where to refer patients (91%). Other forms of assistance desired were physician education in specific subjects (85%), physician education in behavior modification (81%), and training for support staff (76%).

Primary care physicians have expressed a need to learn more about helping patients promote their own health and are looking for assistance to do so. That they may need encouragement in addressing the elderly is suggested by the fact that only 30% of those over 65 in the Rodale/Harris survey said they had been counseled in prevention during the previous 5 years.[49]

This book represents an attempt to fill the gap in information for physicians concerning preventive care for the elderly. Health-related problems of the elderly are many and can be complex in their origin. This book offers clinicians explicit, practical strategies for achieving health and lifestyle changes with elderly patients. Specific recommendations are offered for improved screening, anticipation of problems, and focused counseling. Because, today, there is increasing concern about the burgeoning cost of health care and a recognition that care decisions are often influenced by economic considerations, discussions address the cost implications of recommendations for the provider, the patient and society, and a full chapter is devoted to a review of current analyses of cost effectiveness and cost benefit. Equally important is the fact that recommendations are made with the busy practitioner in mind. Wherever possible, chapter authors have made an attempt to provide concrete suggestions for countering that ever-pressing enemy of effective preventive practices—time.

Time constraints are frequently cited by clinicians as a reason for not living up to their own preventive practice ideals. Included in the book are selected screening tools that can facilitate and standardize data collection and a flow-sheet that can be inserted in the patient chart as a prevention reminder system. Approaches to the development of community support and referral networks are discussed. Perhaps most important is the repeated suggestion that clinicians develop effective collaborative relationships with other health professionals. Health problems associated with aging are multi-factorial and the interdisciplinary team has consistently proven the most effective way to address and manage multiple needs of the elderly.[55,56,57,58] Useful collaborative relationships range from those between physicians, nurses and nurse practitioners in the office, who can share data collection and counseling actiivities, to, as suggested in the chapter entitled "The Home Team," a wider network of collaboration that reaches out into the home through the many professionals associated with home health agencies.

In "As You Like It" Shakespeare assembles a diverse group of distinct individuals, insulates them temporarily in a forest, and allows them to devote themselves to the pursuit of happiness. In this case, the forest is medicine and the pursuit is of independence in old age. This book, like all attempts to describe how things might be better, is meant to be idealistic, but it is also pragmatic. If the script for aging is to be changed, then this book might be considered suggested stage directions for a play where the clinician alternately is prop manager, acting coach and producer, and the patient is director and actor. What happens in the end depends on whether both play their role as they like it.

REFERENCES

1. Fries JF: Aging; Natural death and the compression of morbidity. N Engl J Med 1980; 303:130–5.
2. U.S. Department of Health and Human Services: Healthy People: The Surgeon General's Report on Health Promotion and Disease Prevention. Washington, D.C., Government Printing Office, 1979.
3. National Center for Health Statistics: Vital and Health Statistics: Data from the National Health Survey. Disability Days 1975. U.S. Dept. HEW, Public Health Service, Series 10 - No. 118, DHEW Pub. No. PHS 78–1586.
4. National Center for Health Statistics: Vital and Health Statistics: Data from the National Health Survey. Disability Days 1980. U.S. Dept. HHS, Public Health Service, Series 10 - No. 143, DHHS Pub. No. DHS 83–1571.
5. Williams TF: Comprehensive functional assessment: An Overview. J Am Geriatr Soc 1983; 31(11):637–641.
6 Aging America: Trends and Projections. 1985–86 Edition. Prepared US Senate Special Committee on Aging; AARP; FCDA; AOA. Printed U.S. DHHS PF #3377 (1085).
7. Padula WV: Low vision related to fundamental service delivery for the elderly. In Sekular R, Kline D, Dismukes K (eds): Aging and Human Visual Function. New York, Alan R. Liss, 1982, pp 315–323.
8. Fisch L: Special senses: The aging auditory system. In Brocklehurst JC (ed): Textbook of Geriatric Medicine and Gerontology, 2nd ed. Edinburgh, Churchill Livingstone, 1978, pp 276–290.
9. Hearing impairment and elderly people: Background paper. Office of Technology Assessment. Congress of the United States OTA-BP-BA-30. Washington, D.C., U.S. Government Printing Office. May, 1986.
10. Koopman C: Symposium of Geriatric Otolaryngology. Otolaryngol Clin North Am 1982; 15(2).
11. Stultz BM: Preventive care for the elderly. West J Med 1984; 141(6):832–45.
12. Rubenstein LZ: Falls in the elderly: A clinical approach (Topics in Primary Care Medicine). West J Med 1983; 138:273–5.
13. U.S. National Center for Health Statistics: Episodes of Persons Injured: United States, 1975. Advance date No. 18. DHEW Publications No. (PHS) 78–1250. Hyattsville, MD. U.S. Department of Health, Educationa and Welfare, 1978.
14. Cummings SR, Kelsey JL, Nevitt MC, O'Dowd KJ: Epidemiology of osteoporosis and osteoporotic fractures. Epidemiol Rev 1985; 7:178–208.
15. Physical fitness and exercise. Public Health Reports Supplement. 1983; Sep–Oct: 155–7.
16. Valbona C, Baker SB: Physical fitness prospects in the elderly. Arch Phys Med Rehabil 1984; 65:194–200.
17. Council on Scientific Affairs, American Medical Association: Exercise programs for the elderly. JAMA 1984; 252:544–6.
18. Fuller E: Exercise: Getting the elderly going. Patient Care 1982; 16:67–114.
19. Seidel LG, et al: Studies on the epidemiology of adverse drug reactions III: reactions in patients on a general medical service. Bull Johns Hopkins Hospital 1966; 119:299–315.
20. Klein L, et al: Medication problems among outpatients. Arch Intern Med 1984; 144:1185–8.
21. Caranosos GJ, et al: Drug induced illness leading to hospitalization. JAMA 1974; 288:713–7.
22. Gurland B, Dean L, Cross B: The epidemiology of depression and dementia in the elderly: the use of multiple indicators of these conditions. In Cole JD, Barrett JE (eds): Psychopathology in the Aged. New York, Raven Press, 1980.
23. Arie T: Prevention of mental disorders of old age. J Am Geriatr Soc 1984; 32:460–5.
24. Williamson J, Stokoe IH, Gray S, et al: Older people at home: their unreported needs. Lancet 1964; 1:1117–20.
25. Gallagher DE, Thompson LW: Effectiveness of psychotherapy for both endogenous and non-endogenous depression in older outpatients. J Gerontol 1983; 38:707–12.
26. Weiner RD: The role of electroconvulsive therapy in the treatment of depression in the elderly. J Am Geriatr Soc 1982; 30:710–12.
27. Koch-Weser J: Psychotropic drug use in the elderly (Part 2). N Engl J Med 1983; 308:194–99.
28. Waxman HM, Carner EA, Klein M: Underutilization of mental health professionals by community elderly. The Gerontologist 1984; 24:23–30.
29. Riddiough MA, Sisk JE, Bell JC: Influenza vaccination. JAMA 1983; 249:3189–95.
30. Shank RE: In Adres R, Bierman EL, Hazzard NR (eds): Principles of Geriatric Medicine. New York, McGraw-Hill, 1985, pp 444–460.
31. Russell RM, Sahyoun NR, Whinston-Perry R: In Calkins E, Davis PJ, Ford AB (eds): The Practice of Geriatrics. Philadelphia, W.B. Saunders, 1986, pp 135–145.

32. Remington PL, et al: Current smoking trends in the United States. JAMA 1985; 253:2975–8.
33. Sachs DPL: Cigarette smoking: Health effects and cessation strategies. Clin Geriatr Med 1986; 2:337–62.
34. National Center for Health Statistics, United States, 1984. DHHS Pub. No. (PHS) 85–1232. Public Health Service. Washington. U.S. Government Printing Office, Dec. 1984.
35. Weinstein MC, Coxson PG, Williams LW, et al: Coronary heart disease morbidity, mortality and cost for the next quarter-century. Clin Res 1986; 34:386A.
36. O'Malley K, O'Brien EO: Management of hypertension in the elderly. N Engl J Med 1980; 302:1397–1401.
37. Amery A, Birkenhager W, Brixko P: Mortality and morbidity results from the European Working Party on High Blood Pressure in the Elderly trial. Lancet 1985; 1:1349–54.
38. Christiansen C, Riis BJ, Rodbro P: Prediction of rapid bone loss in postmenopausal women. Lancet 1987; 5:16.
39. National Center for Health Statistics: Advance Data from Vital and Health Statistics 1985 Summary National Hospital Discharge Survey. Hyattsville, MD Public Health Service, 1986. U.S. Public Health Service Publication No. (PHS) 86–1250.
40. Lewinnek G, Kelsey J, White A, et al: The significance and comparative analysis of the epidemiology of hip fractures. Clin Orthop 1980; 152:35–43.
41. Yarnell JWG, Leger AS: The prevalence, severity and factors associated with urinary incontinence in a random sample of the elderly. Age Aging 1979; 8:81–85.
42. House Select Committee on Aging, Subcommittee for Health and Long-term Care. 1985, May 10. Elder abuse: A national disgrace (Executive Summary).
43. National Center for Health Statistics (1979a): Acute conditions: incidence and associated disability, United States, July 1977 - June 1978. (Public Health Services Series 10 - No. 132) US Government Printing Office, Washington, D.C.
44. National Center for Health Statistics (1979b): Physician visits: volume and interval since last visit, United States - 1975. (Public Health Service Series 10 - No. 132) US Government Printing Office, Washington, D.C.
45. Belloc NB, Breslow L: Relationship of physical health status and health practices. Preventive Medicine 1972; 409–21.
46. Breslow L, Enstrom JE: Persistance of health habits and their relationship to mortality. Prev Med 198; 9:469–83.
47. Harris DM, Guten S: Health-protection behavior: An exploratory study. Journal Health Soc Behav 1979; 20:17–29.
48. Steel JL, Broom WH: Conceptual and empirical dimensions of health behavior. J Health Soc Behav 1972; 13:382–92.
49. Prevention Index '87: A Report Card on the Nation's Health. Summary Report. Consumers' survey by Louis Harris and Associates, November 1986. Emmaus, PA, Rodale Press, 1987.
50. Prohaska TR, Leventhal EA, Leventhal H, Keller ML: Health practices and illness cognition in young, middle-aged and elderly adults. J Gerontol 1985; 40(5):569–78.
51. Leventhal E, Prohaska TR: Age, symptom interpretation and health behavior. J Am Geriatr Soc 1986; 34:185–91.
52. Haug M: Age and medical care utilization patterns. J Gerontol 1981; 36:103.
53. Simon S, Wilson L: Medical school and nursing school education in disease prevention, health promotion and aging. Presentation at the Annual Scientific Meeting, Gerontological Society of America, San Francisco, 1983.
54. Valente CM, Sobal J, Muncie HL, et al: Health promotion: Physicians' beliefs, attitudes, and practices. Am J Prev Med 1986; 2(2):82–8.
55. Allen CM, Becker PM, McVey LJ, et al: A randomized controlled clinical trial of a geriatric consultation team: Compliance with recommendations. JAMA 1986; 255:2617–2621.
56. Teasdale TA, Schuman L, Snow E, et al: A comparison of outcomes of geriatric cohorts receiving care in a geriatric assessment unit and on general medicine floors. J Am Geriatr Soc 1983; 31:529–534.
57. Rubenstein LZ, Josephson KR, Wieland GD, et al: Effectiveness of a geriatric evaluation unit: A randomized clinical trial. N Engl J Med 1984; 311:1664–70.
58. Lefton E, Bonstelle S, Frengley JD: Success with an inpatient geriatric unit: A controlled study. J Am Geriatr Soc 1983; 31:149–155.

2
PRINCIPLES OF SCREENING

Susan C. Day, MD, MPH

Over the past 15 years, considerable attention has been paid in the medical community to the importance of screening. Virtually every prominent medical organization, including the American Medical Association, the American Cancer Society, and the American College of Physicians, has made a series of recommendations regarding the appropriate timing and frequency of screening.[1,15,16] The underlying assumption behind all these recommendations is that identifying risk factors and pursuing early detection of disease lead to an intervention in either lifestyle or disease process that subsequently improves the quality or duration of an individual's life.

Review of the various expert recommendations, however, reveals little agreement about the specifics of screening. Who should do the screening, in what setting, how often, and for what diseases are all controversial areas. Figure 1 is taken from the American College of Physicians' 1981 review of expert recommendations for screening. Recommendations for patients over the age of 60 are shown.

The four expert recommendations that were reviewed[1,4–6] agreed about the need to adjust the screening interval and target population according to the prevalence of disease. However, a quick review of the screening tests listed reveals little or no consensus as to the frequency with which tests ought to be performed. For example, only Breslow and Somers recommend a biannual complete history and physical between the ages of 60 and 64, increasing to yearly after age 65. Erratic recommendations in terms of the frequency of pelvic, rectal, and breast examinations similarly support a lack of clarity as to how often even routine evaluation should be performed. While this lack of consensus in part reflects a lack of concrete epidemiologic data on which clear guidelines can be established, it may also reflect the uncertain attitudes of both providers and patients towards screening in the elderly. This chapter will review the rationale for screening in the elderly as well as provider and physician attitudes towards preventive practices and will conclude with recommendations for implementing preventive strategies.

CRITERIA FOR EVALUATING
A SCREENING PROGRAM FOR THE ELDERLY

What kind of medical conditions are appropriate for screening in the elderly population? Frame and Carlson's criteria for justifying screening for a given disease are listed in Table 1. Considering these criteria provides a basis for constructing a screening program for the older patient.

FIGURE 1. Screening recommendations for patients over the age of 60. Reprinted with permission from the Medical Practice Committee, American College of Physicians: Periodic health examination: A guide for designing individualized preventive health care in the asymptomatic patient. Ann Intern Med 1981; 95:729–732.

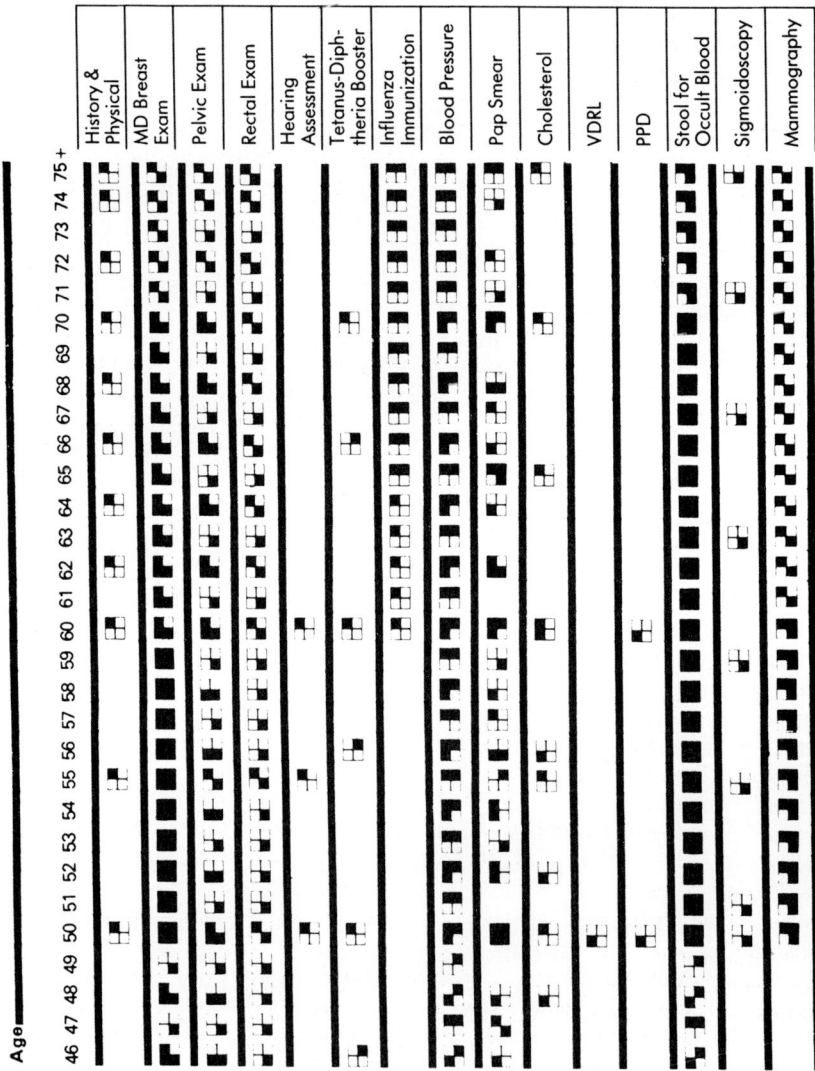

| F | B & S | Frame and Carlson / Breslow and Somers |
| ACS | CTF | American Cancer Society / Canadian Task Force on the Periodic Health Examination |

F   Frame and Carlson
B & S   Breslow and Somers
ACS   American Cancer Society
CTF   Canadian Task Force on the Periodic Health Examination

Age: 46 47 48 49 50 51 52 53 54 55 56 57 58 59 60 61 62 63 64 65 66 67 68 69 70 71 72 73 74 75+

- History & Physical
- MD Breast Exam
- Pelvic Exam
- Rectal Exam
- Hearing Assessment
- Tetanus-Diphtheria Booster
- Influenza Immunization
- Blood Pressure
- Pap Smear
- Cholesterol
- VDRL
- PPD
- Stool for Occult Blood
- Sigmoidoscopy
- Mammography

TABLE 1. Criteria to Justify Screening for a Disease

1. The disease must have a significant effect on quality or quantity of life.
2. Acceptable methods of treatment must be available.
3. The disease must have an asymptomatic period during which detection and treatment significantly reduce morbidity and/or mortality.
4. Treatment in the asymptomatic phase must yield a therapeutic result superior to that obtained by delaying treatment until symptoms appear
5. Tests must be available at reasonable cost to detect the condition in the asymptomatic period.
6. The incidence of the condition must be sufficient to justify the cost of screening

From Frame PS, Carlson SJ, 1975, with permission.[6]

First and foremost, the disease sought must have a significant effect on the quality or quantity of a patient's life. For the elderly, considerations of functional status and quality of life become increasingly important and may outweigh the importance of prolonging life per se, since the elderly face a limited number of future years and often experience comorbid disease that affects the quality of their life. Particularly for the extreme elderly or individuals with functional impairment, screening programs should aim to prolong the period of optimum function and work to minimize handicapping and discomfort from the onset of chronic conditions.[25] For example, it would not be reasonable to screen an 85-year-old woman with severe congestive heart failure for cervical cancer, which has a very long preclinical stage. The patient's cardiac disease will limit her expected survival far more than her carcinoma in situ. On the other hand, screening for decreased visual acuity might result in an intervention that would improve the patient's eyesight and allow her to enjoy more sedentary activities such as reading.

Acceptable methods of treatment must be available. In the elderly patient, consideration must be given to what would be the clinical course of action if a disease is discovered. For example, consider the elderly patient with cancer. Some elderly patients may indicate a reluctance to undergo aggressive chemotherapy or surgery. In determining the best type for therapy for a given elderly patient, different goals for cancer treatment should be discussed; remission, alleviation of pain, or return to normal functional status may be more realistic and acceptable therapeutic goals than "cure." The definition of "acceptable methods of treatment" may vary according to the age, disease and preferences of the patient. It is logical that detecting a disease for which there is no effective therapy does not provide adequate benefit to justify screening. Early treatment, therefore, should **yield a therapeutic result superior to that obtained by delaying treatment.** All interventions carry some risk—financial, social, or medical—and must be of clear benefit to justify screening.

If a treatment does exist, **the disease must have an asymptomatic period during which detection and treatment significantly reduce morbidity and/or mortality.**

This criterion relates to the concept of primary versus secondary and tertiary prevention. The difference between the three levels of preventive effort are demonstrated in Figure 2.

Primary prevention is targeted toward identifying and reversing risk factors that may predispose individuals to developing a disease in the future. Nutrition, exercise, and accident prevention are examples of areas in which the elderly may be encouraged to make fundamental lifestyle changes that may result in

```
                                       Preclinical or
            No Disease              Asymptomatic Disease        Symptomatic Disease

     ─────────┬──────────────────────────┬────────────────────────┬──────────────────────────  Outcome
      Exposure/                     Onset of                 Symptoms
      Risk Factors                  Disease

            |---Primary------| ------Secondary------| -------Tertiary-----|
               Prevention              Prevention              Prevention
```

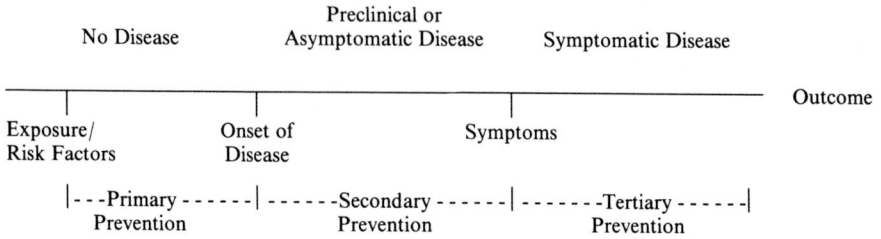

FIGURE 2.   Differences among three levels of prevention

improved function or survival. These topics, along with the issue of immunizations, will be addressed later in this book.

Most screening programs are aimed at secondary prevention (i.e., detecting a disease during the preclinical or asymptomatic phase). Blood pressure detection programs are good examples of secondary prevention. For disease states that are appropriate for screening, early detection leads to earlier diagnosis and, therefore, to more rapid initiation of treatment and subsequently to improved function or survival. In the elderly population, screening programs that include case finding, i.e., detecting symptomatic but unreported disease, may be equally important.[17,12] This type of prevention effort is considered tertiary prevention. The concept of screening programs targeted toward tertiary prevention or maximizing functional status is particularly appropriate for the "older" elderly where long-term survival is less important than maintaining an independent life. Table 2 lists potential geriatric preventive health measures as defined by Stults.[25] The assignment to different categories is somewhat arbitrary; for example, glaucoma screening may result in detection of an elevated ocular pressure before any visual loss has been noted by a patient (secondary prevention) or after a significant field cut has developed and resulted in loss of vision (tertiary prevention). In the latter case, the physician's efforts would be directed towards preventing further progression of disease and helping the patient maintain the usual activities of daily living.

Tests must be available at reasonable cost to detect the condition in the asymptomatic period. The cost addressed by this criterion includes both the cost of the initial screening test/program and the cost of the subsequent evaluation that is performed in response to a positive test. The elderly who exist with fixed income and who may have limited insurance coverage are often unable to afford the costs of screening programs not paid for by their insurance policy. Screening mammograms, for example, are not covered by Medicare. Cost can rapidly add up—the recommended strategy for assessing a positive stool test for occult blood may include a sigmoidoscopy, barium enema, endoscopy and upper GI x-ray. Hidden costs, such as the cost of transportation and the time of a companion who accompanies the patient, must also be considered.

In addition to the dollar costs of the screening test, the morbidity of the initial and follow-up procedures must be considered. While the stool test for occult blood, for example, is a harmless and simple procedure, lower bowel endoscopy carries a small but significant risk of colonic perforation, and obtaining an adequate bowel preparation for a high-quality double contrast barium enema may lead to dehydration with its attendant risks in the elderly patient.

Finally, **the incidence of the condition must be sufficient to justify the cost of screening.** Certainly, the elderly may be considered a high-risk, high-prevalence population for most screening tests. The majority of cancer occurs in

TABLE 2.   Potential Geriatric Health Measures

Primary Prevention

Immunization	Health promotion
influenza	accident prevention
pneumococcus	physical fitness
tetanus	nutrition

Secondary Prevention—Early Detection and Treatment

Hypertension	Mental health
diastolic	dementia
systolic (isolated)	depression
	alcoholism
Cancer	
breast	Social support system
colon	
cervix	Iatrogenic disease: drug therapy
Sensory deficits	Miscellaneous
vision	urinary incontinence
hearing	podiatric disorders
	hypothyroidism

Tertiary Prevention—Rehabilitation

Comprehensive assessment of function: physical, psychological, social
— every 2 years for ages 65-74
— yearly for age 75 and older

From Stults BM: Preventive health care for the elderly. West J Med 1984; 141:6:832, with permission.

patients over 65 years old; 59% of all cancer in men and 52% of all cancer in women occurs after the age of 64.[2] Hypertension (defined as a blood pressure of $> 140/90$) is present in 64% of non-institutionalized individuals; an additional significant percentage of the population will have isolated systolic hypertension ($\geq 25\%$ of men and women over 80 years).[7a] The other conditions listed in Table 2 have a similarly high prevalence. By screening a high risk population, the predictive value of a positive screening test increases as the number of false-positive test results decreases. Thus, the elderly represent an ideal population for screening.

This review of the criteria for evaluating individual diseases suitable for screening may be applied to assessing an entire screening program. Rogers et al. evaluated their own screening program for the elderly and modified these criteria to emphasize the importance of case finding and tertiary prevention. They also emphasize the importance of integrating the screening program into the individual patient's health care as part of a comprehensive plan to maximize functional status.[20]

Another consideration in putting together a screening program is which tests to use. Factors influencing the choice of an optimal test include cost, safety, convenience, patient acceptability and test characteristics (e.g., how well does the test detect disease in early stages, while minimizing false positive results in healthy individuals). These aspects of choosing a screening test will be discussed in depth in the chapter on cancer screening.

THE VALUE OF SCREENING IN THE ELDERLY

With these criteria in mind, recent reports of screening programs directed towards the elderly can be reviewed. Screening programs targeted towards the community-dwelling elderly consistently demonstrate a high "yield" in terms of treatable conditions identified. Most such broad-based screening programs have been implemented by nurses, nurse practitioners, and other paramedical personnel. In one study, 94% of patients had at least one positive finding detected by a program that included a history, physical exam, and routine laboratory tests performed by three nurse practitioners operating out of a senior citizen community center.[23] Fifty-four percent of the 261 patients who were screened were referred to a physician for further evaluation. The most common reasons for referral were urologic problems (14%) and hypertension (10%). Ultimately, 15% of patients were treated for problems identified by this screening program.[23] While some of the problems identified were known to the patients, they were not currently receiving the appropriate treatment for the conditions. This finding emphasizes the importance of tertiary prevention in improving health care for this population.

Further evidence of benefit comes from long-term studies of the effect of regularly scheduled programs of preventive intervention. Hendrickson et al. demonstrated that individuals involved in a regular screening program had a reduced need for nursing home placement, fewer acute care visits, hospitalizations, and overall decreased mortality when compared to individuals who were not regularly screened.[8]

The number of important new problems detected by a screening program targeted toward nursing home patients is lower than that reported for the community elderly.[7,9] This observation is not surprising since these patients are already in contact with health care providers who routinely assess their problems and look for reversible conditions. A screening program in this setting will predictably demonstrate a high prevalence of medical problems but may not result in important, or measurable, changes in the patients' functional status or quality of life.

It is important to note that there are additional psychological benefits related to an active screening program. Elderly individuals who participate report that their overall sense of well-being and self-confidence was improved by the program simply because the regular attention made them feel that somebody cared.[26,8]

If the elderly represent a high-prevalence, high-risk population that is ideal for screening, why do studies of current screening efforts indicate inadequate performance of screening tests?[14,27] First of all, physicians overestimate their performance of screening tests. A recent review of cancer screening in a university general internal medicine practice demonstrated that providers estimated that they performed screening procedures three times as frequently as they were actually observed to do but often only half as frequently as expert panels recommended.[14] This poor compliance with screening recommendations is noted for patients of all ages.[27,21] Other factors that contribute to poor compliance with screening recommendations can be related to a number of variables reflecting behaviors of both providers and patients, which will be discussed below.

PHYSICIAN FACTORS AFFECTING SCREENING

When McPhee et al. asked physicians practicing in their general internal medicine practice why they did not perform the recommended screening tests, the physicians gave four main reasons: (1) they forgot, (2) they didn't have time, (3) the screening test was inconvenient or logistically difficult, or (4) the patient refused.[14] Interviews with the physicians demonstrated that, in addition, they were often unfamiliar with recommended screening parameters.[14] Specific reasons varied according to the type of screening procedure. For example, issues of physician time were particularly prominent for tests such as the pelvic examination that require longer physician encounters, whereas patient discomfort played a role in the reason providers performed fewer sigmoidoscopic and pelvic examinations than were recommended.

The need for increased physician education about generally recommended screening procedures is often cited.[21] Lack of knowledge about screening intervals in the elderly can be assumed to be even greater. Beyond education, however, there are a number of practical suggestions that can facilitate screening activities. Use of a reminder system can help "prompt" providers to perform tests in a timely fashion. An age-sex specific flow sheet can be inserted in each patient's chart (see Appendix B). More sophisticated computerized medical information systems can make screening part of a patient's permanent record.

Involvement by the entire health care team in providing preventive services is also important for both community-dwelling and nursing-home patients. Nursing staff can collect detailed information relating to functional status and medical symptomatology; office staff can assess the home situation. The ways in which a health care team approach can improve preventive care are discussed in depth in Chapter 16.

A more difficult issue to define is the physician's fundamental attitude towards the value of screening in the elderly patient. Physicians may judge that, for a given individual, detecting a problem that requires further intervention, that is potentially painful and costly to treat, is not "justified." Often physicians may make such a decision without fully educating the patient about the relative benefits and risks of screening, and without adequately eliciting the patient's preferences. Physicians may, incorrectly, assume patients would be reluctant to undergo screening.[3] It is possible that physicians perceive a higher level of reluctance than actually exists on the part of the patient—and may not spend the time necessary to identify patient preferences because they themselves are not convinced of the value of a given screening procedure.

PATIENT FACTORS AFFECTING COMPLIANCE WITH SCREENING PROGRAMS

Numerous studies confirm that elderly patients are more likely than younger individuals to pursue healthy behaviors such as regular blood pressure checks, dietary modifications (low salt, fat, cholesterol diet), and preventing accidents.[3,13] The elderly also appear to have a greater belief in the importance of lifestyle modification (diet, exercise, smoking) in reducing the risk of future morbidity.[3]

Not surprisingly, the elderly also perceive themselves to be more vulnerable to the development of serious disease and to have less control over their future health.[3,19] They are willing to accept an increasing number of symptoms as part of normal aging. This acceptance may lead to an under-reporting of symptoms and delay in diagnosis.[22] This accepting attitude probably results in many elderly being less likely to request screening despite a desire for a healthy lifestyle. Therefore, patient education about the efficacy of screening for disease in preclinical and early stages is important in improving acceptance of a screening program.

The emotional response to screening must also be considered. Anger, fear and shame are common responses to illness that are experienced by patients of all ages.[13] An individual may be reluctant to enter into a screening program that might confirm fears of illness. Many elderly are particularly concerned about maintaining their dignity when undergoing medical procedures such as sigmoidoscopy, pelvic examinations, or mammography. Others may see the possible identification of a serious illness as presaging an increased dependence on family or friends. By anticipating and addressing these types of emotional concerns, a provider can improve a patient's participation in a preventive care program.

Patients may also have a number of practical concerns that, if addressed, would increase compliance. Such concerns might include the uncovered costs of screening procedures, as well as the availability (and cost) of transportation to and from the testing site. Discussion of the patient's insurance coverage and availability of social service support may allay his or her concerns. Many elderly may depend on friends or family to bring them to the hospital or doctor's office; availability of these individuals may play a role in determining if and when a patient returns for recommended screening procedures.

Finally, many elderly have been cared for by physicians who have themselves retired from practice. Others have lost touch with, or have never been part of, the health care system. The lack of a primary care physician who knows and understands the patient may reduce their participation in a regular screening program. Table 3 summarizes patient factors affecting compliance with screening. These factors should be taken into consideration in devising a screening program which addresses the special situation of a given individual.

ETHICAL CONSIDERATIONS OF SCREENING

There are a number of ethical concerns that may be raised by instituting a screening program for the elderly. While it may seem obvious that a program designed to improve the quality and duration of a patient's life is in the patient's best interests, the implications of such a program may not be as straightforward.

Pellegrino has argued that large scale preventive efforts should focus on interventions where the causal connection between behavior (e.g., smoking) and disease (e.g., lung cancer) is well-documented and where the proposed method for changing behavior is known to be effective.[18] In general, this argument applies to the selection of a screening program for an individual as well, although the societal issues relating to resource allocation are less persuasive when considering an individual's best interests. Screening for colon cancer is an example of how recommendations for society as a whole may differ from those for an individual. The American Cancer Society has not made a formal recommendation for mass screening for colon cancer with tests for occult blood in the stool because (1) the test characteristics (e.g., sensitivity and specificity) remain imperfect for such large scale screening and (2) epidemiologic evidence does not yet justify the investment of the sort of resources that would be required to follow up on a positive test. On the other hand, the American Cancer Society recognizes that an individual practitioner may be willing to screen individual patients for occult blood in the stool, recognizing the imperfections in the test, because of perceived benefits for that individual.[1]

Other ethical issues relate to a patient's right to decide whether or not he or she wants to undergo screening. Some patients may feel strongly that they would not undergo further diagnostic procedures or therapeutic interventions if a disease was detected by means of a screening program. This decision may be

TABLE 3. Patient Factors Affecting Compliance

Health-seeking behavior
Belief in the efficacy of screening
Cost of screening program (and subsequent testing)
Anticipated feelings of anger, fear, shame
Availability of transportation
Availability of companion
Lack of regular physician

---

based on their personal health belief system and have roots in religious or ethnic beliefs. If the patient is competent, ethical and legal precedents support the patient's right to make his or her own decision as long as he or she has been fully informed about the risks and benefits of screening.[10,17]

Providers may find it difficult to accept a patient's decision to act in either a more or less aggressive fashion in detecting disease than they feel is indicated. This ethical dilemma may be minimized if a pre-existing relationship exists between physician and patient, which helps the physician understand a patient's preference. Unfortunately, as mentioned above, many elderly patients lack a regular physician and so the provider must make an extra effort to understand the patient's decision-making process.

The questions of informed consent and competence must also be addressed. In general, for decisions that involve non-life-threatening diseases (such as result from screening), the standard for informed consent requires that patients not only be told but comprehend the advantages and disadvantages of proceeding with a certain course of action.[10] For the elderly patient with cognitive impairment, there may be a limited ability to understand the implications of screening recommendations and to weigh the pros and cons of proceeding. Does this mean that screening is only appropriate for the competent, well individual? The elderly population is heterogenous, even from a strictly medical perspective. Non-intervention may be appropriate in one patient and inexcusable in another. Pneumonia has been called "the old man's friend"; are there therefore incidences where immunization against pneumonia may not be indicated? Such a situation might arise in a patient with marked disability and limited quality of life.[12]

The answers to these difficult questions must be addressed with the individual patient in mind. It may not be appropriate even to suggest an aggressive program of cancer screening in an elderly patient with multiple co-existing diseases and limited life expectancy. However, for this same individual, screening measures directed at improving functional status might be considered not only appropriate but medically and ethically mandatory.[11,17]

CONCLUSION

This chapter has addressed some of the factors which influence the choice of a screening program for the elderly. The specific components of the screening program will be discussed in depth throughout the remainder of this book. The flow sheet included in Appendix B summarizes the approach recommended by the authors. In order to optimize the appropriateness and effectiveness of a screening program the following recommendations should be followed:

PRACTICE RECOMMENDATIONS

1. Be sure your patient understands, and agrees to, the screening program that you propose for him or her. If appropriate, include family members in the discussion to help identify problem areas that the patient may be overlooking and to help reinforce the importance of screening after the patient leaves your office.

2. Explore the patient's reaction to screening in order to identify questions and improve compliance. Educate the patient regarding the pros and cons of a screening program.

3. Integrate screening into routine visits. Nursing personnel can help make use of the physician's time more efficient by performing preliminary screening of functional status and assessment of social supports, diet, and so forth.

4. Coordinate required testing to minimize the number of visits that must be arranged. For example, a mammogram or audiogram can be scheduled on the same day as the office visit so that the results are available at the time of consultation.

5. Develop a reminder system to help you remember what you need to do for a given patient. A simple flow sheet, such as provided in Appendix B, inserted in the front of the chart, may accomplish this; more sophisticated computerized medical information systems are available to help to keep track of what should be done for a specific patient.

REFERENCES

1. American Cancer Society: ACS report on the cancer related checkup. CA 1980; 30:194–232.
2. Baranovsky A, Myers MH: Cancer incidence and survival in patients 65 years of age and older. CA 1986; 26:1:26–41.
3. Bausell RB: Health-seeking behavior among the elderly. The Gerontologist 1986; 26:556–559.
4. Breslow L, Somers AR: The lifetime health-monitoring program. N Engl J Med 1977; 296:601–608.
5. Canadian Task Force on the Periodic Health Examination: The periodic health examination. Can Med Assoc J 1979; 121:1193–1254.
6. Frame PS, Carlson SJ: A critical review of periodic health screening using specific screening criteria. J Fam Pract 1975; 2:29–35, 123–129, 189–194.
7. Gambert SR, Duthie EH, Wiltzius F: The value of the yearly medical evaluation in a nursing home. J Chron Dis 1982; 35:65–68.
7a. General Working Group on Hypertension in the Elderly: Statement on Hypertension on the Elderly. JAMA 1986; 256:70–74.
8. Hendriksen C, Lund E, Stromgard E: Consequences of assessment and intervention among elderly people: a three year randomized controlled trial. Br Med J 1984; 289:1522–1524.
9. Irvine PW, Carlson K, et al: Long-term care: The value of annual medical examinations in the nursing home. J Am Geriatr Soc 1984; 32:540–545.
10. Jonsen AR, Siegler M, Winslade WJ: Clinical Ethics. New York, Macmillan Publishing Co., 1986.
11. Kee CC: A case for health promotion with the elderly. Symposium on Health Promotion.
12. Kennie DC: Perspectives: health maintenance of the elderly. J Am Geriatr Soc 1984; 32:4:316–322.
13. Leventhal EA, Prohaska TR: Age, symptom interpretation and health behavior. J Am Geriatr Soc 1986; 34:185–191.
14. McPhee SJ, Richard RJ, Solkowitz SN: Performance of cancer screening in a university general internal medicine practice. J Gen Intern Med 1986; 1:275–281.
15. Medical evaluation of healthy persons. Council Report. JAMA 1983; 249:1626–1633.
16. Medical Practice Committee, American College of Physicians: Periodic Health Examination: A guide for designing individualized preventive health care in the asymptomatic patient. Ann Intern Med 1981; 95:729–732.

17. Muir Gray JA: Prevention of Disease in the Elderly. Edinburgh, Churchill Livingstone, 1985.
18. Pellegrino ED: Health promotion as public policy: The need for moral groundings. Prev Med 1981; 10:371–378.
19. Prohaska TR, Leventhal EA, Leventhal H, Keller ML: Health practices and illness cognition in young, middle aged, and elderly adults. J Gerontol 1985; 40:569–578.
20. Rogers J, Supino P, Grower R: Proposed evaluation criteria for screening programs for the elderly. The Gerontologist 1986; 26:564–570.
21. Romm FJ, Fletcher SW, Hulka BS: The periodic health examination: comparison of recommendations and internists' performance. South Med J 1981; 74:265–271.
22. Rowe JW: Health care of the elderly. N Engl J Med 1985; 312:827–835.
23. Rubenstein LZ, Josephson KR, et al: Comprehensive health screening of well elderly adults: an analysis of a community program. J Gerontol 1986; 41:3:342–352.
24. Spitzer WO, Bayne RD, Charron KC, et al: Task Force Report: The periodic health examination. Can Med Assoc J 1979; 121:3–45.
25. Stults BM: Preventive health care for the elderly. West J Med 1984; 141:6:832–845.
26. Tulloch AJ, Moore V: A randomized controlled trial of geriatric screening and surveillance in general practice. J R Coll Gen Pract 1979; 29:733–742.
27. Woo B, Cook EF, Weisberg M, Goldman L: Screening procedures in the asymptomatic adult. JAMA 1985; 254:1480–1484.

3
SCREENING FOR CANCER IN THE ELDERLY

Susan C. Day, MD, MPH

While early detection and treatment of cancer has been the focus of many preventive medicine programs, few of these programs have been designed specifically for the elderly patient. In this chapter, the value of cancer screening in older patients will be discussed and screening criteria for the most common forms of cancer in this age group will be reviewed.

The emphasis in this discussion will be on secondary prevention, i.e., the detection of asymptomatic or early cancer. This is not to imply that identification of risk factors for the development of cancer (primary prevention) is not important in the elderly. For example, patients should be reminded of overexposure to the sun as a risk factor for skin cancer and encouraged to use sun screen. Likewise, a patient's occupational history may be key in alerting the practitioner of the need to screen for related carcinoma, e.g., lung cancer or mesothelioma in the patient with asbestos exposure. The management of patients with advanced cancer is also an important topic. The current rise in hospice programs and home care services has provided an important new dimension in maintaining the quality of life of patients with terminal illness. However, the hypothesis here is that by educating patients about the value of screening and by implementing a screening program tailored to the individual patient, the clinician may have a major opportunity for impact on his or her patients' health.

EPIDEMIOLOGY

Figure 1 lists the most common causes of cancer in patients between 65 and 74 years and over 75 for the years 1979-1981.[5] Several facts highlight why the elderly are a particularly important group to consider for cancer screening. First of all, the elderly have a relatively increased incidence of developing cancer and, therefore, may be considered at high risk when compared to a younger cohort; the risk of developing cancer is 20% between the ages of 65 and 85.[5] Second, patients who die from cancer are more likely to be elderly; 60% of all cancer deaths occur in the 11% of the population over 65.[5] Third, epidemiologic evidence suggests that cancer in the elderly is often detected in a more advanced stage when compared to the younger population.[19] This is particularly true of cancer of the bladder, breast, cervix, ovary, and uterus. This highly positive relationship between advanced stage and years suggests that the diagnosis of cancer is often delayed in the elderly. Patients wait to seek medical attention for subtle symptoms and may be less concerned about minor changes in body function than when they were younger. Since some of these cancers are among

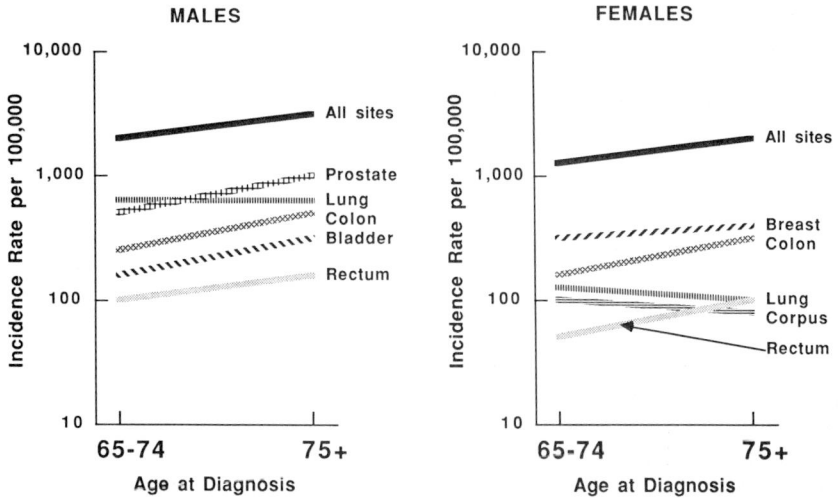

FIGURE 1.   The most common causes of cancer in patients between 65 and 75 years of age for the period 1979–1981. Modified from Baranovsky A, Myers M. Cancer incidence and survival in patients 65 years of age and older. CA 1986; 36:26–41.

those that can be best detected by screening (e.g., cervical and breast cancer), a screening program that includes the elderly should increase early detection of cancer and, thereby, lead to both an improved survival and decreased morbidity.[32]

Of note is the observation that lung cancer is an exception to the generally positive relationship between patient age and stage of cancer at the time of detection. Elderly patients who develop carcinoma of the lung tend to have the disease detected in an earlier stage than their younger counterparts.[19] Since lung cancer is an area in which the value of screening has been questionable,[2] the reasons for this finding need to be further explored. Possible explanations include less aggressive disease in older patients (thus increasing the prevalence of cancer in an earlier stage that might be detected by screening) or increased detection due to more frequent use of chest radiographs in this population for other, unrelated, medical conditions. Since lung cancer is the second most common form of cancer in men and increasingly frequent among women, the potential value of an effective screening program that detects lung cancer at an earlier, possibly curable, stage requires further investigation.

FACTORS IN ASSESSING
A CANCER SCREENING PROGRAM

When considering implementing a cancer screening program, further consideration of the screening criteria discussed in Chapter 2 is appropriate. First is the question of whether earlier diagnosis will lead to a prolongation of life.[13] If the natural history of a particular form of cancer is characterized by a long latent period prior to the development of overt symptoms, there may be less rationale for an aggressive screening program in the extreme elderly. For example, dysplasia characteristically precedes the development of cervical carcinoma by 8–30 years.[32]

Similarly, it is estimated that colonic adenomas may precede the development of adenocarcinoma by 5–10 years.[40] An 80-year-old woman with severe, end-stage Alzheimer's disease and congestive heart failure would not be a logical candidate for a colon or cervical cancer screening program, both because her prognosis is already limited by her existing disease and because the quality of her life is unlikely to be improved by early detection of these cancers. Few would advocate surgical intervention for an asymptomatic lesion in the presence of marked functional limitation. On the other hand, since the average life expectancy of a 60-year-old woman is 18 years and a 60-year-old man 14 years, many healthy elderly may benefit from an effective cancer screening program in terms of both quality and number of years of life saved. The program must be adjusted for the individual.

Second, an acceptable and efficacious method of treatment must be available to justify screening for cancer.[13] The elderly patient's ability to tolerate chemotherapy and surgery for different forms of cancer is currently being investigated, since many earlier trials excluded the elderly from study protocols. This means that there is still limited data about the value of treatment of cancer in the older patient. However, elderly patients with good functional status do not appear to experience increased toxicity secondary to chemotherapy for lung, breast or colorectal carcinoma, the most common malignancies, when compared to a younger cohort entered into the same protocols.[20] On the other hand, the elderly may not do as well when treated intensively for malignancies such as leukemia.[36] The treatment response rate for malignancies that may be detected by screening will vary according to cancer type and functional status, and should be taken into consideration when discussing options for screening with the older patient.[4,20]

Equally as important as the efficacy of treatment is its acceptability to patients. Misconceptions and lack of knowledge about cancer and its treatment may lead patients to be unnecessarily reluctant to undergo screening. Elderly patients may be more likely to have heard misinformation, such as cancer is spread by surgery, or chemotherapy is worse than the disease. Such beliefs will obviously affect the patient's motivation to participate in a screening program, or to mention early symptoms of disease to their physician. Patient education may, therefore, improve compliance with a screening program.

Financial constraints should also be considered as a factor that may influence the acceptability of a cancer screening program for the elderly. Often, older patients receive a fixed income. Medicare does not currently reimburse for such basic tests as screening mammography. As with many of the procedures discussed in this book, patient compliance might be improved if the provider identifies cost obstacles in advance and becomes familiar with each patient's particular insurance program.[32]

Finally, the screening test to be used must be a good test. There are a number of criteria that are useful in assessing the utility of a test in screening for cancer: is it inexpensive? safe? acceptable to patients? Perhaps most importantly, the test should perform well, that is, have a high sensitivity, specificity and predictive value. The standard method for determining these test characteristics is shown in Table 1; a more complete description can be found in any general textbook of epidemiology.[14,28]

The sensitivity of a screening test reflects its ability to identify patients who have the disease being sought, one hopes at the earliest point in time that the disease can be detected. A highly sensitive test will pick up all existing cases of disease and have few false negative results when applied to individuals with

TABLE 1. Test Characteristics

		Disease Present	Disease Absent	
Test	Positive	True Positives $\quad$ a	b $\quad$ False Positives	a + b
	Negative	c $\quad$ False Negatives	d $\quad$ True Negatives	c + d
		a + c	b + d	

Sensitivity = True positives/All patients with disease = $\dfrac{a}{a+c}$

Specificity = True negatives/All patients without disease = $\dfrac{d}{b+d}$

Predictive value positive = True positives/All patients with positive test = $\dfrac{a}{a+b}$

Predictive value negative = True negatives/All patients with a negative test = $\dfrac{d}{c+d}$

known disease. A screening test that fails to identify all individuals who might potentially have asymptomatic, early cancer would provide little reassurance to patient or clinician.

The specificity of a test reflects its ability to correctly identify individuals who do not have the disease, e.g., are normal. A test with low specificity will generate a large number of false positive results; when screening for a rare disease, such as most cancers in the general population, this means that many patients will incur the financial and emotional cost of further evaluation. In cancer screening, false positive results may be particularly worrisome, as for example, in the woman with a positive mammogram who must undergo breast surgery to excise a possibly suspicious, nonpalpable lesion.

The predictive value of a test is the test characteristic that is most meaningful to patients and clinicians, because it allows interpretation of the test results by answering the following question: if a test result is positive (or negative), how likely is it that the patient does (or does not) have the disease for which the patient is being screened. The predictive value of a test is dependent on the prevalence of the condition being sought in the population. Therefore, for a given stage of disease, the predictive value of a positive test will be much lower in the general population than in a high-risk group where the prevalence of disease is elevated. Often, cancer screening tests are first studied in a high-risk setting where the predictive value looks promising, but when the test is applied to the general population, it no longer seems as useful. A dramatic example of this is the use of RIA-prostatic acid phosphatase in screening for prostate cancer. The positive predictive value of this test fell from 93% when applied to patients with a palpable prostate to .41% when applied to the general population.[38] Since the prevalence of cancer in the older population is relatively high, the predictive value of cancer screening tests in this group should be higher than in the general population.

SCREENING RECOMMENDATIONS
FOR SPECIFIC FORMS OF CANCER

COLORECTAL CANCER

Colorectal cancer is a good example of a cancer well-suited to screening in the elderly. Colon cancer is the second most frequently diagnosed cancer in women and third most common in men. The incidence of the disease peaks at age 80 and natural history data indicate that colorectal cancer is less aggressive in the elderly.[17] In addition, patients over 64 years with colon cancer have a relative survival comparable to younger cohorts.[5] Both men and women have an almost 50 percent five-year survival rate for colon cancer, regardless of their age. Five-year relative survival rates are somewhat lower for rectal cancer (45%) in both sexes and all age groups.

The 1980 American Cancer Society recommendations for screening for colon cancer included yearly digital examinations for patients over the age of 40, and yearly six-slide stool sampling for patients over the age of 50 to test for occult blood.[2] Sigmoidoscopy is also recommended every three to five years for all patients over the age of 50, after two negative exams one year apart. There is no upper age limit on the recommendations and patients with a high risk for developing colorectal cancer (e.g., familial polyposis, ulcerative colitis, history of polyps or previous colon cancer, or family history of colorectal cancer) should be screened more frequently.

There remain some unanswered questions about the accuracy of the tests being considered to screen for colon cancer. For example, fecal occult blood testing has had variable results in large trials. Table 2 is taken from a review of the results of six large studies of fecal occult blood testing.[25] Almost 91,000 patients were enrolled in these studies, although on average only 38% of patients returned the guaiac cards for testing. Compliance rates were variable between studies and ranged from 26 to 91%. Of the patients who underwent the screening procedure, 3.6% of responders had positive tests for occult blood. Only 46% of these patients underwent follow-up examination; and of these, an average of 8.2% were found to have cancer. Cancers tended to be found in early stages (Dukes' stage A and B) and incidental adenomas were frequently detected.

These studies suggest significant problems with patient compliance with the fecal occult blood testing procedure. The predictive value of a positive test (e.g., the percentage of patients testing positive for blood in the stool who have cancer) may be as low as 5 to 10%. In addition, Winawer has shown that as many as 76% of patients with rectosigmoid adenomas greater than 0.5 cm may test negative for occult blood intermittently.[41] This high false-negative rate may lead to false reassurance and is a limitation of fecal occult blood testing as a screening test.

These test characteristics were obtained in studies of the general population. What can be expected in the elderly? First of all, fecal occult blood testing is more likely to be positive in the elderly. This is due to the higher prevalence of not only colon cancer in the elderly but other disease that may cause blood in the stools, such as diverticular disease, adenomas, angiodysplasia, and so forth. The effect of this increased prevalence of positive tests on the predictive value of the test will depend on the value to the provider of detecting these diseases. For example, the identification and early removal of potentially precancerous lesions such as adenomas might be considered a valuable outcome from early screening for colon cancer.[33] Therefore, the work-up for a positive fecal occult blood test that

TABLE 2. Results of Screening with Gualac-Impregnated Cards for Colorectal Cancer*

Location	No. initially Registered**	No. (%) Responding†	No. (%) of responders positive for occult blood	No. (%) w/ complete follow-up examination	No. (%) of cancers in positive responders	Dukes' A and B	Adenomas
Mercer Cty., NJ[41]	2,272	1,835 (80.8)	114 (6.2)	41 (36.0)	5 (4.4)	3	Not stated
New York City[37]	13,127	9,709 (74.0)	242 (2.5)	242 (100.0)	43 (17.8)	Not stated	Not stated
Honolulu[40]	1,682	1,529 (91.5)	53 (3.4)	32 (60.4)	3 (5.7)	2	3
Nottingham, England[36]	10,253	3,613 (36.8)	77 (2.1)	77 (100)	12 (15.6)	11	27
Evanston, IL[42]	54,101	14,101 (26.1)	617 (4.38)	66 (10.7)	30 (4.9)	19	40
Cook Cty., IL[43]	9,550	3,531 (37.0)	146 (4.1)	117 (80.1)	10 (6.8)	5	18
Total	90,985	34,328 (37.7)	1,249 (3.6)	575 (46.0)	103 (8.2)	—	—

* From Moore JR, LaMont JT: Colorectal cancer: risk factors and screening strategies. Arch Intern Med 1984; 144:1819–1823.
** Those registered in a study were given gualac-impregnated test cards and instructions.
† Responders were persons who returned gualac-impregnated cards for testing.

yielded an adenoma, although "negative" for cancer, actually could be considered to have a valuable outcome.

A study of screening for colon cancer in an elderly nursing home population confirms the relatively high yield on follow up evaluation of stool samples that test positive for blood.[24] In this study, 450 residents of a long-term care facility had three stool specimens tested for occult blood, and all patients with one or more stools testing positive underwent barium enema, upper GI radiography and, if all these were negative, complete colonoscopy. Twenty-one patients had positive results; of these, two patients were found to have colon cancer and one had gastric cancer. Five patients had duodenal ulcers, and one had esophagitis. Overall, 17 of the 21 patients with positive tests had clinically significant disease detected as a result of screening.[24] Since detection of these diseases generally led to changes in management, and presumably improved health status for these patients, the benefit of the screening test was increased by a broader definition of its yield.

The negative implications of increased detection of fecal occult blood become evident when the morbidity of working up a positive Hemoccult test in the elderly is considered. The complete bowel preparation required for a high quality barium enema or colonoscopy to be performed has the potential risk of causing dehydration, while colonoscopy carries the risk of perforation in one of 250.[6] Several trips back and forth to the hospital for testing are often required; these trips may require enlisting the help of an individual to accompany the patient or coordinating ambulance service.

These considerations of increased costs and morbidity of screening for colorectal carcinoma in the elderly might discourage a clinician from recommending routine fecal occult blood screening to this age group. However the potential benefit of screening for colon cancer in elderly has been estimated at between a one-third and two-thirds reduction in mortality,[9] and most expert panels now favor an ongoing screening program.[12,13] Most of the decrease in mortality is related to early detection and removal of adenomatous polyps. Winawer et al., studying patients older than 70 who tested positive on stool testing for occult blood, noted that 83% had either adenomas or colorectal cancer; adenomas were three times more common than cancer.[41]

One reasonable strategy to screen for colorectal carcinoma, as advocated by Stults, is to obtain two annual sigmoidoscopies.[33] Flexible sigmoidoscopy, with a 30 cm sigmoidoscope, can be performed by primary care physicians. Studies have shown that most non-endoscopists can be easily trained to insert the flexible sigmoidoscope to the near full depth.[39] The flexible sigmoidoscope is more comfortable for patients and will detect the 55% of lesions that arise in the distal 25 cm of bowel.[40] If these two examinations are negative, annual fecal occult blood testing is recommended, with air contrast barium enema and/or colonoscopy being performed for evaluation of positive tests.[33] This strategy, as outlined in Figure 2, should result in detection of adenomas that have developed since the initial negative screening with sigmoidoscopy. Given the 5- to 10-year lead time required for carcinoma to develop in an adenoma, such a strategy in patients over 70 would seem quite reasonable.

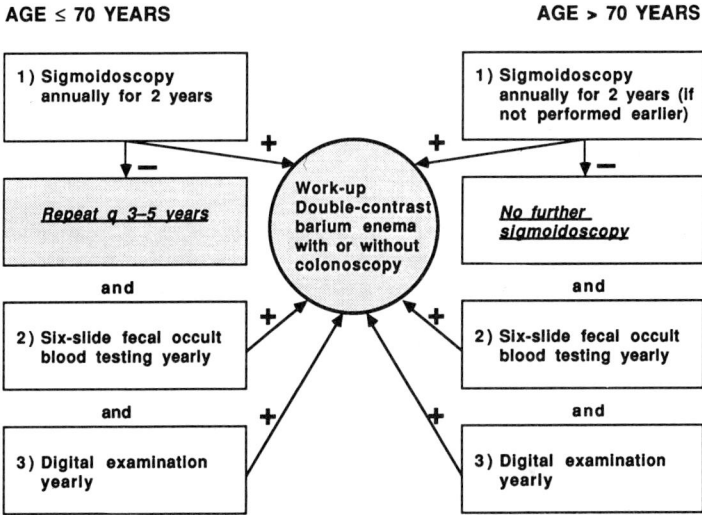

FIGURE 2. Screening for colorectal cancer.

BREAST CANCER

As with colon cancer, early detection and treatment of breast cancer can reduce mortality and morbidity. Fifty percent of breast cancer occurs in women over the age of 65.[5] The prognosis of older women with breast cancer is difficult to predict. Some studies have shown that women over 75 have a lower survival rate than younger women.[1] On the other hand, the proportion of hormonally responsive carcinomas is increased in the elderly; these cancers carry a more favorable prognosis and can be treated with few side effects.[17] Other studies have demonstrated that 5- to 10-year survival rates are as good in patients over the age of 70 undergoing surgery for breast cancer as younger patients.[18] Therefore, patients should be reassured that their age alone will not limit the choice of appropriate therapy for management of their breast cancer.

In April 1987, the United States Preventive Services Task Force published their recommendations for breast cancer screening.[35] Based on a careful review of well-designed cohort or case control trials, which included patients over the age of 60, their consensus was that patients over 60 should undergo annual mammogram and clinical breast examination by a health care provider. The sensitivity of these combined modalities in detecting breast cancer in women over 60 is estimated at 81%.[26] Of the lesions which are detected, one-third of the lesions in the elderly will be detected by a mammogram only, one-third on clinical exam only, and another third by clinical examination and mammography.[30]

There continues to be a paucity of long-term data regarding the efficacy of mammography in screening for breast cancer in the elderly. The Health Insurance Plan data that first demonstrated the efficacy of mammography was limited by an upper age cut off at entry of 64 years. However, an ongoing study in Sweden appears to demonstrate a reduction of mortality of almost 40% in patients aged 50–74,[26] and results in younger individuals are so encouraging that there is little reason to doubt the benefit of screening with mammography in the elderly.[27] If anything, the yield of mammography improves in the older patient in whom the breasts are less dense and better internal visibility can be obtained.[29]

There may still be, however, a reluctance on the part of patients to undergo regular mammographic examinations. This reluctance comes from several sources. First is the inconvenience of returning for separate testing, which can be overcome by scheduling mammography at the same time as a regular office visit. Second are concerns about cost, since screening mammograms in asymptomatic women, as of 1988, are not covered by Medicare and out-of-pocket costs may be high. Other elderly patients may fear the possibility of lack of privacy while undergoing the test and having unfamiliar technicians handle such intimate parts of their bodies. These fears should be addressed by assuring the patient about the discretion and tact of the radiology staff, which is often entirely female.

Finally, many patients have heard about possible risks associated with the radiation exposure involved in mammography. They should be reassured that current exposure levels are minimal (0.2 to 0.6 rad) and only slightly increase the risk of developing breast cancer. The American College of Obstetricians and Gynecologists estimated that a 50-year-old woman who received a yearly mammogram for 20 years would increase her theoretical risk of cancer from 7% to 8.4%.[10] In the elderly, the already minimal risk of irradiation induced malignancy is further reduced because of the latency period for developing a secondary breast cancer, which may well exceed the predicted life expectancy of the patient.

The actual frequency with which mammography should be performed in the elderly is not clear. Most official panels, such as the US Preventive Services Task Force,[35] have not placed an upper limit on obtaining yearly mammograms. The epidemiologic evidence cited above would support annual mammographic exams through the age of 74. Increasing the interval between exams at that point to every two or three years would seem reasonable until further data are available, although annual breast examination by a physician or other health care provider should continue.

The utility of combining breast self-examinations with mammography and clinical examination by a physician or other health care provider has been debated.[26] The Breast Cancer Detection Demonstration Project estimated that only 21% of cancers in patients over 60 years old were detected on monthly self-examination.[3] This somewhat low sensitivity should be contrasted with other earlier studies that suggested that regular breast self-examination leads to detection of earlier lesions that have a more favorable prognosis.[11] Patients may be taught to perform breast self-examination; however, the provider should be aware that older patients may be unfamiliar with the rationale for self-examination and be more reluctant to examine their breasts both for reasons of modesty and lack of confidence in their ability to perform a proper exam.[32] Arthritis and changes in sensation may also impede a proper exam.[32] For these reasons, breast self-examinations should be considered as an adjunct to the regular screening program of mammogram and clinical examination described above.

CERVICAL AND UTERINE CARCINOMA

Cervical carcinoma has historically been a form of cancer where the benefit of screening is considered to be well-established.[2] However, since the natural history of cervical carcinoma is remarkable for a decreased conversion of negative Pap smears to positive in the elderly, this population has been considered a low priority group for screening. In fact, the American Cancer Society in 1980 recommended all asymptomatic women age 20 and over have an annual Pap test for two negative exams, and then every three years until age 65.

A review of the epidemiology of cervical cancer provides a different perspective, however, because even though carcinoma in situ is rare, the prevalence of cervical cancer is higher in elderly women.[22,23] In fact, in 1976 25% of cervical cancer was diagnosed over the age of 65, and 41% of all cervical carcinoma deaths were reported in women over the age of 65.[5] These incidence rates can be attributed to the fact that elderly women are less likely to have received regular screening with Pap smears. In a survey of elderly patients in an outpatient medical clinic, 15% of women over the age of 65 had never had a Pap smear, whereas 64% had either never had a Pap smear or not had one in the preceding three years.[22,23] In addition, one third of women who reported a previous history of hysterectomy had a cervix in place when a pelvic examination was performed.[22]

Another reason for the underscreening of the elderly with Pap smears is that the Pap smear was developed in 1948 and was not actively promoted until the 1960s.[2] Therefore, many of the current elderly may have completed their childbearing years prior to the time regular screening for cervical cancer became the standard of care. These patients should be carefully questioned about previous Pap smears and provided with information about the rationale for such a procedure. It can be hoped that the number of "unscreened" elderly will be reduced as patients who received regular screening in their youth age and continue regular contact with their gynecologist or primary provider. In the meantime, dates and results of previous Pap smears should be documented, and efforts to convince patients to undergo pelvic examination continued.

Adequacy of previous Pap smears should also be documented. False negative rates for Pap smears may range as high as 20–30%, due to a combination of factors. One major cause is inadequate sampling of the squamocolumnar junction, where malignant transformation occurs. In the elderly, atrophic vaginal mucosa and osteoarthritis that limits hip rotation may both contribute to increased difficulty in adequate visualization and sampling of the transformation zone. Drying artifact and a variety of laboratory factors can also result in an inaccurate result.[42] The incidence of false negative Pap smears is one reason why repeated examinations are recommended to reduce the chance of missing an early cervical carcinoma.

The Pap smear is not a reliable method for detecting endometrial cancer. Endometrial tissue sampling is a more sensitive method for detecting this form of uterine cancer, with up to 90% sensitivity reported.[7] It is recommended by the American Cancer Society that endometrial biopsy be performed at the time of menopause and in high-risk individuals.[2] For example, endometrial biopsy should be considered as a way of monitoring patients receiving estrogen therapy for prevention of osteoporosis (Chapter 9).

Annual pelvic examinations are currently recommended by the American Cancer Society for all women.[2] The reason for continuing regular pelvic examinations in the elderly woman is that there are multiple problems that can be identified and addressed. First, changes in the size of the uterus or ovaries can be detected. An enlarged ovary is always abnormal in the elderly and deserves further evaluation to exclude the presence of ovarian cancer. In addition, elderly women often have genitourinary symptoms related to aging that can be diagnosed by an internal examination (see Chapter 14). For example, atrophic vaginitis and stress incontinence are two common problems that should initially be evaluated by pelvic examination.

It should be noted that both patient and physician may find performing a pelvic examination in the lithotomy position more difficult and/or uncomfortable in the elderly patient who suffers from underlying arthritis or musculoskeletal or neurologic problems. The patient should become familiar with other positions that can be used for the pelvic examination, such as the left lateral Sims position.[32] By reassuring the patient, being sensitive to concerns of modesty, and acknowledging possible apprehension about the examination, the provider may also alleviate some patients' reluctance to proceed with the procedure.

PROSTATE CANCER

There is still no sensitive, cost-effective, screening test that can detect prostate cancer in early stages (A or B) when cure rates are reasonable.[21] As a result, most cases of prostate cancer are advanced at the time of diagnosis[2] and the utility of screening is much debated. Methods for screening that have been evaluated most closely are the rectal examination and prostatic acid phosphatase measurements (by radioimmunoassay and enzymatic measurement).[37,38] Guinan et al. evaluated 10 diagnostic procedures in 300 elderly men who presented with symptoms of bladder outlet obstruction.[16] The prevalence of prostate cancer on biopsy in this group was 23%. The results of the screening tests they compared are presented in Table 3. There are several points to note. First of all, the sensitivity of all tests ranged from 17 to 69%, a discouragingly low figure. The stage of disease at the time of diagnosis was not given, but it would be expected that the test would have a lower sensitivity in patients with earlier disease.

Rectal examination was the most sensitive test for detecting prostate cancer, with a positive predictive value in this population of patients of 67%. Put another way, 67% of patients with an abnormal rectal exam were ultimately diagnosed as having cancer. Enzymatic determination of the prostatic acid phosphatase was next most sensitive, with a comparable predictive value to digital exam. A subsequent study by Vihko et al. in an unselected population of male veterans also found that rectal examination and immunoassay of prostatic acid phosphatase had comparable, although considerably lower, predictive values (22 versus 17%) in this group where the prevalence of prostate cancer was 9/771.[37]

TABLE 3.   Results of Screening Tests for Prostate Cancer*

Test	No. of Patients	Sensitivity	Specificity	Predictive Value	
				Positive Test	Negative Test
Rectal examination	300	0.69	0.89	67	91
Acid phosphatase—enzyme	300	0.56	0.94	72	88
Acid phosphatase—RIA	100	0.20	0.85	29	78
Acid phosphatase—CIEP	100	0.20	0.95	56	80
Urine cytology before massage	202	0.17	0.98	67	80
Prostatic-secretion cytology after massage	211	0.29	0.98	78	82
Urine cytology after massage	209	0.22	0.98	71	81
Aspiration cytology	200	0.55	0.91	65	88
Lactic dehydrogenase V/I ratio	132	0.47	0.82	44	83
Leukocyte-adherence inhibition	113	0.50	0.79	43	83

* From Guinan PI, et al: The accuracy of the rectal examination in the diagnosis of prostate carcinoma. N Engl J Med 1980; 303:499–503.

The very low predictive value of both rectal exam and serum assay for prostatic acid phosphatase (PAP) as screening tests makes it difficult to recommend mass screening with these techniques.[38] A preliminary study of prostate-specific antigen as a marker for prostate cancer shows this serum assay to be more sensitive than the PAP, but still limited by a low specificity.[31] Since the rectal examination is already recommended annually in patients over 40 as a test for colon cancer, it should be performed to screen for prostate disease as well.

Endorectal ultrasound examination of the prostate is a technique that can be used to evaluate prostate size and parenchyma. Initial studies have demonstrated that a per-rectal probe can provide information about the size and texture of the gland; since the probe can image the entire prostatic capsule, better visibility of the anterolateral part of the capsule can be obtained than with the digital examination.[8] The methodology clearly has advantages in guiding needle biopsy of palpable nodules, staging known prostate cancer, and following patients receiving treatment.[15] The application to general screening has yet to be carefully studied and subjected to cost-effectiveness analysis. Therefore, prostatic ultrasound cannot be recommended as part of the routine screening of elderly men.

SUMMARY AND RECOMMENDATIONS

Recent evidence suggests that the elderly are at high risk for developing cancer, are currently underscreened, and may do very well with treatment. Therefore, for patients who have a good functional status, incorporating the basic elements of cancer screening into a program of periodic examination may lead to earlier detection of treatable malignancy.

Our recommendations follow for screening of individuals over the age of 60. As the information available on the efficacy of existing tests increases and new screening techniques are developed, these recommendations may change and the clinician is advised to watch for updates.

PRACTICE RECOMMENDATIONS

1. Women should have a careful clinical breast examination and pelvic examination together with rectal examination annually and stool testing for occult blood annually. Pap smears should be performed and results documented every three years, at least until age 75.

2. For men, a careful rectal examination with prostate exam and stool test for occult blood should be performed annually.

3. Mammography, performed every year, is clearly justified for screening for breast cancer through the age of 75. At that point, the benefit of detecting a slow-growing, non-palpable, mass through mammography becomes less certain and the clinical breast examination becomes the mainstay of breast cancer screening.

4. For both men and women sigmoidoscopy should be performed every three to five years, after two negative exams one year apart, up to the age of 70. At that point, testing the stool for occult blood each year becomes the primary method of screening.

5. There is no clear evidence that chest x-rays are of any value in screening for lung cancer; however, recent studies, which indicate detection of lung cancer in earlier stages in the elderly, may lead to reconsideration of periodic screening for high risk individuals, i.e., patients with occupational exposures or heavy smoking histories.

6. Remember that cancer screening needs to be individualized for specific patients. Patient preferences, functional status, and the presence of comorbid disease may all impact on the type of program which is appropriate for a given individual.

7. Many patients will be receptive to screening if the reasons for recommending a procedure are explained in advance. Patient education materials may help reduce fear and irrational beliefs.

8. The use of flow charts (such as provided in Appendix B) will help to keep a screening program on schedule and facilitate advance planning to integrate appropriate testing and physical examination into regular office visits.

REFERENCES

1. Adami H, Malker B, Holmberg L, Persson I, Stone B: The relation between survival and age at diagnosis in breast cancer. N Engl J Med 1986; 315:559–563.
2. American Cancer Society: Guidelines for the cancer-related checkup: recommendations and rationale. CA, 1980. 30:4–47.
3. Baker LH: Breast cancer detection demonstration project: five-year summary report. CA 1982; 32:194–225.
4. Balducci L, Phillips M, Wallace C, Hardy C: Cancer chemotherapy in the elderly. Am Fam Phys 1987; 35:133–143.
5. Baranovsky A, Myers M: Cancer incidence and survival in patients 65 years of age and older. CA 1986; 36:26–41.
6. Berci G, Parish JF, Schapiro M, Conlin R: Complications of endoscopy and polypectomy. The Southern California Society for Gastrointestinal Endoscopy. Gastroenterology 1974; 67:584–585.
7. Boone MI, Calvert JC, Gates HS: Uterine cancer screening by the family physician. Am Fam Phys 1984; 30:157–166.
8. Brooman JC, Peeling WB, Griffiths GJ, et al: A comparison between digital examination and per-rectal ultrasound in the evaluation of the prostate. Br J Urol 1981; 53:617–620.
9. Eddy D: Screening the "well elderly." CA 1986; 36:318–319.
10. Executive Board of ACOG: Mammography Statement. Washington, D.C., American College of Obstetricians and Gynecologists, 1979.

11. Foster RS, Lang SP, Costanza MC, et al: Breast self-examination practices and breast-cancer stage. N Engl J Med 1978; 299:265–270.
12. Frame PS: A critical review of adult health maintenance: Part 3: Prevention of cancer. J Fam Prac 1986; 22:511–520.
13. Frame PS, Carlson SJ: A critical review of periodic health screen using specific screening criteria. respiratory, cardiovascular and central nervous systems. J Fam Prac 1975; 2:29–36.
14. Friedman GD: Primer of Epidemiology. New York, McGraw-Hill, 1980.
15. Griffiths GH, Clements HR, Jones DR, et al: The ultrasound appearances of prostatic cancer with histological correlation. Clin Rad 1987; 38:219–227.
16. Guinan P, Bush I, Ray V, et al: The accuracy of the rectal examination in the diagnosis of prostate carcinoma. N Engl J Med 1980; 303:499–503.
17. Hall SW: Cancer: Special considerations in older patients. Geriatrics 1984; 39:74–78.
18. Herbsman H, Feldman J, Seldera J, et al: Survival following breast cancer surgery in the elderly. Cancer 1981; 47:2358–2363.
19. Holmes FF, Hearne E: Cancer stage-to-age relationship: implications for cancer screening in the elderly. J Am Geriatr Soc 1981; 29:55–57.
20. Lipschitz DA, Goldstein S, Reis R, et al: Cancer in the elderly: basic science and clinical aspects. Ann Intern Med 1985; 102:218–228.
21. Love RR, Fryback DG, Kimbrough SR: A cost-effectiveness analysis of screening for carcinoma of the prostate by digital examination. Med Decis Making 1986; 5:263–278.
22. Mandelblatt JS, Hammond DB: Primary care of elderly women: Is pap smear screening necessary? Mt Sinai J Med 1985; 52:284–290.
23. Mandelblatt J, Gopaul I, Wistreich M: Gynecological care of elderly women: another look at Papanicolaou smear testing. JAMA 1986; 256:367–371.
24. Mangla JC, Pereira M, Murphy J: Diagnosis of occult gastrointestinal lesions by stool guaiac testing in a geriatric hospital. J Am Geriatr Soc 1981; 29:473–475.
25. Moore JR, Lamont JT: Colorectal cancer: Risk factors and screening strategies. Arch Intern Med 1984; 144:1819–1823.
26. O'Malley MS, Fletcher SW: Screening for breast cancer with breast self-examination: A critical review. JAMA 1987; 2197–2203.
27. Rodes ND, Lopez MJ, Pearson DK, et al: The impact of breast cancer screening on survival: A 5- to 10-year follow-up study. 1986; Cancer 57:581–585.
28. Sackett DL, Haynes RB, Tugwell P: Clinical Epidemiology: A Basic Science for Clinical Medicine. Boston, MA, Little, Brown and Co., 1985.
29. Sadowsky NL, Kalisher LL, White G, et al: Radiologic detection of breast cancer: Review and recommendations. N Engl J Med 1976; 294:370–373.
30. Shapiro S, Venet W, Strax P, et al: Ten to fourteen year effects of breast cancer screening on mortality. J Nat Cancer Inst 1982; 69:349–355.
31. Stamey TA, Yang A, Hay AR, et al: Prostate-specific antigen as a serum marker for adenocarcinoma of the prostate. N Engl J Med 1987; 317:909–916.
32. Stromborg M: Early detection of cancer in the elderly: problems and solutions. Int J Nurs Stud 1982; 19:139–156.
33. Stults BM: Preventive cancer care for the elderly. Front Radiat Ther Oncol 1986; 20:182–191.
34. Stults BM: Preventive health care for the elderly. West J Med 1984; 141:832–845.
35. US Preventive Services Task Force: Recommendations for breast cancer screening. JAMA 1987; 257:2196.
36. Vaughan WP: Cancer: What's special about the elderly? Geriatrics 1984; 39:15–16.
37. Vihko P, Kontturi M, Lukkarinen O, et al: Screening for carcinoma of the prostate. Rectal examination and enzymatic and radioimmunologic measurements of serum acid phosphatase compared. Cancer 1985; 56:173–177.
38. Watson RA, Tang DB: The predictive value of prostatic acid phosphatase as a screening test for prostatic cancer. N Engl J Med 1980; 303:497–499.
39. Weissman GS, Winawer SJ, Baldwin MP, et al: Multicenter evaluation of training of non-endoscopists in 30-cm flexible sigmoidoscopy. CA 1987; 37:26–29.
40. Winawer SJ, Andrews JM, Flehinger B: Progress report on controlled trial of fecal occult blood testing for the detection of colorectal neoplasia. Cancer 1980; 45:2959–2964.
41. Winawer SJ, Sherlock P, Schottenfeld D, Miller DG: Screening for colon cancer. Gastroenterology 1976; 70:783–789.
42. Zuna RE: The Pap smear revisited: controversies and recent developments. Postgrad Med 1984; 76:36–46.

4
IMMUNIZATION IN THE ELDERLY

Richard V. Sims, MD

The elderly are vulnerable to a variety of infectious processes. Of particular concern are the potentially preventable infections caused by influenza A and B, *Streptococcus pneumoniae* and *Clostridium tetani*. In this chapter, the epidemiology of these diseases and the etiologic factors underlying this special vulnerability are reviewed. Consideration of the clinical and financial benefits likely to accrue from programs dedicated to wider immunization of the aged will follow. Finally, recommendations aimed at redressing the current under-utilization of these vaccines will be discussed.

EPIDEMIOLOGY

Epidemiologic data collected over a 10-year period (1969–1978) reveal that of the 120,000 excess deaths attributed to influenza, 82% occurred in elderly persons.[1] A report on a series of influenza A epidemics in Texas documented hospitalization rates exceeding 115 per 10,000 and mortality rates of 187 per 100,000 in persons 65 years old and older. Among people aged 45–64 years old, these rates were reported to be 25 per 10,000 and 13 per 100,000, respectively. Because mortality figures in this study were based on death certificates, which may under-report specific causes of death, real mortality rates attributable to influenza may have been three times greater than those published.[2] Among residents of nursing homes, morbidity data are more striking: a review of lower respiratory tract infections during an influenza epidemic in one such facility documented a 35% annual incidence. In those instances in which an etiologic agent was isolated, influenza A was a common pathogen; however, *Haemophilus influenzae* and *S. pneumoniae* were also frequently identified.[3]

Less is known about the epidemiology of pneumococcal infections, which present 80% or more of the time as pneumonias. Current estimates of incidence rates for pneumococcal pneumonia range from one to two cases per 1000, overall, with roughly 20% of cases complicated by bacteremias.[4] Among the eldest and youngest subjects, incidence rates are probably much higher.[5] Despite the application of ICU technologies and appropriate antibiotics, 30–45% of adults over age 65 succumb to bacteremic pneumococcal pneumonias. Predisposing conditions, especially cardiopulmonary disorders, are present in almost 90% of such patients. Case fatality rates were highest in one study among persons with chronic renal insufficiency, malignancies, coronary artery disease, and alcoholism.[5] While the prevalence of chronic disorders increases with age, it is by no means clear whether the risk of acquiring pneumococcal pneumonia is increased among the "healthy" elderly, who are presumably without conditions predisposing to it. Ruben and co-workers reviewed the independent predictors of death among pneumococcal bacteremia patients at one institution over a 5-year period. Age per se did not appear to increase mortality in the absence of acute or chronic disorders, asplenia, complications, or inappropriate use of antibiotics.[6]

In addition to predisposing acute and chronic diseases, elderly subjects with pneumonia may present with lower fevers and nonfocal symptoms, which can delay diagnoses and lead to higher mortality.[7] Signs such as lethargy, change in mental status, or hypophagia may, at times, be the only clues to an acute respiratory infection. Unless physicians and caregivers recognize these as potential signs of serious disease, diagnosis and treatment may be needlessly delayed.

As a public health concern, tetanus has declined in importance relative to influenza and pneumococcal pneumonia; therefore, it will not be discussed in depth. It should be noted, however, that a majority of the 75 to 100 cases that occur annually in the United States develop in those 65 years of age and older.[8]

Despite the increased incidence, mortality and morbidity from pneumococcal infection, influenza, and tetanus, patients at high risk remain largely unimmunized. In 1985, in several settings fewer than 50% of elderly outpatients had received the trivalent influenza vaccine. Among residents of nursing homes, who may be at highest risk from influenza and pneumonia, average immunization rates of only 60% of eligible subjects have been documented.[9] Rates of pneumococcal vaccine use are also low: one study of more than 500 persons admitted to a hospital with high-risk conditions found that none had been immunized with the polyvalent vaccine.[10]

Surveys of protective antibody titers among adults document that 11% of persons 18–39 years old and more than half of those 60 years old and older lack adequate circulating levels of the tetanus antitoxin.[8]

Thus, underutilization of these vaccines remains an important and ongoing public health concern.

INCREASED SUSCEPTIBILITY TO INFECTION IN THE ELDERLY

The special susceptibility of aged persons to infectious diseases may in part be attributed to the physiologic and immunologic concomitants of "normal" aging. The increased prevalence of chronic diseases and the resulting therapeutic interventions, such as tracheostomies or chronic indwelling Foley catheters, that accompany them further add to this susceptibility.

The chief physiologic manifestations of aging on lung function are related to changes in lung and chest wall compliance. The chest wall becomes stiffer with age, and the muscles of respiration—the diaphragm, intercostal muscles, and accessory muscles—decline in strength, resulting in a decrease in inspiratory force. There is also a progressive loss of pulmonary elastic recoil. The clinical correlate of these changes is "senile emphysema," and standard spirometric measurements of lung functions (FEV_1, PEFR, and VC) diminish with age. Total lung capacity is unchanged, but at the expense of an increased residual volume. RV increases nearly 50% between childhood and age 70. A less effective cough and reduced respiratory reserve result. Other alterations include a fall in arterial oxygen tension from ventilation-perfusion mismatching and a less vigorous ventilatory response to hypoxia and hypercarbia. The ciliary action of columnar cells lining the trachea and bronchi and local IgA secretion are reduced. Alveolar macrophages clear foreign material less efficiently. The frequent imposition of cardiac disease, which is quite prevalent among the elderly, on the aged pulmonary system further compromises the host's ability to resist pulmonary infections.[11]

Adding to the effects of age, the burden of underlying disease increases the risk of acquiring influenza and pneumonia. As the population matures, the proportion of individuals free of chronic disease decreases. Among geriatric populations, most have between 5–8 chronic diseases. Chronic diseases, such as renal failure, cancer, and arteriosclerotic heart disease, are central to high mortality rates due to influenza and pneumonia.[5]

Institutionalization, which affects up to 5% of older persons, may be a particular risk factor for both influenza and pneumonia. The institutionalized elderly are likely to have severely impaired mobility, many to the point of being bedridden. In such a population, pooling of secretions and atelectasis is not uncommon. They are prone to malnutrition and senile dementia. Furthermore, the sedative and anticholinergic effects of the psychotropic medications used to treat dementia-related behavioral disturbances may also inhibit the ability to clear secretions. All these factors, along with the closed character of these populations, increase the risk of communicable disease and make prophylactic immunization a highly desirable strategy.

The elderly may be less immunologically competent both to fend off acute infectious diseases and to respond to standard vaccines against influenza A and B, *S. pneumoniae,* and clinical tetanus. The involution of the thymus gland and the loss of thymic hormones with age have been identified as central to changes in immunocompetence. The number of thymocytes that differentiate into functionally mature T lymphocytes is reduced, but consistent changes in lymphocyte subpopulations have not been documented. Functional changes among B and T cell lines have been demonstrated, as in impaired lymphocyte blastogenesis due to decreased responsiveness of some cells and an attenuated delayed hypersensitivity response. Cytotoxic and natural killer T-lymphocytes, which defend against virus-infected and cancer cells, are generated less prolifically. Abnormal regulation of antibody production is manifested by the increased prevalence of auto-antibodies and of benign gammopathies.[12]

A less robust response to type-specific antigens has been documented in a variety of studies. Recent work has attributed the reduction in phytohemagglutinin-induced blastogenesis and anti-influenza antibody production to decreased interleukin-2 production by aged helper (T4) cells.[12] In the future, higher than normal doses of the influenza vaccine may be suggested for elderly patients. A major immunological response—a hemagglutination inhibition titer greater than 1:40—could be achieved in 70% of subjects (age range 71 to 74) in one study only by administering three times the usual dose. Other workers have documented considerable declines in antibody titers within six months, contributing to outbreaks of influenza in the spring.[24]

In summary, elderly patients experience an increased incidence of infectious diseases as well as disproportionate morbidity and mortality due in part to physiologic and immunologic changes of normal aging. Furthermore, the elderly are even more susceptible because of the effects of institutionalization, chronic diseases, impaired mobility, and other deficits characteristic of this population.

BENEFITS OF IMMUNIZATION

The ability to respond to immunization is impaired even in the healthy, well-nourished elderly. What evidence is there, then, that vaccination will be beneficial to them or to the frailer, institutionalized older person? Studies of the efficacy of the influenza vaccine have consistently demonstrated values from 0% to 36%. However, in a study of influenza-related illness and complications among 1,082 clients in seven Michigan nursing homes, significant reductions in influenza-like illnesses (risk ratio [RR] comparing magnitude of risk in unvaccinated versus vaccinated patients = 2.6), hospitalization (RR = 2.4), roentgenographically proven pneumonia (RR = 2.9), and deaths (RR = 5.6) were documented among vaccinated patients.[13]

Further, Levine and colleagues reported cumulative seroconversion rates (a fourfold or greater rise in hemagglutinin-inhibiting antibody against the influenza virus) of 70% in a sample of elderly men from a chronic care facility. While antibody titers reached putative protective levels in the majority of responders by the fourth week after vaccination, 18–28% of seroconversions occurred after the fourth week.[14]

The first evidence of the effectiveness of the pneumococcal vaccine in preventing pneumococcal pneumonia among the institutionalized elderly was reported in 1947. More than 5,000 subjects were immunized with a trivalent vaccine (against capsular antigens from types 1, 2, and 3) and were compared with an equal number of unvaccinated controls for the development of disease. Several-hundred-fold elevations in protective antibody levels were measured in vaccinated persons, and overall the vaccine reduced the incidence of pneumonia by 39% and of mortality by 32% in this population. Efficacy trials among young healthy South African gold miners for a newer 12-valent vaccine revealed a greater than 75% reduction in vaccine serotype disease among vaccinated subjects. The results of subsequent trials involving elderly patients have been less conclusive. A 1986 case-control study found a crude efficacy rate of 70% among patients 55 years old and older.[15] Other workers, using methodology in which the frequencies of pneumococcal bacteremias caused by vaccine and non-vaccine serotypes were compared in a population of vaccinated and unvaccinated subjects, documented 61% efficacy among healthy elderly subjects and those with chronic cardiopulmonary disease and diabetes mellitus.[16]

Patients with multiple myeloma, leukemia, hypogammaglobulinemia, treated lymphomas (particularly Hodgkin's disease), and organ transplantation may not respond to vaccine antigens, but are otherwise at high risk. Such patients should be offered the vaccine, provided they are educated about its reduced effectiveness in this setting. If possible, patients should be immunized two weeks prior to splenectomy or beginning chemotherapy.

Therefore, despite a less striking rise in antibody titer in response to specific antigens, the elderly appear to benefit from immunization at least with the influenza and 14-valent pneumococcal vaccine. A 23-valent vaccine, which includes serotypes responsible for more than 85% of all pneumococcal bacteremias, was introduced in 1983, and should therefore have a higher rate of vaccine efficacy.

As well as helping to reduce disease in older patients, wider use of the influenza and pneumococcal vaccines and the tetanus toxoid should assist in reducing hospitalization and often associated functional decline, the need for custodial care, and financial hardship.

COST IMPLICATIONS OF IMMUNIZATION

To the extent that vaccination programs prevent death and disability, preventive immunization can be thought of as a money-saving strategy. However, depending on the point of view (patient, hospital administrator, or society at large), such a formulation can be considered simplistic. For society, for example, prolongation of years of life may necessitate greater expenditures for health care and retirement benefits for elderly citizens in the long term. On the other hand, more years of productivity by otherwise healthy elderly might be expected to enhance revenues generated by taxes.

A cost-effectiveness study carried out by the U.S. Office of Technology Assessment found that, for the years 1971 through 1978, vaccination of persons 65 years old and older against influenza saved net medical care costs and improved health. Assuming annual vaccination rates of 22%, immunization of elderly patients saved about $6.6 million in medical costs associated with epidemic influenza in 1971 and produced a gain of about four weeks of healthy life. When expected medical costs for additional years of life saved are included, the net annual cost per year of quality life gained by immunizing high-risk elderly approximates $4,000—a low relative cost when compared to other preventive efforts. This estimate does not take into account additional productivity generated by vaccinees who continue to work because of reduced disability and death from influenza.[17]

Using new estimates of key variables, Sisk and Riegelman re-examined the cost-effectiveness and costs to Medicare of subsidizing pneumococcal vaccinations. Taking into account a lower expected incidence of pneumococcal pneumonia (10% of all pneumonias), higher physician's fees, and a three-year duration of immunity, vaccination of an elderly person would gain one year of healthy life for about $6,000 (1983 dollars). This result was compared with the costs of screening women 30 to 39 years of age for cervical cancer every three years, which would require about $16,000 (1979 dollars) per year of healthy life saved. Net costs to Medicare would range between $4,400 to $8,300 per year of life saved, depending in part on the cost per vaccination. If the duration of immunity were proved to be eight years or more, the authors point out that vaccination of the elderly *en masse* would be cost saving if the vaccine were provided by a public program. In light of these findings, the authors of the study concluded that current utilization rates of the pneumococcal vaccine are "wastefully low."[18]

STRATEGIES FOR INCREASING IMMUNIZATION

It is clear that the influenza, pneumococcal, and tetanus vaccines are underused. To understand why this should be so, we will examine how attitudes among physicians and among patients, as well as the current medical care milieu, influence the use of these agents.

THE PHYSICIAN

Perhaps the chief obstacle to the widespread use of vaccines is the current climate, which undervalues prevention in general. Training and reimbursement patterns favor acute in-hospital care and the use of sophisticated technologies, but slight preventive strategies that are relatively cheap and associated with few side effects. Physicians' own fascination with technology has been termed the technological imperative by observers of our profession. While this technological imperative has driven the behavior of many individual physicians, as well as policy makers, there is increasing pressure to use appropriate technology to stay our hand. Nowhere is this more relevant than in geriatrics.

Side effects exist for all therapies, including the influenza and pneumococcal vaccines. However, they are minor for these two vaccines and, with rare exceptions, should not deter physicians from recommending vaccination. It is estimated that 10% of elderly given the trivalent influenza vaccine experience local erythema and swelling. Systemic reactions with fever and myalgias are uncommon, occurring in 1% to 2% of those vaccinated.[25] Mild, local reactions are described among 30–40% of elderly who were administered the 14-valent pneumococcal vaccine; fever, arthralgia, and rash developed in less than 7%. Three cases of anaphylaxis may have occurred among the first 4 million doses.[4] The newer 23-valent vaccine with less total polysaccharide is expected to cause significantly fewer ill effects. Similar local reactions with the administration of the combined tetanus and diphtheria toxoids are described, but fever and systemic reactions are typically rare.[8]

Fear of vaccine-drug interactions may contribute to low use rates by some physicians. However, current evidence suggests that for two implicated drugs, warfarin and theophylline, adverse reactions following influenza vaccinations are unlikely and should not dissuade physicians from inoculating elderly people at risk for influenza.[27] The absence of randomized clinical trials proving efficacy of the pneumococcal and influenza vaccines in particularly healthy aged and the relative rarity of clinical tetanus may have adversely affected physicians' practice patterns. One 1985 study found that although physicians had a strong belief in the utility of the influenza vaccine, all methods of reminders to physicians failed to improve the low rates of vaccine use.[28] In another report, both patient behavior and the failure by health care providers to promote vaccination appeared to contribute to this trend.[27]

A large nationwide survey of private primary care providers found that, despite the high degree of agreement that the pneumococcal vaccine was indicated for the high-risk groups, more than half of the survey respondents immunized only patients with cardiorespiratory diseases.[29] Daily chart audits in a family practice residency revealed significant underuse of the pneumococcal vaccine, primarily because the physicians' knowledge about vaccine indications was inadequate, and they failed to consider vaccination during the physician-patient encounters.[30] Uncertainties about the local and systemic effects, which are minor in adults, and concerns about inadvertent reimmunization with the pneumococcal vaccine further discourage its use.

Since the potential benefit of influenza and pneumococcal immunization clearly outweigh the risks for all but a few patients, workable strategies for increasing immunization rates must be developed by individual physicians and health service organizations. While the particular strategy must be tailored to the individual setting, three principles are important:

1. Choose a clear method of identifying patients.
2. Institute a reminder system for both patients and physicians.
3. Expand the sites for immunization beyond the patient-physician encounter.

Know the Vaccination Status. Uncertainty regarding the vaccination status of a patient is often given as a reason for not immunizing, especially in the case of the pneumococcal vaccine. Therefore, good record-keeping is essential. Flow sheets and stickers for the chart are probably the most practical methods for individual and small groups of physicians. Such charting tasks may escape the busy practitioner; however, the nurse, medical assistant, or even secretary could be responsible for documenting the immunization. Large group practices or HMOs can make use of computerized medical-records packages that incorporate billing data in the medical record, so that an immunization that is billed becomes a part of the medical record.

Implement Office Practices to Increase Immunization. Actively promote immunization with mailings and educational literature and by involving other health professionals. In a randomly chosen group of elderly attending a general internal medicine practice, 56% of 91 patients received the pneumococcal vaccine. Those who received the vaccine were more likely than those who did not to have received the previous year's influenza vaccine, to have a medical-problem list attached to the clinic chart, to have been seen by clinic physicians in the year before the study, and to have more than two medical problems recorded in the clinic computer file. When unimmunized patients were sent letters urging vaccination, the inoculation rate improved significantly. Interestingly, those patients who were up-to-date with their influenza and tetanus vaccines proved the most likely to respond to the mailings.[21]

Other interventions found to be effective in increasing the delivery of influenza and pneumococcal vaccines were collection of immunization histories and distribution of printed educational literature by medical clinic secretaries,[22] and coordination of a vaccination program by clinic pharmacists.[23] Other innovative strategies might include posting a reminder notice in the waiting room or exam room, instructing the medical assistant or secretary to put a reminder on every elderly patient's chart before giving the chart to the physician, incorporating a reminder into taped telephone answering machine messages, or sending reminders to caregivers of elderly patients.

Identify Sites Other Than Physician-Patient Encounters in Private Practice Offices that Are Appropriate for Immunization. Vaccinate hospitalized patients. Previous hospitalization has been found to be a risk factor for acquiring serious pneumococcal infections. The Shenandoah study, which used a computerized data base on 72,000 Medicare enrollees discharged from 14 northern Virginia hospitals, reported that 52% of 1,227 elderly with discharge diagnoses of pneumonia had been hospitalized within the previous three years. As many as 60% to 70% of patients with pneumococcal bacteremia had been hospitalized within the previous five years, and high-risk conditions were evident in 69% of these patients on an earlier hospital admission. It is clear from these findings that hospitals should assume a larger role in preventive vaccination.[20]

Annual influenza vaccination among the especially vulnerable custodial care community has been recommended since 1981. An institutional policy regarding a standing order for the vaccine resulted in the inoculations of 95% of patients in one hospital-based extended-care facility.[24]

In addition, some physicians have found that the establishment of a day or evening exclusively for immunizations, when patients can come without an appointment and receive immunizations from the nurse or medical assistant, are effective. Similarly, encouraging patients to seek immunizations at convenient places such as senior centers may remove some obstacles and improve immunization rates.

THE PATIENT

Although the attitude of the physician may have some influence on the extent to which the influenza, pneumococcal, and tetanus vaccines are used, other factors may shape the readiness of patients to accept immunization. Frank, Henderson, and McMurray undertook to identify the determinants of acceptance of the influenza vaccine among 273 elderly people living in the community. Persons who had previously experienced ill effects or found the vaccine lacking in effectiveness were less inclined to accept vaccination subsequently. Although the active encouragement of physicians tripled vaccination rates in this instance, 50% of persons originally found to be unwilling remained so because of the perceived risks.[28] More recently, a decision model predicting influenza vaccination compliance was tested on an ambulatory clinic population composed of the elderly and the chronically ill. The model accurately distinguished vaccine compliance versus noncompliance 82% of the time (sensitivity, 96%; specificity, 44%). Shot "takers" differed significantly from "non-takers" in regard to concerns about the complications and side effects of the vaccine, the discomfort and complications of the infection, and the likely impact of the influenza on activities of daily living and independence. Anxieties about the side effects of flu shots correctly identified patients who intended to receive the vaccine but ultimately failed to be inoculated.[31] Information about patient attitudes and behavior is not available for either the pneumococcal vaccine or the tetanus toxoid. It is likely, however, that the attitudes of primary care provider and client toward these preventive therapies are similarly responsible for the low rates of use.

Thus, it is important to provide readable information to patients that will reduce their concerns.

TIME AND MONEY

As we have seen, the vaccines have few, if any, major side effects. They are cheap (approximately $5 for a pneumococcal vaccine injection) and are reimbursable through Medicare for persons 65 years old and older.

The willingness of the care provider to promote immunization will improve vaccination rates among a proportion of his or her patients. In certain settings, such as the busy solo medical or subspecialty practice, the time commitment necessary to educate and assure clients offers a true challenge. However, there are effective settings from which to manage immunization for high-risk patients.

PRACTICE RECOMMENDATIONS

1. Check the influenza, pneumococcal, and tetanus immunization status of all elderly patients.
2. Give the 23-valent pneumococcal vaccination to all elderly patients once. Routine booster immunization is not recommended in patients who have already received the 14-valent vaccine.[18]
3. If it is impossible to document a patient's pneumococcal vaccine history, the risk of serious complication due to repeat vaccination is low enough to justify giving the vaccine.
4. Immunize all elderly patients against influenza in the late fall. Studies have documented considerable declines in antibody titers within six months, contributing to outbreaks of influenza in the spring and leading to the recommendation that vaccinations be provided as late as possible (late October) before the start of influenza season.[23]
5. Give all elderly patients a tetanus toxoid booster every 10 years. For adults who have not completed the primary immunization course, a 0.5 ml

injection of the combined toxoid is suggested. Some authors have suggested that boosters be given on mid-decade birthdays (65, 75, etc.).

6. Test for immediate hypersensitivity to tetanus toxoid on any patient in whom a history of an allergic reaction is suspected. A severe hypersensitivity reaction or neurologic reaction following a previous dose is the only contraindication to the use of the tetanus toxoid.

7. Document all immunizations using some system which will remind you of vaccination status as well as the time for tetanus boosters. (See Prevention Checklist in Appendix B).

8. Institute a reminder system for patients that will let them know when it's time to have their influenza vaccination and tetanus booster.

9. Actively promote immunization with mailings and educational literature, by involving other members of the office staff, and through other professionals, such as pharmacists.

10. Identify sites other than your practice office, such as hospitals, that are appropriate for offering immunizations.

11. Take extra time to explore reasons for non-compliance among "non-takers." Clear information about side-effects and relative risks of immunization versus nonimmunization can often allay unnecessary anxieties.

REFERENCES

1. Tillet HE, Smith JW, Gooch CD: Excess deaths attributable to influenza in England and Wales: Age at death and certified cause. Int J Epidemiol 1983; 12:344–352.
2. Glezen WP: Serious morbidity and mortality associated with influenza epidemics. Epidemiol Rev 1982; 4:25–44.
3. Andrews J, Chandrasekaran P, McSwiggan D: Lower respiratory tract infections in an acute geriatric male ward: A one-year prospective surveillance. Gerontology 1984; 30:290–296.
4. Schwartz SJ: Pneumococcal vaccine: Clinical efficacy and effectiveness. Ann Intern Med 1982; 96:208–220.
5. Mufson MA, Oley G, Hughey D: Pneumococcal disease in a medium-sized community hospital. JAMA 1982; 248:1486–1489.
6. Ruben FL, Norden CW, Korica Y: Pneumococcal bacteremia at a medical/surgical hospital for adults between 1975 and 1980. Am J Med 1984; 77:1091–1094.
7. Finklestein MS, Petkun WM, Freedman ML, Antopol SC: Pneumococcal bacteremia in adults: Age-dependent differences in presentation and in outcome. J Am Geriatr Soc 1983; 31:19–27.
8. Committee on Immunization, Council of Medical Societies, American College of Physicians: Guide for Adult Immunization. Philadelphia, PA, American College of Physicians 1985.
9. Kendal AP, Patriarca PA, Arden NH: Policies and outcomes for control of influenza among the elderly in the U.S.A. Vaccine 1985; 3:274–276.
10. Klein KS, Adachi N: Pneumococcal vaccine in the hospital: Improved use and implications for high-risk patients. Arch Intern Med 1983; 143:1878–1881.
11. King TE, Schwartz MI: Pulmonary function and disease in the elderly. In Schrier RW (ed): Clinical Internal Medicine in the Aged. Philadelphia, PA, WB Saunders Co., 1982.
12. Delafuente JC: Immunosenescence: Clinical and pharmacologic considerations. Med Clin North Am 1985; 69:475–486.
13. Patriarca PA, Weber JA, Parker RA, et al: Efficacy of influenza vaccine in nursing homes. Reduction in illness and complications during an influenza A epidemic. JAMA 1985; 253:1136–1139.
14. Levine MA, Beattie BL, McLean DM, Corman D: Characterization of the immune response to trivalent influenza vaccine in elderly men. J Am Geriatr Soc 1987; 35:609–615.
15. Shapiro ED, Clemens JD: A controlled evaluation of the protective efficacy of pneumococcal vaccine for patients at high risk of serious pneumococcal infections. Ann Intern Med 1984; 101:325–330.
16. Bolan G, Broome CV, Facklam RR, et al: Pneumococcal vaccine efficacy in selected populations in the United States. Ann Intern Med 1986; 104:1–6.
17. Riddiough MA, Sisk JE, Bell JC: Influenza vaccination. JAMA 1983; 249:3189–3195.

18. Sisk JE, Riegelman RK: Cost effectiveness of vaccination against pneumococcal pneumonia: An update. Ann Intern Med 1986; 104:79–86.
19. Health and Public Policy Committee, American College of Physicians: Pneumococcal vaccine. Ann Intern Med 1986; 104:118–120.
20. Fedson DS: Improving the use of pneumococcal vaccine through a strategy of hospital-based immunization: A review of its rationale and implications. J Am Geriatr Soc 1985; 33:142–150.
21. Siebers MJ, Hunt VB: Increasing the pneumococcal vaccination rate of elderly patients in a general internal medicine clinic. J Am Geriatr Soc 1985; 33:175–178.
22. Ratner ER, Fedson DS: Influenza and pneumococcal immunization in medical clinics, 1978–1980. Arch Intern Med 1983; 143:2066–2069.
23. Spruill WJ, Cooper JW, Taylor WJR: Pharmacist-coordinated pneumonia and influenza vaccination program. Am J Hosp Pharm 1982; 39:1904–1906.
24. Setia V, Serventi I, Lorenz P: Factors affecting the use of influenza vaccine in the institutionalized elderly. J Am Geriatr Soc 1985; 33:856–858.
25. Reisenberg DE: Influenza immunization changes for elderly? JAMA 1986; 255:177.
26. Busby J, Caranasos GJ: Immune function, autoimmunity and selective immunoprophylaxis in the aged. Med Clin North Am 1985; 69:465–474.
27. D'Arch PF: Vaccine-drug interactions. Drug Intell Clin Pharm 1984; 26:101–103.
28. Frank JW, McMurray L, Henderson M: Influenza vaccination in the elderly: The economics of sending reminder letters. Can Med Assoc J 1985; 132:371–375.
29. Patriarca PA, Schlech WF, Hinman AR, et al: Pneumococcal vaccination practices among private physicians. Public Health Rep 1982; 97:406.
30. Brownlee HJ, Brown DL, D'Angelo RJ: Utilization of pneumococcal vaccine in a family practice residency. J Fam Pract 1982; 15:111–114.
31. Carter WB, Beach LR, Inui TS, et al: Developing and testing a decision model for predicting influenza vaccination compliance. Health Serv Res 1986; 20:897–932.

5
PREVENTING ADVERSE DRUG REACTIONS IN THE ELDERLY

Risa Lavizzo-Mourey, MD, MBA

Iatrogenic disease related to adverse drug reactions increases steadily after age 50,[1] making it one of the most common preventable diseases among the elderly. Adverse reactions to medications can result from side effects of the medication, drug interactions, or medication misuse. Nearly one-third of elderly patients report adverse drug reactions,[1,2] and these reactions are more likely to cause significant morbidity or mortality among the elderly than among younger patients. Adverse drug reactions, particularly those due to drug-drug interactions, account for as many as 10% of hospitalizations.[1,27] One study found 65% of drug-drug interactions to be definitely avoidable and another 36% probably avoidable. The reasons for this increase in adverse drug reactions are multifactorial and are related to clinical as well as social factors.

The clinical factors that increase the elderly's risk of adverse drug reactions relate to the aging process and the disease burden seen in the elderly. While all medications have side effects, physiologic changes related to age and particular disease states may potentiate some side effects and lessen others. For example, total body water decreases by 10–20% between the ages of 20 and 80, and there is an associated 35–40% decrease in extracellular fluid volume. Concomitantly, total body fat increases, going from 18% to 36% in men and from 33% to 45% in women. Therefore, lipophilic medications have a larger volume of distribution, lower serum levels for a single dose, but a longer elimination time.[5] The clinician can expect side effects due to peak levels to be lessened and those due to accumulated doses to be potentiated. Other age-related changes and their clinical implications are shown in Table 1. Serum albumin decreases from a mean of 4.7 mg/dl in the young to 3.8 mg/dl in the elderly.[6] Since albumin is the major binding protein for medications, protein binding of many medications commonly prescribed among the elderly is affected. Reduced protein binding is associated with increased free-drug levels, an altered volume of distribution, and an increase in certain kinds of drug-drug interactions.[5] Medications with known alterations in protein binding are shown in Table 2. The aging process affects both the liver[6-8] and the kidney,[6-9] and therefore has implications for drug elimination. Changes in creatinine clearance can be estimated in men and women using the following formula:

$$\text{Creatinine clearance} = \frac{(140 - \text{age}) \ (\text{Body weight in kg})^*}{72 \times \text{Creatinine mg}/\%}$$

---

* This refers to men. To estimate the creatinine clearance in elderly women, multiply by 0.85

TABLE 1. Clinical Implications of Age-Related Changes*

Effect	Age-Related Alteration	Clinical Importance
Absorption	Elevated gastric pH Reduced gastrointestinal blood flow ? Reduced number of absorbing cells ? Reduced gastrointestinal motility	Available studies indicate little effect of age
Distribution	**Body composition:** Reduced total body water Reduced lean body mass/kg body weight	Higher concentrations of drugs distributed in body fluids
	Increased body fat	? Longer duration of action of fat-soluble drugs
	Protein binding Reduced serum albumin	Higher free fraction of highly protein-bound drugs
Elimination	**Hepatic metabolism:** ? Reduced enzyme activity Reduced hepatic mass	Apparently slower biotransformation of some drugs
	Reduced hepatic blood flow	Influenced by environmental factors (nutrition & smoking)
	Renal excretion: Reduced glomerular filtration rate Reduced renal plasma flow Altered tubular function	Slower excretion of some drugs and metabolites

* Reprinted with permission from Vestal R: Geriatric Clinical Pharmacology: An Overview. Sydney, ADIS Health Science Press, 1984.

Changes in elimination by the liver are due to reductions in blood flow and oxidative enzyme levels[5,10] but are less quantifiable. Medications with age-related reductions in hepatic elimination are shown in Table 3. So while side effects exist for every medication, they are not always equated with adverse reactions and can be potentiated or lessened by physiologic changes.

    Since many adverse reactions are related to interactions among medications and medication misuse, the potential for adverse reactions would, logically, increase with the number or regularly consumed medications. The elderly have multiple chronic diseases. Ambulatory, community-dwelling elderly have, on average, 3.5 chronic illnesses.[14] This number increases with age, as does the number of disabilities.[13] Therefore, people over 85 not only have more chronic diseases but also are likely to have one major disability, such as inability to see or walk. Multiple chronic diseases beget multiple medications. Surveys indicate that the elderly take between five and eight prescription medications regularly, and may take as many or more nonprescription medications.[12–19] Given the documented positive correlation between number of medications and risk of

TABLE 2. Altered Protein Binding

Carbenoxolone	Fluphenazine	Phenylbutazone	Tolbutamide
Chlormethiazole	Lorazepam	Phenytoin	Warfarin
Diazepam	Meperidine		

TABLE 3. Altered Hepatic Metabolism in the Elderly*

Hepatic Extraction Ratios of Selected Drugs		
High	Intermediate	Low
Isoproterenol	Aspirin	Amobarbital
Lidocaine	Desipramine	Diazepam
Meperidine	Nortriptyline	Digitoxin
Morphine	Quinidine	Isoniazid
Nitroglycerin		Phenobarbital
Pentazocine		Phenylbutazone
Propoxyphene		Phenytoin
Propranolol		Procainamide
		Salicylic acid
		Theophylline
		Tolbutamide
		Warfarin

* Reprinted with permission from Lang P: Modifying drug dosage in elderly patients. In Covington P, Walker J (eds): Current Therapy in Geriatrics. Philadelphia, WB Saunders Co., 1984.

adverse reactions,[2] it is not surprising that the elderly, with their high burden of illness and consumption of medications, have an increased incidence of adverse drug reactions.

Social factors frequently increase the risk of medication misuse. Cost is a major factor. The elderly use a large part of their income for medications: $700 or $800 per year on the average.[20] This cost has been largely unreimbursed until recently. Only a few states (e.g., New York, Pennsylvania, and New Jersey) have pharmaceutical assistance programs, but catastrophic insurance legislation passed in 1988 does partially cover prescription medications. Like inadequate funds, lack of transportation to and from the pharmacy can prompt an elderly person to "stretch" a prescription or otherwise misuse their medications. Lastly, social isolation can contribute to poor compliance and medication misuse. Supervision of medication use has been shown to increase compliance. Fedder[23] has developed a profile of patients at high risk for medication misuse that summarizes these social factors. High-risk patients were found to be elderly women of low socioeconomic status who lived alone. While each of these social and clinical factors leads to adverse drug reactions, in the young as well as the old, they result in many more adverse reactions in the elderly. When the multitude of chronic diseases, prescription and nonprescription medications, and social problems are added to the age-related alterations in pharmacokinetics and pharmacodynamics, the multifactorial nature of the problem can be appreciated.

COSTS AND BENEFITS

Iatrogenic illness related to adverse drug reactions results in hospitalizations and changes in functional and mental status.[24] The estimated cost related to adverse drug reactions in 1979 was $3 billion. Among demented elderly, it has been shown that eliminating adverse drug reactions results in an improvement in both subjective and objective functional status.[25,26,26a] Studies of hospitalized elderly indicate that up to 10% are admitted to medical services because of drug-related complications.[1,27] A pilot study that evaluated the efficacy of a drug utilization review program indicates that inappropriate outpatient therapy contributes to the need for hospitalization.[28] While it has not been definitively proven, preventing adverse drug reactions should reduce hospitalizations and hospitalization costs. However, these cost implications extend further.

Homebound elderly take complicated medication regimens, yet these regimens can be simplified without significantly increasing the cost. It has yet to be shown that simplifications designed to avert adverse reactions also reduce cost to the elderly. However, it seems logical that if the total number of medications is reduced, so too should the cost.

The cost implications for the physician must be viewed in light of the changing health care environment. As capitation and risk-sharing between physicians and third-party payers become increasingly common, physicians will have strong incentives to prevent adverse reactions. The major cost to physicians of attempting to reduce adverse reactions is time. It takes more time to investigate potential interactions, design alternate medication regimens, and explain these regimens to the patient. However, if these efforts result in a true reduction in adverse reactions, this cost should be outweighed by the savings resulting from a reduction in the use of hospital and other medical care services. A Health Care Finance Administration sponsored study indicates that inappropriate drug use results in increased medical care services, an increase which is even more marked in the aged.[28] Under a capitation system, this increase in medical services is a cost to the physician. Similarly, hospitalizations resulting from iatrogenic illness are a direct and preventable cost to HMO physicians in managed care settings.

OBSTACLES TO IMPLEMENTING PREVENTIVE PRACTICES

Even physicians' best intentions to prevent drug-related iatrogenic illness are often thwarted. Three factors are important to consider here: 1. inadequacy of information, 2. common physician behaviors, and 3. patient resistance. There is an increasing awareness of the importance of drug interactions in the elderly; however, the specific information needed to effectively reduce these iatrogenic illnesses lags behind.

Inadequate Information. Preventing any illness or condition is predicated on a clear understanding of the etiologies of the illness. In the case of iatrogenic illness, one must know the side effects and how those side effects differ in various situations. It is this kind of specific information that is often lacking with regard to the elderly.

Although this is changing, in the past, pre-marketing drug trials often had limited numbers of elderly participants. Therefore, there is frequently uncertainty about the side effects of particular medications in the elderly. Identification of these side effects during the post-marketing phase depends on individual reporting. As a result, a considerable time may elapse before adequate data on side effects among the elderly are obtained and disseminated.[29] For example, a recently published article links propranolol with depression in the elderly.[30] Propranolol has been available for many years and is frequently used for cardiovascular diseases that plague the elderly.

Even among older medications, where the side-effects in the elderly are well described, there are few guidelines on how to individualize medications in the elderly. When medications that are cleared by the kidney are being used, age-, weight- and sex-adjusted nomograms can be helpful in guiding decisions about the initial dose. However, few medications are exclusively handled by the kidney. In a few specific cases, such as theophylline and quinidine, studies have been done that generated specific guidelines.[31,32] For the most part, individualization of medications for the elderly is based on a knowledge of age-related changes in pharmacokinetics and pharmacodynamics, physiology, and good clinical judgment.

The lack of knowledge is compounded because the elderly take, on average, between three and five prescription medications. There are publications that specifically address the potential interactions between two medications;[31-33] however, the most commonly used pharmaceutical reference, the *Physician's Desk Reference,* does not contain comprehensive information about drug interactions. In seeking information about drug interactions, the physician may be successful in obtaining drug interaction data about two medications. However, information relating three or more potentially interacting medications is virtually impossible to find. Therefore, every level of information related to adverse drug reactions among the elderly is limited, which curtails the physician's ability to successfully prevent this form of iatrogenic illness. Nevertheless, many adverse reactions can be prevented.

Physician and Patient Behaviors.   While it would seem that the easiest way to prevent this form of iatrogenic illness would be to limit the number of medications the elderly take, there are several factors that act to perpetuate the reliance on medications. Physicians traditionally favor pharmacologic therapies over nonpharmacologic therapies. For example, weight reduction is an effective means of reducing blood pressure in overweight hypertensives; however, in reality, medications are the mainstay of therapy. Physicians are not totally to blame for the "favorite son" position pharmacologic therapy holds. Patients, too, play a role. Patients have come to expect a prescription for a medication in response to a complaint. Insomnia, a complaint of nearly half of those over 65, responds poorly to the long-term use of sedatives, yet this is precisely what patients request. Nonpharmacologic therapies often require more effort and a sustained commitment to the therapy. For example, Kegel exercises to strengthen the pelvic floor are an effective treatment for stress incontinence in women. Once the exercises are learned, only a few minutes each day are required to maintain the tone of the pelvic floor and maintain continence. However, if the exercises are stopped, the positive effects are lost and incontinence returns. The ongoing involvement required of many nonpharmacologic therapies is often an obstacle but should be turned into a useful way to promote healthful behaviors among the elderly.

Physician Time Constraints.   Finally, the time constraints physicians face probably act to limit their involvement in preventing iatrogenic illness related to adverse drug reactions. Busy practitioners have little time to take a comprehensive drug history, verify that history, and then systematically review the patient's prescribed and nonprescribed medications. These same limitations of time make nonpharmacologic therapies less attractive. The explaining and rehearsing of nonpharmacologic therapies is time-consuming. It may not require any more time than adequately attempting to reduce adverse drug reactions through carefully reviewing historical data, thoughtfully limiting the number of medications, adjusting dosing schedules, and attempting to minimize interactions with each patient.

In short, the dearth of information about medications, their interactions, their pharmacokinetics and pharmacodynamics in the elderly, coupled with well-established behaviors and expectations, are the major obstacles to widespread use of practices which should reduce adverse drug reactions.

Specific Recommendations. The potential benefits of reducing iatrogenic illness secondary to medication reactions warrant increased effort by physicians towards preventing these problems. Despite the limitations in our knowledge, attention to optimizing the dosing schedule and monitoring potential interactions and side effects can help to prevent adverse drug reactions in the elderly.

1. Simplify medication regimen and optimize dosing schedule

Since the number of interactions and adverse drug reactions increases with the number of medications, limiting the number of medications is a crucial first step toward preventing adverse drug reactions. While studies indicate as many as 50% of patients can have some medications eliminated,[20] it is the minority who can have all medications eliminated. Therefore, optimizing the dosing schedule of essential medications, coupled with judiciously eliminating non-essential medications, becomes vital in preventing iatrogenic illness related to drugs. In considering the optimal dosing schedule, adjustments that will limit the number of times per day medications must be taken should be based on age-related changes in the pharmacokinetics of the drug and on social factors influencing compliance.

The total number of times per day medications are to be taken is inversely related to compliance.[16,34] Ideally, a once-a-day dosing schedule for all medications should be prescribed, However, since the half-lives of most medications do not allow for this kind of dosing schedule, every effort should be made to prescribe medications that can be given concurrently. Increasing the dosing intervals and choosing drugs with similar half-lives are the common ways to simplify a medication regimen. Sometimes a long-acting preparation of the same medicine can be used, and other times a similar medication with a longer half-life must be substituted.

Even among once-a-day medications, the dosing schedule can be important. If the taking of a medication interferes with part of the patient's daily activities, compliance may decrease. By knowing the patient's activities, the physician can optimize the dosing schedule. Practical and seemingly obvious suggestions for dosing should be discussed with the patient. For example, it should be suggested that sedating medicines be taken before bedtime or an afternoon nap, that diuretics be taken in the late afternoon after the errands have been run, and that sympathomimetics not be taken close to bedtime.

Adjusting the dosing schedule to ensure some supervision may also increase compliance. Studies have indicated that compliance is better among patients for whom supervision can be provided.[22,23] Therefore, if a dosing schedule can be adjusted to coincide with a visiting nurse encounter, a family member's routine check, or a daily visit to the senior center, compliance may improve. In addition, other reliable sources of information will be gained.

Finally, in determining the optimal dosing schedule, remember that it may be necessary to individualize a particular patient's dosing interval. The half-life of a medication is dependent on the dosage of the medication and its clearance. Since the clearance of medications is frequently decreased in the elderly, it is necessary to make adjustments in either the dose or the dosing interval. Reducing the dose rather than increasing the interval seems to be the more popular strategy. By increasing the dosing interval, one has the potential not only to reduce the risk of overdosage but also to increase compliance. Among highly toxic medications, such as digoxin, quinidine, lithium, tricyclic antidepressants, and aminophylline preparations, drug levels are particularly useful in making these decisions.

The following rules, which were developed to guide researchers in decisions about the simplification of medication regimens, may help the busy clinician determine the potential to simplify a particular patient's medication regimen.[20] The medication regimen can probably be simplified if:

    a. The medical regimen has more than one medication of the same class and the medications are not complementary; e.g., nadolol and propranolol but not spironolactone and furosemide.

    b. A medication can be substituted with a long-acting preparation of the same medication; e.g., Inderal and Inderal-LA.

    c. A medication can be substituted with a long-acting preparation of the same class; e.g., nadolol and propranolol.

    d. A medication can be given less often with the same efficacy; e.g., phenytoin 400 mg qd versus phenytoin 100 mg qid.

    e. More than one medication is being given for the same indication where one is proven to be effective; e.g., cimetidine and antacids.

2. Keep in mind that drug interactions have patterns

Monitoring the potential for drug-drug interactions in an elderly person taking five to eight medications is a formidable task that can be managed through a systematic approach to prescribing and monitoring medications. The elderly take multiple medications because of multiple diseases. The patterns of these diseases, in fact, dictate the patterns of medications. Therefore, the most frequently used medications are cardiovascular medications (including antihypertensives), hypnotics and sedatives, antibiotics and analgesics. Although there are hundreds of medications that fall into these categories, only a few are commonly used. Fifty prescription medications in Pennsylvania represented half of all prescriptions that were filled under a pharmaceutical assistance program for the elderly during 1984. The implication of this observation is that it is relatively easy to devise a table of common interactions (Table 4). This, of course, does not address the problem of actions between active metabolites or interactions between two or more drugs and another drug or set of drugs.

It should also be kept in mind that most of these interactions are "potential" interactions. Even though there may be well-documented reports of interactions in the literature, the individual physician may not see the interactions in each and every patient prescribed that medication. The probability of an adverse outcome is certainly not 100%, nor is it constant. The probability of digoxin and quinidine interacting is greater if there is an intercurrent illness leading to a change in the level of carrier protein and therefore the volume of distribution. Therefore, prescribing medications that have a potential for interacting falls into the category of a relative contraindication. These interacting medications can frequently be given together if appropriate periodic monitoring is also incorporated.

An understanding of the mechanisms and time courses involved in some common interactions provides basic guidance on monitoring.

Table 5 summarizes information about known drug-drug interactions among some medications commonly used by the elderly. The most common mechanisms of drug interactions result from changes in volume of distribution

TABLE 4. Summary of Drug Interactions

	Benzodiazepines	Beta Blockers	Captopril	Chlorpropamide	Cimetidine	Clonidine	Digoxin	Diltiazem	Ethanol	Indomethacin	Prazosin	Procainamide	Quinidine	Salicylate	Theophylline	Thiazide	Tolazamide	Warfarin
Benzodiazepines					•			•					•	•				
Beta Blockers					•					•	•				•			
Captopril										•								
Chlorpropamide									•					•		•	•	
Cimetidine	•	•					•					•	•		•			•
Digoxin								•					•			•		
Clonidine															•			
Diltiazem							•											
Ethanol	•			•	•													
Indomethacin		•	•															
Prazosin		•																
Procainamide					•													
Quinidine	•				•		•											•
Salicylate	•																•	•
Theophylline		•		•	•													
Thiazide				•			•										•	
Tolazamide					•									•				
Warfarin					•								•	•				

and elimination. The majority have delayed onset of the interaction ranging from a few days to—as in the case of digoxin–tetracycline—to a few months. In most cases, monitoring drug levels of therapeutic effects during the initiation period can avoid serious consequences of the interactions.

The majority of common, well-documented drug–drug interactions have involved prescription medications. However, interactions between nonprescription and prescription drugs do exist. Fortunately, most of these interactions are minor. For example, antacids taken with aspirin may result in a lowered effectiveness of aspirin. While this is not a severe interaction, it might explain a patient's complaint that a previously effective aspirin dose is no longer effective. There are a few serious drug interactions involving nonprescription medications. Two particularly important examples in the geriatric age group are aspirin–warfarin and digoxin–anticholinergics. The effects of these interactions are discussed in Table 5. Some medications with anticholinergic effects such as scopolamine, chlorpheniramine, and diphenhydramine are available over the counter. A complete assessment of a patient's medications, prescription and

TABLE 5. Drug Interactions Involving Prescription Drugs

Drug	Onset	Severity	Effect	Mechanism	Management
Antacids, iron salts	Delayed	Minor	↓ Hematologic response to Fe	↓ Absorption of Fe due to high gastric pH	Give Fe several hours before antacids, liquid preferred
Benzodiazepines; ethanol	Rapid	Minor	↑ Effects of both → ↑ Psychomotor dysfunction and sedation	Synergistic effects and ↓ VD; ↑ elimination of benzodiazepines	Avoid ETOH
Beta blockers; prazosin	Rapid	Moderate	↑ Severity and duration. Hypotension associated with the 1st dose of prazosin	Blocked cardiovascular reflex due to orthostatic hypotension	1st prazosin dose at qhs. Monitor orthostatic BP
Beta blockers; indomethacin	Delayed	Moderate	↓ Antihypertensive effect of B-blockers; BP + 5-10 mm Hg	Inhibition of prostaglandin synthesis	Check BP after 7-10 days
Captopril; indomethacin	Rapid	Moderate	↓ Effect of captopril	Inhibition of prostaglandin synthesis	Check BP day 1 of indomethacin Rx. Discontinue if BP too high
Cimetidine; procainamide	Rapid	Moderate	↑ Effect of procainamide including GI toxicity, weakness hypotension; ↑ C.O., arrhythmias	↓ Renal clearance of procainamide	Decrease procainamide 25-35% before starting cimetidine; check procainamide & NAPA levels 24 hrs. after cimetidine
Clonidine; tricyclic antidepressants	Rapid	Moderate	↓ Antihypertensive effect of clonidine. Hypertensive crisis possible	Unknown	Avoid concomitant use, or increase clonidine dose. Beware of risks of high dose clonidine
Digoxin; quinidine	Delayed	Major	↑ Toxic effects of digoxin < 10% of pts.	↓ VD, ↓ renal and non-renal elimination of digoxin	Check EKG, digoxin level & effect 27-72 hrs after starting combination; again 3-5 days; adjust if needed
Digoxin; tetracycline	Delayed	Major	↑ Digoxin toxicity seen in	↑ Bioavailability of digoxin; ?-degree change in GI flora	Check digoxin level 507 days after starting antibiotic & again in 3-4 mos. Adjust dose accordingly
Digoxin; anticholinergics	Delayed	Major	↑ Digoxin toxicity	↑ Bioavailability of slow dissolving digoxin preparation	Use liquid or rapidly dissolving digoxin preparations
Digoxin X Thiazide + Loop	Delayed	Major	↑ Digoxin toxicity, esp. arrhythmias	Diuretic induced hypokalemia potentiates arrhythmias	Maintain K of 4-4.5 with potassium supplementation
Lithium; thiazide	Delayed	Major	↑ Levels & toxicity of lithium; polyuria, weakness, lethargy, EKG changes	↓ Renal excretion of lithium	Use loop diuretics or more carefully monitor lithium levels and reduce dose accordingly

C.O. = cardiac output; VD = volume of distribution.

Table 5 continued

TABLE 5. *Continued.*

Drug	Onset	Severity	Effect	Mechanism	Management
Quinidine; rifampin	Delayed	Moderate	↓ Effect of quinidine	↑ Metabolism of quinidine	Monitor quinidine levels 1 wk after starting rifampin; review 3-5 days after discontinuing rifampin
Salicylates; warfarin	Delayed	Major	↑ Anticoagulant effect	Synergistic effect	Avoid combination
Salicylates; antacids	Delayed	Minor	↓ Effect of salicylate	↑ Renal excretion of salicylate	↑ Dose of salicylate; check levels
Sulfonylureas; thiazide diuretics	Delayed	Minor	↓ Hypoglycemic effect	Thiazide-induced glucose intolerance	Monitor glucose, ↑ dose of sulfonylureas
Theophyllines; erythromycin	Delayed	Moderate	↓ Effect of erythromycin; ↑ Effect of theophylline	Hepatic metabolism of theophyllines inhibited	↓ Dose or ↑ dosing interval of theophyllines by 60%; monitor levels
Theophyllines; B-blockers	Delayed	Moderate	↓ Effect of theophylline	↑ Bronchial resistance caused by B-blockers	Avoid B-blockers in pts w/reactive airway diseases
Warfarin; thyroid hormone	Delayed	Major	↑ Hypothrombinemic effect; bleeding	Unknown	Adjust dose according to patient results
Warfarin; quinidine	Delayed	Major	↑ Hypthrombinemic effect	↓ Vitamin K dependent factor synthesis	↓ Anticoagulant dose. Check pt 5-7 days after starting combination

nonprescription, together with an understanding of the mechanism of inter-action, is important in predicting changes in the probability of interaction.

3. Ask patients about over-the-counter drugs

Patient education and monitoring become especially important with regard to over-the-counter medications. Nineteen percent of adverse drug reactions are caused by over-the-counter medications. Yet the elderly do not regularly discuss these medications with their physicians, and physicians rarely ask about them. **The importance of asking about over-the-counter medications cannot be overemphasized.** Eighty-three percent of elderly take over-the-counter medications, yet few discuss them with their physician or pharmacist unless asked. Analgesics (particularly aspirin), antacids and laxatives are the most common sources of drug interactions among over-the-counter medications. In one study, 18% of adverse reactions were due to over-the-counter medications. However, the most common nonprescription agent leading to drug interactions is ethanol. Table 6 lists over-the-counter medications with active ingredients that may interact with medications commonly prescribed in the elderly.

Attention to side effects is, of course, necessary if this form of iatrogenic disease is to be prevented. Just as the elderly under-report many symptoms of diseases, they also under-report the side effects of medications.[2] The elderly are less likely to stop a medication or to adjust its dose because of perceived side effects than other age groups. The physician's clinical skill is further tested in this area because side effects in the elderly often differ from those in the young and frequently are nonspecific. Anorexia, lassitude, and change in mental status frequently herald adverse drug reactions in the elderly.

TABLE 6. Over-the-counter Medications with Ingredients
Potentially Interacting with Prescription Medications

Aspirin:	Chlorpheniramine:	Diphenhadramine:
Alka Seltzer	Alka Seltzer Plus	Benadryl
Anacin	Allerest	Benylin
Arthritis Pain Formula	Cheracol Plus	Nervine
Ascriptin	Chlor-Trimeton	Sleepeze
Bufferin	Comtrex	Sominex
Ecotrin	Contac	Excedrin PM
Ecaprin	Coricidin	
4-Way Cold Tabs	Dristan	Theophylline:
Momentun	Novahistine	Bronkaid
Sine-Off Sinus Tablets	Sine-Off	Bronkolixer
Triaminicin Tablets	Sudafed Plus	Primatene
	Triaminic	

Many of the commonly-used medications produce side effects not readily reported by the elderly. The elderly under-report symptoms related to cognitive or mental status change, incontinence, sexual dysfunction, and mobility. When using medications, one must be particularly diligent about monitoring for side-effects. In short, **take an active approach.** Ask the elderly regularly about **all** medications and symptoms that may be caused by side effects or interaction.

4. **Review medications regularly**

Many physicians have a place in their medical records for medications to be recorded, but these lists are often out of date. The contribution of nonprescription medications to this problem has already been discussed. In addition, patients frequently get prescriptions from more than one physician and do not mention the added medication to their primary care provider. The best way to avoid this is to review all of the medications at each visit. Insisting that the patient bring in the bottles of all medications used since the last visit works well in our practice. Another health care provider, a nurse or medical assistant, can record and check the accuracy of the labeling. This often provides the opportunity to assess the patients' understanding of their medications, to check for the presence of outdated medications, and to assess compliance with some degree of objectivity. Having the bottle in the office while discussing medication changes with the patient can enhance communication. Rather than having the patient try to relate your instructions to the white pill or the heart pill, you can actually *show* him or her the medication to be changed and change the label. On an initial home visit, I noted three bottles of the same medication, each with different dosing instructions. Such a situation could only add to a patient's confusion and potential for medication misuse, and is avoidable by in-office medication review.

The key to successfully incorporating regular medication review into a practice is to use other health care providers and to make the procedure routine. Medical assistants keep the patient flow moving by assisting patients to an exam room, weighing them, recording blood pressure, and helping them disrobe. An additional few minutes to record the medications is time well spent.

Incorporate the help of other office personnel or team members in obtaining a schedule of patient activities, educating patients about potential side effects, and assessing compliance and monitoring side effects. Patients may feel less threatened in talking about these things with nonphysicians. In addition, involving other team members helps to lessen the impact of time constraints on providing this kind of preventive care.

5. Individualize

The individualization of therapy is a central theme in geriatrics. This is a concept that is intuitively obvious. If a medication regimen that is tailored to the patient can be designed, one can reasonably hope that compliance will increase and adverse reactions decrease. Even though most physicians are sensitive to the importance of choosing the right match between the medication and the patient, the number of factors involved makes effective individualization difficult unless a systematic approach is taken. Asking the following six questions lets you consider all the factors, even though you may not be able to address all the issues they raise.

1. **What is the patient's profile?** The profile should include the patient's diagnoses, medications, anthropomorphic characteristics, social supports, and economic situation. The patient's diagnoses determine not only the specific indications for each medication but also which side effects may or may not be tolerated. In addition, problems related to renal and hepatic function affect elimination, volume of distribution, and therefore dosing schedules. The other medications have bearing on potential interactions and the simplicity of the regimen. Height, weight, and lean body mass influence the volume of distribution and therefore the dosage. Lastly, the patient's economic and social situation will partially determine his or her ability to obtain, pay for, and comply with medications.

2. **What drug best fits the patient's profile?** Of primary importance is efficacy in treating the symptoms or disease under consideration. Given that a drug is effective, other properties—including its absorption, elimination, protein binding qualities, and bioavailability—become important. The ideal drug has the characteristics described in Table 7. Since few drugs are "ideal," the patient profile must be meshed with the medication profile. For example, the patient on several medications with high protein binding may be at risk for altered drug effects if another highly protein bound medication is added. In addition, potential drug interactions related to other mechanisms and side effects must be considered. The patient with peripheral neuropathy and orthostatic hypotension may not tolerate a drug such as thioridazine, which has the side effect of orthostatic hypotension.

3. **What is the best initial dose?** Often there are few hard data on which to base this decision. Of course, consider the patient's weight and lean body mass. In frail patients who weigh under 45 kg, pediatric dosing schedules may be useful guides. Otherwise, start with one-half to two-thirds of the usual recommended dose, and monitor the effectiveness carefully.

4. **What preparation and dosing schedule is most appropriate?** Here it is most important to ask the question and let common sense be the guide. The goal is to minimize the number of times per day the patient has to take a medication and the inconvenience associated with the dosing schedule while maximizing the probability that the patient will be supervised. For example, a liquid form may be preferable if the patient has to break or crush a tablet in order to take it. Since liquids are absorbed more quickly, they may be preferable in avoiding certain potential drug interactions (see Table 5).

5. **What should be monitored and how often?** Where drug levels correlate well with therapeutic effect and are easily obtained, drug levels are the best choice. Otherwise, monitor specific, measurable effects of the drug—for example,

TABLE 7. Characteristics of the Ideal Drug

Characteristic	Therapeutic Advantage
Complete absorption	Less scatter in drug response Low oral dose
High bioavailability	Low daily dose
Low first-pass effect	Little effect of hepatic extraction and hemodynamics Low daily dose; no saturation effect
Low protein binding	Plasma levels and drug effects relatively insensitive to concurrent multiple-drug therapy, disease, malnutrition
Balanced clearance by kidney and liver	No accumulation in patients with renal or hepatic impairment

Reprinted with permission from Lang P: Modifying drug dosage in elderly patients. In Covington P, Walker J (eds): Current Therapy in Geriatrics. Philadelphia, WB Saunders Co., 1984.

heart rate in the case of B-blockers or weight in the case of diuretics. Set up a schedule for monitoring known side effects and signs of drug interactions (Table 8). Timing varies with the specific interactions and mechanisms of the side effects (see Interactions, Table 5). However, in most cases, it is appropriate to make the first measurement coincide with reaching steady state.

6. **What other medications should be eliminated or changed?** This question can be thought of as a final checkpoint. It ensures that the new medication regimen is as simple and free of interactions as possible (refer back to the Guidelines for Simplification).

PATIENT EDUCATION

Most physicians use a relatively small number of prescription medications; therefore, each physician should develop a personal formulary based on his or her prescribing patterns and one or two alternatives to his or her most commonly prescribed medications. Inform patients about the medicines you commonly prescribe as well as nonpharmacologic therapies that might be used in conjunction with, if not instead of, those medications. Make this a part of your therapeutic plan. This is best done through brochures or pamphlets that are prepared by the physician and distributed as one would an individual prescription. Providing a patient with easy access to a wide variety of pamphlets or brochures, only a few of which may be relevant, is probably less effective in changing patient behavior. Large type and a concise style similar to that in the National Institute of Aging's *AGE PAGE* make the literature easy to read and understand.

The physician who is not inclined to write his or her own information sheets can rely on United States pharmacological publications *Advice for the Patient* or *About Your Medications.* Consumer Union puts out guides to both prescription and nonprescription medications. In addition, the AMA has a *Patient Medical Information* program that makes information sheets available to physicians at a reasonable cost. Such patient information sheets have also been developed by pharmaceutical companies and are often available at little or no cost.

An even more basic form of patient education is to write—or instruct the pharmacist to write—the medication's indication on the label; e.g., "Digoxin .25 mg every day for heart failure" conveys basic but essential information about the patient's illness and medications.

TABLE 8.   Commonly Used Medications Requiring Monitoring in the Elderly

Medication	Reason(s) to Monitor
Analgesics:	
Morphine	Increased pain relieving effect.
Pentazocine	Lower dosages may be necessary.
Sedatives:	
Benzodiazepines	Decreased clearance.
	Increased depressant effect.
	Lower dosages may be necessary
Antibiotics:	
Aminoglycosides and others renally excreted	Increased half-life.
	Increased dosing interval.
	Monitor levels.
Tricyclic Antidepressants:	Increased sedative and anticholinergic effects; more frequent cardiovascular side effects; starting dose 12.5 mg.
Halperidol	Increased extrapyramidal effects.
	Start with small doses .5 mg B.I.D.
Lithium	Decreased excretion.
	Monitor drug level frequently, and watch for interactions.
Anticoagulants:	Increased anticoagulant effect of heparin and warfarin; reduce initial dose.
Diuretics:	Increased risk of postural hypotension.
Propranolol:	Increased risk CNS side effects, especially depression; monitor symptoms.
Digoxin:	Half-life prolonged.
Theophylline:	Decreased clearance; reduce dose 25%.
Quinidine:	Decreased clearance; monitor levels.
Nonsteroidal antiinflammatory:	Reversible renal impairment.
	Mental status changes.
	Monitor symptoms

PRACTICE RECOMMENDATIONS

1. Update medications list at regular intervals. This is especially important if the patient has more than one provider of care.

2. Suggest that patients bring in all their medications periodically so that they can be checked for accuracy against your medication list. This will also allow assessment of medication compliance and of the expiration date.

3. Ask about self-prescribing with over-the-counter medications.

4. Involve other office personnel in obtaining and updating the medication history and reinforcing the therapeutic plan.

5. Review medications for potential interactions, keeping in mind that there are often patterns of interactions.

6. Simplify medication regimen and optimize dosing schedule.

7. Individualize therapy based on the following questions:
   - What is the patient profile?
   - What drug best fits the patient's profile?

- What is the best initial dose?
- What preparation and dosing schedule is most appropriate?
- What should be monitored and how often?
- What other medications should be eliminated or changed?

8. Use medications parsimoniously. Avoid empiric treatment of symptoms with medications before the symptom and its etiology are fully understood.

9. Develop your personal formulary and know the age-related properties of those medications (especially potential side-effects and drug-drug interactions).

10. Develop and distribute patient education materials about medication interactions and side-effects.

REFERENCES

1. Seidel LG, et al: Studies on the epidemiology of adverse drug reactions III: reactions in patients on a general medical service. Bull Johns Hopkins Hosp 1966; 119:299–315.
2. Klein L, et al: Medication problems among outpatients. Arch Intern Med 1984; 144:1185–1188.
3. Grosney M, Tallis R: Prescription of contraindicated and interacting drugs in elderly patients admitted to hospital. Lancet September 8, 1984.
4. Borbes GB, Reina TC: Adult lean body mass declines with age: some longitudinal observations. Metabolism 1978; 19:653–663.
5. Cohen J: Pharmacokinetic changes in aging. Am J Med 1986; 80 (Suppl 5A):31–38.
6. Greenblatt DJ: Reduced serum albumin concentration in the elderly: a report from the Boston Collaborative Drug Surveillance Program. J Am Geriatr Soc 1979; 27:20–22.
7. Lamay P: Comparative pharmacokinetic changes and drug therapy in an older population. J Am Geriatr Soc 1982; 511–519.
8. Greenblatt DJ: Drug disposition in old age. N Engl J Med 1982; 306:1081–1088.
9. Rowe J, et al: The effect of age on creatinine clearance in man: a cross-sectional study and longitudinal study. J Gerontol 1976; 31:155–163.
10. Schmucker D: Drug disposition in the elderly: a review of critical factors. J Am Geriatr Soc 1984; 31:144–149.
11. Cockcroft DW, Gault MH: Prediction of creatinine clearance from serum creatinine. Nephron 1976; 16:31–41.
12. Vener A, et al: Drug usage and health characteristics in non-institutionalized retired persons. J Am Geriatr Soc 1979; 28:83–90.
13. Verbrugge L: Longer life but worsening health? Trends in health and mortality of middleageds and older persons. Milbank Memorial Fund Quarterly 1982; 62:475.
14. Ouslander JG, Beck J: Defining the health problems of the elderly. Am Rev Public Health 1982; 3:55–83.
15. Aoki F, et al: Aging and heavy drug use: a prescribed survey in Manitoba. J Chron Dis 1983; 36:75–84.
16. Bergman U, Wholin BE: Patient medication on admission to a medical clinic. Eur J Clin Pharm 1981; 20:85.
17. Cupit G: The use of non-prescription analgesics in an older population. J Am Geriatr Soc 1982; 30:576–580.
18. Kendrick R, Bayne JR. Compliance with prescribed medication by elderly patients. CMA Journal 1982; 127:961–962.
19. May F, et al: Prescribed and non-prescribed drug use in an ambulatory elderly population. South Med J 1982; 75:522–528.
20. Lavizzo-Mourey R, et al: Medication usage among homebound elderly. Unpublished manuscript, 1985.
21. Adkinson L, et al: An investigation into the ability of elderly patients to take prescribed drugs after discharge from the hospital and recommendations for improving the situation. Gerontology 1978; 24:225–234.
22. Libow L, Mehl B: Self administration of medications by patients in hospitals or extended care facilities. J Am Geriatr Soc 1970; 18:81–95.
23. Fedder D: Managing medication and compliance—physician-pharmacist-patient interactions. J Am Geriatr Soc 1982; 30:5113–5117.
24. U.S. Senate Special Committee on Aging. Drugs in Nursing Homes: Misuse, High Cost and Kickbacks. Washington, DC, 1986.

25. Larson EB, et al: Diagnostic evaluation of 200 elderly outpatients with suspected dementia. J Gerontol 1985; 40:536–548.
26. Larson E, et al: Dementia in elderly outpatients: a prospective study. Ann Intern Med 1984; 100:417–423.
26a. Larson EB, et al: Adverse drug reaction associated with global cognitive impairment in elderly persons. Ann Intern Med 1987; 107:169–173.
27. Caranosos GJ: et al: Drug induced illness leading to hospitalization. JAMA 1974; 288:713–717.
28. Morse ML, et al: Reducing drug therapy-induced hospitalization: Impact of drug utilization review. Drug Information Journal, October/December, 1982.
29. Wegner F: Post marketing surveillance and geriatric drug use. In Moore and Teal (eds): Geriatric Drug Use: Clinical and Social Perspectives. New York, Pergamon Press, 1985.
30. Avron J, Ever HD, Weiss S: Increased antidepressant use in patients prescribed B blockers. JAMA 1986; 255:357–360.
31. Jusko WJ, Gardner M, Mangione A, et al: Factors affecting theophylline clearance. J Pharm Sci 1979; 68:1358–1366.
32. Ochs RH, Greenblatt D, Woo E, et al: Reduced quinidine clearance in elderly persons. Am J Cardiol 1978; 43:481–485.
33. Hansten PD: Drug Interactions, 4th ed. Philadelphia, Lea & Febiger, 1979.
34. Solomon F, et al: Sleeping pills, insomnia and medical practice. N Engl J Med 1979; 300:803–808.
35. Maly BS: Rehabilitation principles in the care of gynecologic and obstetric patients. Arch Phys Med Rehabil 1980; 61:78–81.
36. Evaluations of Drug Interactions, 2nd ed (Suppl). Washington, DC, American Pharmaceutical Association, 1978.
37. Mangini R (ed): Drug Interaction Facts. St. Louis, J.B. Lippincott Company, 1985.
38. Darnell J, et al: Medication use by ambulatory elderly: an in-home survey. J Am Geriatr Soc 1986; 37:1–4.

6
REDUCING CARDIOVASCULAR RISK
IN THE ELDERLY

Thomas H. Lee, MD, MSc

For the last 20 years, mortality from ischemic heart disease in the United States has been steadily declining, a trend that has been apparent among blacks and whites, men and women, and in all age groups. Coronary artery disease nevertheless remains the leading cause of death among individuals older than age 65, with malignancies of all kinds still a distant second.[1] However, while risk factors and preventive strategies are increasingly well-defined for middle-aged people, considerable controversy persists about whether these findings and recommendations are relevant to the elderly.

One reason why the impact and practicality of preventive strategies among the elderly is so uncertain is that many landmark trials excluded this population. The Lipids Research Clinics Coronary Primary Prevention Trial only recruited men aged 35–39 years.[2] The Multiple Risk Factor Intervention Trial (MRFIT) enrolled men 35–57 years old.[3] Koch-Weser has observed that only 10% of patients included in 41 published trials of antihypertensive drugs were over the age of 60.[4]

Even if these studies had included more elderly patients, an important principle of epidemiology implies that they would still have had difficulty demonstrating a beneficial impact from risk-factor interventions. This principle is that the effect of a risk factor (or an intervention aimed at that risk factor) is most easily demonstrated in a population that is otherwise at low risk for the disease. Thus, the effects of hypercholesterolemia and of cholesterol-reducing drugs were clearly demonstrated among young men in the Lipids Research Clinics trial, but these effects might well have been "lost" had the trial been performed using elderly individuals who would be expected to have a baseline high rate of coronary disease and its complications.

Despite the lack of hard data that directly supports measures aimed at preventing heart disease among the elderly, the fact remains that coronary disease is declining in this age group coincident with population-wide changes in known cardiac risk factors, suggesting that effective preventive measures are already being applied. Consequently, interest in preventing coronary artery disease and its complications among the elderly (as well as younger individuals) continues to grow. This interest can be expected to intensify in the future, since, despite the decline in mortality *rates* from coronary artery disease (i.e., deaths per 100,000 individuals), the absolute *numbers* of new cases of ischemic heart disease and deaths from its complications are expected to rise due to aging of the population as a whole and a subsequent increase in the elderly population at risk. Weinstein et al. have projected that, if risk factors and the efficacy of medical care remain constant, we will see a 40% increase in the incidence, mortality, and costs associated with coronary artery disease by the year 2010.[5] Thus, clinicians can expect to see more of all the chronic diseases in the coming years, including coronary artery disease.

To limit the demands that these diseases will impose upon the health care system, diversified strategies that include preventive approaches must be developed, since realistic expectations for the public health impact of traditional medical interventions must be conservative. One recent analysis concluded that, despite the conspicuousness of technologies such as coronary care units and coronary artery bypass graft surgery, most of the decline in coronary deaths over the last 20 years can be attributed to reductions in serum cholesterol level and cigarette smoking.[6] Looking ahead, some patients will undoubtedly benefit with symptomatic relief and longer life expectancies as a result of newer techniques such as coronary angioplasty, but increasing economic pressures upon the health care system make it unlikely that such technologies will lead to major reductions in coronary mortality.

Finally, and perhaps most importantly from the clinician's perspective, individual elderly patients often want and expect preventive efforts as part of their care. While it is true that cost-effectiveness analyses indicate that treatment of high blood pressure in the elderly is a relatively expensive way to buy a year of life, and that no data demonstrate that tobacco is a risk factor for coronary disease in the elderly, to ignore hypertension or smoking in an elderly patient is to give that patient a message: It is no longer worth "trying." Such a message, though unspoken, can damage the physician-patient relationship and affect compliance on other issues.

Nevertheless, the goals that the clinician should use when treating hypertension or trying to lower cholesterol in elderly individuals are not necessarily the same as those that are appropriate for younger patients. Making informed management decisions requires knowledge of the available data, however scanty. Therefore, this chapter will discuss each of the cardiac risk factors that are most widely accepted in the general population, reviewing what is known and describing possible management strategies, and conclude with a discussion of an overall approach to the elderly patient.

CHOLESTEROL

The Lipids Research Clinics randomized trial seemed to settle most issues about the merits of treating hypercholesterolemia when it was published in 1984.[2] This study demonstrated that reducing total cholesterol by treating men with elevated serum cholesterol levels with the bile acid sequestrant cholestyramine led to decreased incidence and mortality from coronary heart disease. However, as noted above, this study only enrolled males between 35 and 39 years of age. Thus, questions remain regarding the benefits of treating hypercholesterolemia in elderly patients.

Indeed, whether hypercholesterolemia is even a significant risk factor in the elderly is controversial, as published analyses from the Framingham Study have not demonstrated an association between total serum cholesterol level and the risk of death from coronary heart disease in individuals aged ≥ 65 years after adjusting for other variables.[7] These analyses also do not demonstrate an independent contribution to risk of coronary death from diabetes or smoking in elderly men, or from systolic blood pressure in females. More recent data include information on a larger number of elderly patients and therefore have greater statistical power for detecting effects of potential risk factors. One preliminary analysis indicates that cholesterol levels above the 90th percentile are associated with increased risk in women. A similar trend was found among men, although it did not reach statistical significance.[8]

One possible reason for the difficulty of demonstrating an association between high cholesterol levels and coronary disease in the elderly is that individuals with severe hypercholesterolemia do not survive beyond middle age. Consistent with this hypothesis is the common clinical experience that marked elevations of serum cholesterol (> 350 mg/dL) are uncommon in elderly patients. An alternative possibility is that patients with other risk factors but without hypercholesterolemia die at younger ages. If so, high cholesterol levels in the elderly would be present in individuals who were otherwise at relatively low risk, and therefore would have less significance.

However, in all likelihood, the difficulty of demonstrating an increase in cardiac risk with elevated cholesterol levels instead reflects the limited statistical power of even a study as large as the Framingham Study. For older individuals, the overall risk of death from both cardiac and noncardiac causes is so high that the expected small incremental benefit associated with a lower cholesterol level may be overwhelmed. Accordingly, elderly patients who are put on a cholesterol-lowering diet may not survive long enough for this regimen to have any effect on the progression of atherosclerosis. Any study that attempted to reproduce the findings of the Lipid Research Clinics trial among the elderly—i.e., demonstrate a benefit from therapy aimed at lowering cholesterol—would therefore need a study population several orders of magnitude larger than the 3,806 middle-aged men who were actually followed, with a similar exponential increase in cost. This obviously makes such a study prohibitive.

What should the clinician do in its absence? It seems most reasonable to assume that the pathophysiology that has been demonstrated in younger patients is valid in the elderly, even if its effects are less evident. Indeed, data from the National Center for Health Statistics indicate that the decline in coronary mortality rates among the elderly has coincided with a fall in mean total cholesterol levels among men age 65–74 from 230 mg/dL in 1960–62 to 226 mg/dL in 1971–74 to 221 mg/dL in 1976–80, and a fall among women in that age group from 266 mg/dL to 250 mg/dL to 246 mg/dL over the same periods.

Thus, the risk of death from coronary heart disease in the elderly, as in younger individuals, probably has a curvilinear relationship with total serum cholesterol, increasing more rapidly as cholesterol levels rise above 220 mg/dL. An alternative way of expressing this relationship is to assume that everyone has a genetically determined rate of atherogenesis, but that this rate varies with cholesterol level. A man who would have developed angina at age 70 if his cholesterol level during his adult life were 220 mg/dL might develop those symptoms at age 55 if his cholesterol level were 280 mg/dL, and at age 90 if it were 180 mg/dL.

This perspective implies that there is no "safe" cholesterol level—the lower the better—and that there is no patient who does not stand to benefit from attempts to lower cholesterol. A widely quoted rule-of-thumb is that a 1% reduction in the cholesterol concentration decreases the risk of cardiac events over a 7–9 year period by 2%.[9] However, initiating treatment of hypercholesterolemia at age 40 clearly will have a much greater impact on coronary mortality than beginning at age 70. One recent analysis concluded that lowering serum total cholesterol by 20%—about the maximum that could be expected from dietary interventions—would increase the life expectancy of a 60-year-old woman by just 2.5 years, whereas the gain for a 60-year-old man would be only five months.[10] This consideration can markedly influence management strategies and the vigor with which a cholesterol level in "the normal range" is pursued.

Given these caveats, most experts recommend that virtually all patients be screened for hyperlipoproteinemia as part of the initial evaluation with serum cholesterol and fasting serum triglyceride levels.[11] Such screening can be performed with automated chemistry profiles, although some of these assays have been found to yield cholesterol levels about 10 mg/dL higher than the enzymatic assays used in research settings. (These discrepancies probably represent calibration errors.) Cholesterol levels are not significantly affected by whether a patient has recently eaten, but triglyceride levels should be obtained after the patient has not eaten for at least 12 hours. High triglyceride levels are at most only a weak independent risk factor for coronary artery disease, but they can cause or be due to other medical problems and are useful in classifying the patient's hyperlipidemia.

If either cholesterol or triglyceride levels are elevated, both tests should be repeated to ensure that the results were not laboratory errors. If either of these levels is still elevated, further workup is indicated, including, if total cholesterol is increased, measurement of the high density lipoprotein (HDL) fraction of cholesterol, the so-called "good" cholesterol. As is familiar to a surprising number of patients these days, HDL removes cholesterol from cholesterol-engorged cells and transports it back to the liver for removal from the body. Thus, HDL cholesterol is inversely correlated with cardiovascular risk, with each 10 mg/dL increase associated with a 50% decrease in risk.[12]

Excellent algorithms for further evaluation and treatment of hyperlipidemias have been published elsewhere.[11] In evaluating elderly patients with elevated cholesterol, the clinician need not emphasize the search for familial hypercholesterolemia, since virtually all homozygotes and most heterozygotes will have developed and possibly died from coronary artery disease in their middle age. Instead, the immediate goal is to classify patients into moderate- and high-risk groups, since the intensity of any interventions may vary between them.

The total cholesterol level alone provides a crude measure of risk (Table 1). For example, analyses of data from the Framingham Study suggest that a 65-year-old man with a systolic blood pressure of 150, no smoking history, no left ventricular hypertrophy on his electrocardiogram, normal glucose levels, and a total cholesterol < 220 mg/dL has a 9% probability of developing ischemic heart disease within six years. If that man's cholesterol is 220–300 mg/dL, his risk rises to 10%, and if his cholesterol is > 300 mg/dL, his risk is 11%. While this 2% change in risk may appear small, it should really be viewed as a rise in risk above the baseline of 2/9, or 22%.

For more refined estimates of risk, many experts recommend computing the total cholesterol/HDL cholesterol ratio; a ratio of 5.0 is associated with average risk; a ratio of 3.5 is optimal, corresponding to an overall risk of cardiac disease that is about half the national average. Ratios higher than 5.0 place the patient into higher risk categories. Another approach is to estimate the amount of low density lipoprotein (LDL) cholesterol ("bad" cholesterol) by the following equation:

LDH cholesterol = total cholesterol -([triglycerides/5] + HDL cholesterol)

In most cases, this equation is an accurate and inexpensive alternative to direct measurement of LDL cholesterol. LDL values over 175 mg/dL place elderly

TABLE 1. Risk of Coronary Artery Disease
Associated with Lipoprotein Cholesterol Profiles

Test*	Level	Approximate Risk
Total cholesterol (TC)	< 220 mg/dL	Low
	220–300 mg/dL	Moderate
	> 300 mg/dL	High
LDL cholesterol	< 125 mg/dL	Low
	125–185 mgdL	Moderate
	> 185 mg/dL	High
HDL cholesterol	> 65 mg/dL	Low
	35–65 mgdL	Moderate
	< 35 mg/dL	High
TC/HDL cholesterol	< 3.5	Low
ratio	3.5–5.0	Moderate
	> 5.0	High

* LDL = low density lipoprotein; HDL = high density lipoprotein. See text for explanation of how to estimate LDL cholesterol. Risks descriptions are qualitative and are presented to allow crude estimation of the impact of lipoprotein levels on a patient's overall risk of coronary disease.

individuals in a moderate-risk group, while values over 200 mg/dL place them at high risk.

Having made a judgment of the patient's risk, the clinician must now decide what to do with that information. The first step in all moderate and high-risk patients should be dietary therapy, which, to be effective, must involve more than handing the patient some brochures and wishing him or her good luck. Enduring modifications of dietary practices require professional dietary counseling aimed at developing a realistic and specific plan for the individual. If no nutrition clinic is available nearby, the American Dietetic Association (1-800-621-6469) will provide lists of nutritionists for the state in which the patient lives.

Most informed dietary advice is similar to the American Heart Association guidelines.[13] These guidelines emphasize attaining and maintaining ideal body weight, reducing overall fat consumption and replacing saturated fats with polyunsaturated oils, and, of course, reducing dietary cholesterol intake. Translated into the patient's language, these guidelines mean increased consumption of fruits, vegetables, and whole grains, while replacing red meats, pork, and organ meats with poultry and fish. Polyunsaturated vegetable oils should replace saturated fat in cooking and salad dressings. Diary products high in butterfat and eggs should be minimized.

Exercise, cessation of smoking, and fish intake increase HDL cholesterol and should be recommended. In contrast, alcohol, which has also been demonstrated to raise HDL, should be avoided because of its abuse potential, high caloric content, and deleterious effect on triglyceride-rich lipoproteins.

These measures can reduce total serum cholesterol by 10–20% in most patients. This decline is detectable within a few weeks, and early remeasurement can provide patients with psychological reinforcement. A more definitive re-evaluation should take place 3–6 months after dietary intervention begins, and, if total or LDL cholesterol levels have fallen out of the range indicating elevated risk, no further treatment is needed beyond continued dietary measures. The NIH Consensus Development Conference recommends a target range for total cholesterol of 180–200 mg/dL.

The question of which elderly patients should be treated with pharmacological interventions is more complex. While guidelines aimed at the general population recommend drug therapy for anyone whose serum cholesterol is not normalized by dietary therapy within 3–6 months, these recommendations must be tempered by the cost and the toxicities associated with available drugs and the lack of definitive evidence that these agents produce clinical benefits in elderly patients. In the absence of hard data, many clinicians use a higher threshold, such as a total cholesterol level of 300 mg/dL despite serious efforts at dietary modification, for initiating drug therapy in the elderly, and are satisfied if total cholesterol drops below 250 mg/dL.

Although the Lipid Research Clinic trial used cholestyramine to reduce cholesterol, many experts recommend niacin as a first-line drug. In the Coronary Drug Project, niacin reduced the rate of non-fatal myocardial infarction by 21%,[14] and, during long-term follow-up, led to an 11% reduction in death compared with placebo.[15] The choice of niacin over the bile acid sequestrants is based on niacin's lower cost (about a third of the bile acid sequestrants) and toxicity.

To minimize its side effects, niacin should be started at low doses (100 mg three times a day) and increased by 300 mg/day until a maintenance dose of 3–9 gms/day is achieved. Cutaneous flushing and pruritus about 20 minutes after taking the drug occur in most patients during the first several days, but generally decrease over 3–6 weeks with continued administration, especially if an aspirin is taken one hour before the niacin and the niacin is ingested with meals. Many patients find that sustained release preparations of niacin, such as Nicobid, cause fewer side effects. Other complications include nausea, vomiting, diarrhea, a reversible hepatitis, impaired glucose tolerance, and hyperuricemia. Thus, this drug is relatively contraindicated in patients with liver disease, diabetes, or gout.

Alternative agents and guidelines for their use can be found elsewhere.[11] Patients who have elevations of both cholesterol and fasting triglyceride levels may be candidates for treatment with gemfibrozil or probucol as second-line drugs, whereas the next choice for isolated hypercholesterolemia is usually one of the bile acid sequestrants.

Early trials with a qualitatively different agent, mevinolin (lovastatin), suggest that this inhibitor of cholesterol synthesis can reduce total cholesterol by more than 30% while raising HDL cholesterol, with rare side effects.[16] Thus, some clinicians expect that this drug may become the drug of choice in the future for treating hypercholesterolemia, although further experience with it is clearly required.

Already apparent in health food stores and supermarkets are fish oil capsules, which, because of their high content of unsaturated omega-3 fatty acids, may decrease serum cholesterol without affecting HDL cholesterol, while also inhibiting platelet aggregation. Some epidemiological data supports the hypothesis that fish consumption is associated with lower mortality from coronary disease, but evidence for a beneficial effect from the fish oil capsules on the market is lacking. Furthermore, fish oil has been found to raise LDL cholesterol in some patients. Thus, clinicians should not recommend this approach to patients at this point.

HYPERTENSION

The prevalence of hypertension in the elderly population depends on how hypertension is defined, since blood pressure is a continuous variable that tends to rise with age. Using the somewhat arbitrary definition of 160/95 mmHg as the upper limit of normal, about half of individuals over the age of 65 are hypertensive, many with disproportionately elevated systolic blood pressures, and about 10% have isolated systolic hypertension.[17] In patients age 75 or more, the prevalence of isolated systolic hypertension increases to about 25%. These individuals are clearly at higher risk of coronary artery disease, congestive heart failure, and stroke, regardless of whether the hypertension is diastolic or systolic, fixed or labile. That increase in risk of cardiovascular complications is about 30% for every 10 mmHg increment in systolic blood pressure.

Identifiable curable causes of hypertension—e.g., renal artery stenosis, coarctation of the aorta, hyperaldosteronism—are unusual in elderly patients, though not unknown. Instead the usual culprit is arteriosclerosis, leading to decreased distensibility of the arterial tree and elevated systolic pressures. Since atheromatous plaques can compromise blood flow in major arteries, clinicians should routinely check blood pressures in both arms of elderly patients to ensure that hypertension is not missed because the arm used for the blood pressure cuff has a stenosed vessel. In addition, because of the decreased compliance of the arterial tree, orthostatic changes in blood pressure should be sought before and during treatment. In light of the uninspiring success rates and high complication rates of renal artery angioplasty for atheromatous renal artery stenosis, aggressive searches for this entity are not warranted in elderly patients except in those who have hypertension refractory to multiple drug therapy or sudden marked worsening of their hypertension.

Given the increased cardiovascular risk associated with hypertension in the elderly, does treatment make a difference? Data from elderly patients in several studies indicate that therapy reduces both cardiovascular and cerebrovascular events.[18] Although studies directed at the geriatric population are limited, at least one major study found that treatment reduced cardiovascular mortality by 27% and cerebrovascular events by 52% in patients over age 60 with systolic blood pressures 160–239 mmHg and diastolic blood pressures 90–119.[19] Whether treatment of isolated systolic hypertension reduces risk is unknown, but a clinical trial sponsored by the National Institutes of Health is in progress.[20] As is the case with serum cholesterol, the expected benefit from antihypertensive therapy is sufficiently small that definitive trials require huge numbers of patients.

While the cost per year of life saved by treating hypertension increases markedly as patients age,[21] reasonable recommendations include starting treatment in elderly patients whose blood pressures are greater than 160/90 mmHg on two occasions.[18] In patients with lower diastolic pressures, a systolic blood pressure greater than 180 mmHg is used as the threshold for treatment by some experts.[22]

More controversial is when to stop, as attempts to "normalize" blood pressure can compromise blood flow to vital organs, cause orthostatic hypotension, and induce fatigue by reducing cardiac output. To avoid the risk of iatrogenic hypotension, many geriatricians recommend using a standing (rather than a sitting or supine) blood pressure to guide management. A reasonable goal is systolic pressures of 140–160 mmHg.[22]

If salt restriction and weight reduction do not produce a satisfactory response, pharmacological therapy must be considered. In choosing a drug, the physician must weigh efficacy, side effects, and cost. Thiazide diuretics have long been the first choice of many clinicians;[22] they are inexpensive, and, in the Systolic Hypertension in the Elderly Program, were successful in controlling blood pressure in 88% of patients.[20] However, in recent years, these drugs have lost some of their appeal because of their secondary complications to which the elderly are especially sensitive, including hypokalemia, hyperuricemia, hypomagnesemia, and impaired glucose tolerance. In addition, results from the MRFIT trial[3] have raised questions about whether these complications of diuretics may increase the rate of sudden death due to arrhythmias.

Some experts recommend starting with one of the many available beta-adrenergic blocking agents. These drugs are all considerably more expensive than the thiazide diuretics; are relatively contraindicated in patients with asthma, peripheral vascular disease, or congestive heart failure; and are probably slightly less likely to control hypertension in an elderly patient when used alone. However, they do not have the adverse metabolic consequences of the thiazides and are especially useful if the patient also has symptoms of ischemic heart disease. Consequently, a reasonable approach is to begin with a beta-adrenergic blocking agent and to add a small amount of a diuretic if needed. This approach is sufficient in about 65% of patients.[23]

In patients whose blood pressures remain markedly elevated despite this combination, vasodilators can be considered as a third drug, though, at this point, many patients will complain of orthostatic symptoms, too many pills that need to be taken at too many times during the day, and unbearable costs. The elderly are especially sensitive to the central nervous system depressant effects of methyldopa, reserpine, and clonidine, so these drugs must be used with caution if at all. Often, the clinician and the patient must consider just how aggressively to pursue lower blood pressure. At some point, adding more drugs leads to decreased compliance for the entire regimen.

Although these agents have been developed relatively recently, angiotensin converting enzyme inhibitors such as captopril and enalapril are being used with increasing frequency, sometimes even as first-line drugs. These agents are much more expensive than the beta-adrenergic blocking agents but are relatively free of metabolic complications and, most importantly, seem to permit a better quality of life for the patient. A randomized double-blind trial of men between the ages of 21 and 65 found that, in comparison with methyldopa and propranolol, captopril produced less sexual dysfunction and better results on several scales measuring general well-being.[24] Although these data do not include elderly patients, this class of drugs offers a much-needed alternative for those who are tolerating other regimens poorly.

Calcium channel blocking agents are also successful in achieving normotension in many patients, but are still quite expensive. Like angiotension converting enzyme inhibitors, they have the advantage of avoiding metabolic complications and are associated with fewer central nervous system effects than some traditional first- and second-line drugs. Thus, despite their high cost, they may be the drugs of choice for some elderly.

CIGARETTE SMOKING

While cigarette smoking has been consistently shown to be a powerful independent risk factor for coronary artery disease and peripheral vascular disease, its contribution to cardiovascular risk in the elderly is uncertain. Data from the Framingham Study do not show an independent association between smoking and heart disease after adjusting for other risk factors,[8] raising questions of whether smokers who are susceptible to heart disease die before age 65. However, other studies support increased risks of death from coronary artery disease or lung disease in the elderly and suggest that giving up smoking leads to lower mortality rates.[25] Since smoking is probably the most easily reversible of the major risk factors and because it causes so many other adverse medical consequences, the clinician should make all possible efforts to discourage it.

The advisability of quitting smoking for health reasons will not be new to most patients. Indeed, many individuals will have attempted to quit many times before but failed for a variety of psychological and physiologic reasons. For patients who may be physically addicted to nicotine, nicotine tablets or gums are useful as temporary aids to be used in conjunction with behavioral interventions. Characteristics that have been shown to correlate with nicotine dependence include: (a) smoking more than 15 cigarettes per day; (b) preference for high-nicotine brands (> 0.9 mg); (c) tendency to inhale deeply; (d) smoking a cigarette within 30 minutes of awakening; (e) difficulty in giving up early morning smoking; and (f) smoking even when ill and confined to bed.

Because nicotine has cardiostimulating effects, it is relatively contraindicated in the period immediately following acute myocardial infarction or in patients with unstable angina or significant arrhythmias. Other systemic complications are rare. However, patients who successfully give up smoking with the aid of nicotine substitutes often find themselves unable to give up the substitutes themselves.

DIABETES

While its effects may be less marked than in younger patients, glucose intolerance has been found to make an independent contribution to the risk of developing coronary artery disease in the elderly, with a random glucose level above 175 mg/dL leading to a doubling in cardiac risk.[8] However, evidence that tight control of diabetes leads to a reduction in symptoms or mortality from coronary artery disease does not exist. Therefore, aggressive management with insulin therapy for the purpose of preventing cardiac disease is not justified, though the clinician and patient should attempt to avoid the hemodynamic derangements that may accompany marked hyperglycemia.

OBESITY

The association between obesity and coronary artery disease is often attributed to the relationship between obesity and other risk factors, including hypertension, diabetes, and hypercholesterolemia. However, multivariate analysis indicates that, even after adjusting for these other risk factors, Metropolitan Relative Weight correlates with the risk of developing coronary disease in the elderly.[8] In addition, being obese imposes a physiologic burden on patients who have coronary artery disease and may therefore reduce functional status.

Consequently, efforts should be made to reduce the weight of obese patients through dietary advice and encouraging exercise programs. While clinicians are often skeptical of the ability of elderly patients to undertake exercise programs, considerable data demonstrate that habitual endurance exercise reduces multiple risk factors (obesity, cholesterol, blood pressure, glucose intolerance) and leads to improved cardiac function. These benefits do not depend on the degree of activity during youth and middle age; thus, exercise programs should be considered for even the least athletically inclined patients. Not all individuals will be reasonable candidates for jogging or swimming programs, but daily long walks at the request of the doctor may lead to decreased weight as well as a feeling of well-being (see Chapter 7).

OTHER FACTORS

The value of obtaining information or trying to alter other traditional risk factors in the elderly is less clear. For example, family history is useful as a method of identifying young and middle-aged patients who may have familial hypercholesterolemia and therefore be at risk for myocardial infarction at an early age. Since such patients do not survive without symptoms to old age, the family history has little to offer in the evaluation of cardiac risk of the elderly patient.

In other cases, data indicate an association between a risk factor and heart disease, but whether intervention is effective is uncertain. Hyperuricemia and its best known clinical manifestation, gout, are associated with coronary artery disease, but there is no evidence in younger or older individuals that treatment of asymptomatic hyperuricemia leads to a reduction of cardiac disease. Similarly, Type A personalities, who are characterized by a sense of time-urgency, have been reported to have elevated mortality from coronary disease, but guidelines on which patients warrant intervention do not exist.

Coffee has been occasionally rumored to be a cardiac risk factor, but prospective studies do not support a significant independent effect.

OVERALL APPROACH TO PREVENTION OF CORONARY ARTERY DISEASE IN THE ELDERLY

Given the data reviewed above, efforts to reduce the risk of ischemic heart disease in the elderly should emphasize controlling tobacco use, hypertension, hypercholesterolemia, and obesity. These efforts must be tempered by the knowledge that interventions against these factors have not been demonstrated to produce major clinical or public health benefits. Nevertheless, compared to other risk factors, these variables are more susceptible to intervention, and measures aimed at one of them may have beneficial effects on the others while increasing the individual's sense of well-being.

Thus, regular exercise may lower blood pressure, cholesterol level, and weight at the same time, while raising HDL cholesterol and providing an incentive to stop smoking. Similarly, cholesterol-lowering diets also tend to lead to weight reduction, and, if salt intake is reduced, may lower blood pressure as well.

Consequently, recommendations for most elderly patients should emphasize diet, exercise, and smoking cessation. If blood and cholesterol cannot be controlled with these conservative measures, then pharmacologic interventions can be considered, although the goals of therapy should be more conservative than those used for younger individuals. Some specific recommendations that are based on my interpretation of the literature and personal clinical experience are offered below. These should be considered with the understanding that, due to lack of data, specific thresholds for treatment have not been developed through any formal analysis and must be personalized for individual patients.

PRACTICE RECOMMENDATIONS

1. Ask all elderly patients whether they have symptoms that would indicate cardiovascular disease, such as:
    a. Chest discomfort with exertion.
    b. Syncope or near-syncope.

    c. Waking at night short of breath.

    d. Shortness of breath lying flat.

  2. Check blood pressure in both arms at least once in all patients.

  3. Check for orthostatic changes in blood pressure.

  4. Check a serum total cholesterol level and a fasting triglyceride level in all patients at least once.

  5. If the total cholesterol is high (e.g., > 250 mg/dL) or the triglycerides are elevated, repeat both tests.

  6. If repeat measurements show persistent elevation of total cholesterol, check the serum HDL cholesterol level.

  7. If the ratio of total cholesterol to HDL cholesterol is greater than 5.0, the patient should be referred to a nutritionist for development of a low-cholesterol diet.

  8. If cholesterol abnormalities persist after 3–6 months, with a serum total cholesterol > 300 mg/dL, consider drug therapy. A total cholesterol level below 250 mg/dL is a reasonable goal for most patients.

  9. If hypertension persists despite initiation of a low-salt diet and weight reduction measures, consider pharmacological therapy for a diastolic blood pressure > 100 mgHg or a systolic blood pressure > 180 mmHg.

  10. In treating hypertension, aim for a systolic pressure of 160 mmHg. Ask the patient about side effects including fatigue, mental status changes, and sexual dysfunction.

  11. Encourage smoking cessation, prescribing nicotine tablets or gum for patients with symptoms suggestive of physical dependence.

  12. Encourage weight loss through dietary and exercise interventions.

  13. Tight control of diabetes cannot be justified solely for the purpose of reducing coronary risk.

REFERENCES

1. National Center for Health Statistics: Health, United States, 1984. DHHS Pub. No. (PHS) 85-1232. Public Health Service. Washington, D.C., U.S. Government Printing Office, Dec. 1984.
2. Lipids Research Clinics Program: The Lipid Research Clinics Coronary Primary Prevention Trial Results. I. Reduction in incidence of coronary heart disease. JAMA 1984; 251:351–364.
3. Multiple Risk Factor Intervention Trial Group: Multiple Risk Factor Intervention Trial. Risk factor changes and mortality results. JAMA 1982; 248:1465–1477.
4. Koch-Weser J: Treatment of hypertension in the elderly. In Crooks J, Stevenson IH (eds): Drugs and the Elderly. London, Macmillan, 1979, pp 247–262.
5. Weinstein MC, Coxson PG, Williams LW, et al: Coronary heart disease morbidity, mortality and cost for the next quarter-century. Clin Res 1986; 34:386A.
6. Goldman L, Cook EF: The decline in ischemic heart disease mortality rates. An analysis of the comparative effects of medical interventions and changes in lifestyle. Ann Intern Med 1984; 101:824–836.
7. Kannel WB, Gordon T: Cardiovascular risk factors in the aged: The Framingham Study. In Haynes SG, Feinlieb M (eds): Second Conference on the Epidemiology of Aging. Washington, D.C., DHHS, NIH publication no. 80-969, 65–86, 1980.
8. Harris T, Cook EF, Kannel WB, Goldman L: Proportional hazards analysis of risk factors for coronary heart disease in individuals over the age of 65: The Framingham Heart Study. J Am Geriatr Soc (in press).
9. National Institutes of Health Consensus Development Conference Statement: Lowering blood cholesterol to prevent heart disease. JAMA 1985; 253:2080–2086.
10. Taylor WC, Pass TM, Shepard DS, Komaroff AL: Cholesterol reduction and life expectancy. A model incorporating multiple risk factors. Ann Intern Med 1987; 106:605–614.
11. Hoeg JM, Gregg RE, Brewer HB: An approach to the management of hyperlipoproteinemia. JAMA 1986; 255:512–521.

12. Kannel WB: High density lipoproteins: Epidemiologic profile and risks of coronary artery disease. Am J Cardiol 1983; 52:9B–12B.
13. Gotto AM, Bierman EL, Conner WE, et al: Recommendations for treatment of hyperlipidemia in adults: The Nutrition Committee and Council on Atherosclerosis of the American Heart Association. Circulation 1984; 69:1067A–1090A.
14. Coronary Drug Project Research Group: Clofibrate and niacin in coronary heart disease. JAMA 1975; 231:360–381.
15. Canner PL: Mortality in coronary drug project patients during a nine-year post-treatment period. J Am Coll Cardiol 1985; 4:442.
16. The Lovastatin Study Group II: Therapeutic response to lovastatin (Mevinolin) in nonfamilial hypercholesterolemia. A multicenter study. JAMA 1986; 256:2829–2834.
17. O'Malley K, O'Brien EO: Management of hypertension in the elderly. N Engl J Med 1980; 302:1397–1401.
18. Byyny RL: Hypertension in the elderly. Am J Med 1986; 81:1055–1058.
19. Amery A, Birkenhager W, Brixko P: Mortality and morbidity results from the European Working Party on High Blood Pressure in the Elderly trial. Lancet 1985; 1:1349–1354.
20. Hulley SB, Furberg CD, Gurland B, et al: Systolic hypertension in the elderly program (SHEP): Antihypertensive efficacy of chlorthalidone. Am J Cardiol 1985; 56:913–920.
21. Weinstein MC, Stason WB: Hypertension: A Policy Perspective. Cambridge, MA, Harvard University Press, 1976.
22. Rowe JW: Systolic hypertension in the elderly. N Engl J Med 1983; 309:1246–1247.
23. Wikstrand J, Westergren G, Berglund G, et al: Antihypertensive treatment with metoprolol or hydrochlorothiazide in patients aged 60–75 years. JAMA 1986; 255:1304–1310.
24. Croog SH, Levine S, Testa MA, et al: The effects of antihypertensive therapy on the quality of life. N Engl J Med 1986; 314:1657–1664.
25. Hennekens C, Buring J, Mayrent S: Smoking and aging in coronary artery disease. In Bosse R, Rose C (eds): Smoking and Aging. Lexington, MA, Lexington Books, 1984.

7
EXERCISE

Jeane Ann Grisso, MD, MSc

Most elderly are sedentary. Unless employment necessitates continued activity, in most people a marked decline in activity level occurs over time. The National Health Survey documented that 68% of men and 72% of women over the age of 65 reported *not* exercising regularly in 1985.[35] Prevailing beliefs and attitudes have not been supportive of exercise for the elderly. The stereotype is still commonly held that older people should sit back and take a well-deserved rest, since they have worked all of their lives. The older person should enjoy the "good life." Reinforcing this attitude is the belief that decline is inevitable and irreversible with age.

Evidence is accumulating, however, that fitness *can* be regained and increased in old age. A number of studies have shown that exercise programs for the elderly do result in improvements in both physical and mental functioning.[4-9] The studies consistently show improvement in a number of physical measures, including aerobic capacity, muscle strength, flexibility, range of motion, and coordination. In addition, exercise programs may improve functional status and prolong independence, and enhance an older person's self-image. Thus, it is now generally accepted that physical activity is a very important aspect of obtaining and maintaining optimal health in the elderly. Although a great deal of publicity has been given to the benefits of sustained activity and exercise in the elderly, clinicians have been provided with very little information that would guide them in their exercise prescriptions for elderly patients. Who should be screened before beginning an exercise program? Who is at high risk for adverse effects of exercise? What is a reasonable exercise prescription for someone over 65? This chapter will address the risks and benefits of exercise for elderly individuals and provide guidelines for physicians interested in counseling elderly patients.

BENEFITS AND RISKS OF EXERCISE IN THE ELDERLY

Exercise may result in improvement in coordination, maintenance of independence, and improvement in a general sense of well-being. Psychological benefits have been reported, including improved psychomotor reaction time, better relaxation, improved sleeping, and general elevation of mood and self-image.[1,2,4,9]

Exercise results in improvement in physiological parameters that are associated with stroke and myocardial infarction in the elderly, including decreases in systolic blood pressure and total peripheral resistance and increases in cardiac output and maximal oxygen consumption.[7,8] Exercise has been found to have positive effects on other cardiovascular risk factors, including decreases in cholesterol and triglyceride levels, obesity, and blood glucose levels.[10] Epidemiologic studies have reported a decreased risk of cardiovascular disease in physically active individuals compared to sedentary individuals.[2,23,24]

Just as exercise reduces cardiovascular risk factors, inactivity is associated with increased cardiovascular risks as well as other adverse effects (Table 1). Inactivity causes increased rates of bone loss. Astronauts and people confined to bed lose about 1% of their bone mass each week. Results of few trials have suggested that postmenopausal women can slow the rate of bone loss by walking for periods ranging from 30 to 60 minutes, three times a week.[11,26] Whether regular exercise reduces the risk of fractures is not yet known.

On the other hand, vigorous physical activity may induce adverse effects, such as injuries or cardiovascular complications.[13] Clinical reports suggest that a variety of musculoskeletal injuries occur as a result of exercise. However, a review by Koplan and others concluded that there is very little information about the risks of musculoskeletal injury due to exercise.[14] A study of joggers of all ages found that 1 in 3 was injured per running year and 1 in 10 required medical attention.[25] The risks of fractures, tissue injuries, and accelerated osteoarthritis have not been quantified for the elderly but may be assumed to be higher.

Although no cost-benefit analyses have been carried out to evaluate exercise as a preventive measure, Louise Russell in her book *Is Prevention Better than Cure?* has outlined potential costs to the patient.[18] In general, these expenditures are minor and include the costs of exercise equipment, transportation to facilities for exercise, and membership dues. Some forms of exercise, like walking, would necessitate little, if any, expenditures. Medical costs include charges for medical evaluations before an exercise program is begun. Medical costs would also include those that arise from injury or cardiovascular events. Potential savings include those related to improved function and the possibly reduced risk of coronary artery disease and osteoporosis.

EVALUATION OF CARDIAC RISK

Because of the high incidence of cardiac disease in the elderly, many clinicians suggest that a thorough cardiovascular evaluation is necessary before prescribing an exercise program. The evaluation should include a careful history, physical exam, resting ECG, and possibly an exercise test.

Patients should be asked about cardiac risk factors, as well as about a history of cardiac dysrhythmia, palpitations, angina, exercise-related chest pain or myocardial infarction. The physical exam should include an assessment of blood pressure, resting pulse, and the presence of signs of congestive heart failure. Older persons with one or more cardiac risk factor or symptoms of coronary artery disease should be advised to undergo an exercise stress test before beginning an exercise program. Important cardiac risk factors include: diabetes mellitus, hypertension, significantly elevated cholesterol levels, and cigarette smoking.

Whether to advise an exercise stress test for those older persons without symptoms or cardiac risk factors is controversial. It is increasingly advocated for older adults because of the high prevalence of coronary artery disease in the elderly and because the elderly frequently do not experience the classic signs and symptoms of angina or myocardial infarction. The American Heart Association recommends that an exercise test be carried out for some patient groups before a patient is advised to take up exercise or increase it significantly. They advise an exercise test for sedentary men over 45 and sedentary women over 50 as well

TABLE 1. Effects of Inactivity

Increased systolic blood pressure
Increased total peripheral resistance
Increased total level of cholesterol
Increased risk of glucose intolerance
Increased risk of obesity
Increased rate of bone loss
Decreased cardiac output
Decreased maximal oxygen consumption
Decreased muscle strength, endurance, and coordination

---

as for anyone with heart disease or hypertension.[19] In Great Britain, the Royal College of Physicians and the British Cardiac Society have agreed on a recommendation that minimizes the use of special evaluations, arguing that "most people do not need a medical examination before starting an exercise program" as long as the workout begins at a low level and builds intensity very slowly.[18]

Nevertheless, Cantwell[21] lists eight reasons for performing a stress test prior to initiating an exercise program: (1) to determine the level of fitness; (2) to screen for significant underlying coronary artery disease; (3) to assess chest pain related to exercise; (4) to screen for exercise related cardiac dysrhythmias; (5) to screen patients who will participate in rehabilitation programs; (6) to evaluate exercise-related leg cramps; (7) to assess labile hypertension and antihypertensive therapy; and (8) to measure the response to the exercise program.

The American College of Sports Medicine has an excellent review of the major features of graded exercise testing.[27] It is important to remember some special concerns for older persons. Medications should be given particular attention. Cardiovascular drugs, tranquilizers, diuretics, and sedatives, which account for half of prescribed drugs for older Americans, may affect exercise tolerance and physiologic responses to exercise testing. Elderly subjects often have much more anxiety about exercise testing than younger individuals and should be counseled about the normal discomfort that occurs as one progressively increases work output.

The target for stopping the exercise test can either be symptom limited (maximal fatigue) or heart-rate limited. Most recommendations for exercise test endpoints for the elderly favor a target heart rate of 75% to 85% of the age-adjusted maximal heart rate.[28] The maximal heart rate is conservatively estimated at 220 minus the age. Thus, for a 65 year old, the target heart rate would be between 116 and 132.

EXERCISE STRESS TESTS: TEST-STEP TESTING OR TREADMILL

Step testing is a reasonably familiar activity for exercise testing that requires minimum learning and minimum monetary investment in equipment. The Canadian Home Fitness Test consists of six stages of stepping on two 20 cm steps.[29] Others advocate varying the step height from 4 to 12 inches, depending on the individual's ability. In general, if the person can step up and down 24 to 30 times per minute, he or she should reach 75% to 85% of maximal heart rate in 3 to 5 minutes.

Major problems with step testing include difficulty in taking blood pressure while the participant is stepping up and down and progressive loss of balance as the participant becomes fatigued. It is also not possible to monitor the ECG in a standardized fashion to evaluate ischemic changes.

Several treadmill protocols are available for graded exercise testing; however, the most commonly used Bruce protocol has increments that are too large to be comfortably tolerated by most of the elderly. Smith suggests the Modified Balke Treadmill Test as the most adaptable test for the majority of elderly participants.[30] This uses a constant walking speed of 2 mph with appropriate treadmill grade increments to increase the work stages by approximately 0.5 METs. A number of others have successfully adapted treadmill tests to conform to the special needs of the elderly.[31,32]

Although treadmill walking provides the most familiar skill for testing, it is not without problems. The same balance difficulties that occur in step testing can occur in treadmill testing as well. In addition, many elderly participants may have to terminate the test because of joint pain during weight-bearing.

During exercise testing, the pulse, blood pressure, and ECG tracing should be monitored. Many advocate keeping the product of the systolic blood pressure times the heart rate to around 20,000. That would mean a systolic blood pressure of 180 or less and pulse of 120 or less. If the patient can achieve the target heart rate without chest pain, abnormal ECG changes, or undue fatigue, then the patient may be advised to exercise up to that level without cardiac monitoring. However, in older individuals the exercise ECG is associated with a high proportion of false positive results. The percentage of abnormal electrocardiograms in elderly subjects has been reported in men to range from 17% to 46% and in women from 21% to 100%.[20] The abnormalities often are nonspecific STT-wave changes or the pattern of LVH with strain frequently seen in hypertensive persons. If an elderly person has a positive exercise stress test and the circumstances make it important to know whether the finding is due to coronary artery disease, then a stress-thallium test is recommended. The results of a stress-thallium test are more specific and can be helpful in ruling out significant coronary artery disease.

To prohibit exercise for a patient with exercise-induced angina or stable angina may be a serious disservice to the individual concerned. Inactivity is likely to decrease the quality of life and lead to chronic incapacitation. Under these circumstances it is best to advocate an exercise program in a monitored setting. Cardiac rehabilitation programs in hospitals and physical therapy clinics offer monitored exercise programs. In these programs progressive interval training (where submaximal, low-intensity exercise is performed at frequent intervals) can often break the vicious cycle of angina secondary to deterioration in physical condition. Medication such as nitroglycerin can be taken immediately prior to exercise, and the pace of activity can be slowed if anginal pain occurs. If, however, frequent extrasystoles or other arrhythmias occur during exercise, the patient should be referred to a cardiologist for further evaluation.

In summary, before instituting an exercise program an exercise stress test is recommended for older persons with known cardiac disease, cardiac symptoms, or risk factors for coronary artery disease. Given the prevalence of coronary artery disease, clinicians should consider advocating an exercise stress test even in asymptomatic elderly persons if the persons were previously sedentary. Monitored exercise programs should be advised for those with angina or exercise-induced angina.

GUIDELINES FOR ASSESSMENT
AND PRESCRIPTION OF EXERCISE

ASSESSING THE APPROPRIATENESS OF
AN EXERCISE PROGRAM FOR THE INDIVIDUAL PATIENT

Take into account the patient's desires as well as what you think would be best. It is important that the patient enjoy the activity. Some of the most popular leisure activities for the elderly are walking, gardening, and fishing. Exercise programs can be designed to incorporate a person's favorite recreational activities into a systematic exercise program.

Assess functional impairment and prescribe exercises accordingly. It is important to take a good history of present physical activity patterns and a history of orthopedic problems. Methods to assess functional status are described in Chapter 11.

Evaluate cardiac risk factors as discussed above and consider ordering an exercise stress test. An exercise stress test can provide important information about clinical conditions that are latent at rest, functional capacity for the purpose of measuring an exercise regimen and baseline values that can be used to gauge the success or failure of the exercise program.

PRESCRIBING A PATTERN OF EXERCISE THAT
FULFILLS THE PURPOSE OF THE EXERCISE PROGRAM

Exercise performed by persons of any age can be grouped into two categories: aerobic exercise and low-intensity exercise. Aerobic exercise has come to mean exercise that strengthens the cardiovascular system. Jogging, cycling, and swimming are aerobic exercises. Low-intensity exercise has little effect on the cardiovascular system but is helpful in controlling weight, in improving flexibility and balance, and in halting age-related bone loss. This type of exercise may include yoga, golfing, fishing, or gardening. Exercise that may be low-intensity for a young individual may be aerobic for an older person. For example, walking at an average pace does not increase the heart rate enough to result in cardiovascular conditioning in a young individual but may often result in a heart rate of 110–120 BPM (the target heart rate) for aerobic exercise in an older person.

The type of exercise that one recommends is based on the needs, interest, and medical status of the potential exercise participant. If the main purpose of the exercise program is to improve the patient's well-being and to reduce isolation and depression, then group recreational programs should be recommended. If the main purpose is to reduce excess body fat, then moderate intensity of walking for increasing periods of the day is the most useful exercise. Muscle strengthening exercises have disadvantages, since physiological responses to isometric contractions include increased blood pressure, increased cardiac workload, and development of skeletal muscles without augmentation of cardiac muscle. In general, isometric contractions are not recommended for the elderly. However, there can be an advantage to isometric contractions where strengthening of appropriate muscle groups can stabilize particular joints.

In many instances the clinician will be able to plan an exercise program with a patient based on the patient's goals and health status utilizing published guides and community resources. An exercise pamphlet produced by the American Physical Therapy Association is included in the Appendix. It can be reproduced and given to elderly patients as a guide. At other times it is useful to consult with a physical therapist in planning and monitoring exercise programs. Examples of two individualized exercise prescriptions developed by physical therapists are included in the section that follows:

CASE HISTORIES*

Anna.   Anna C, a 70-year-old female, has a history of arteriosclerotic heart disease (ASHD) and hypertension that are controlled by medications. She currently resides in a board-and-care facility where she is responsible for her own ADL and walking to a common dining area. Evaluation revealed fair-plus strength overall, a walking speed of 27 m/min, marginal ability to walk as far as the dining room (250 feet), and difficulty getting up from a seated position. Anna was fearful of losing her ability to function independently in the board-and-care facility.

Exercise Prescription.   Program weeks 1 and 2: walk 25 feet at a pace of 35 m/min, rest, repeat 4 to 5 times. Do bed exercises of bridging, gently resisted rolling, and lower extremity extension. Weeks 3 and 4: walk 40 feet at 35 m/min, rest, repeat 5 to 6 times. Do bed exercises as above plus supine on elbows and unilateral straight leg raising.

Anna's program ultimately consisted of six to seven longer walks, some at her usual rate of speed, some at a brisk pace. During part of the walk, pushing a wheelchair with telephone books on the seat was added to the program. A few more bed exercises were done, and sitting exercises to assist standing capability were initiated. When on her own, she was instructed to get up from her chair every half hour and move about. After 2 months Anna was walking confidently to the dining room and getting up from her bed, chair, and the toilet without difficulty.

It must be noted that performance varied day to day and Anna's program was modified accordingly. Her blood pressure and heart rate were monitored continuously during the treatment.

Ruth.   Ruth W, a 74-year-old widow, was hospitalized for pancreatitis but during her hospital stay experienced other problems (phlebitis, flu, and embolism) that necessitated almost 4 weeks of bedrest. This previously energetic and independent woman who managed her own home was no longer capable of sitting secondary to hip, knee, and back extension contractures.

Exercise Prescription.   Successful rehabilitation included exercises for improving range of motion. Week 1: bed exercises consisted of neck flexion and rotation, rolling and reaching to the right and left, active straight leg raising and leg circling, bringing knee toward chest, and walking. At the end of each exercise or warm-up session, the bed back was elevated to her tolerance level, and pillows were placed under her knees. This position was maintained for 20 to 30 minutes and often during this time period the bed was raised a few more degrees and another knee pillow was added. By the end of the first week Ruth was transferred to a reclining wheelchair with elevating leg rests. After 20 to 30 minutes of sitting, leg rests were lowered and the seat back brought a little closer to the upright. After 2 weeks of exercise and positioning, the client was able to sit in a regular chair, stand, and walk by herself.

Ruth is now coming to an exercise class for seniors that meets twice a week. Her flexibility exercises include (sitting position) (1) reaching toward the ceiling, then bending forward to touch the floor; (2) hands on hips and trunk twisting; (3) lateral bends; (4) upper extremity ballet-type movements; and (5) knee to chest. Each session, exercises start slowly and are confined to a small arc within the available range of motion. After approximately 15 minutes, the pace of exercise is quickened and activities incorporating the full arc of available range of motion initiated. Exercises sometimes are performed to music, but the tempo never reaches that of a typical jazz or aerobics class.

---

* From Brown M, Rose SJ: The effects of aging and exercise on skeletal muscle. In Smith EL: Effects of Aging and Exercise. Topics in Geriatric Rehabilitation 1985; 1(1):26–29, with permission.

EXERCISE PRESCRIPTION

Shepard recommends the following principles for a physician prescribing exercise for an elderly person.[20] To be most effective, a prescribed program should provide written instructions for the type, intensity, duration, and frequency of exercise:

- **Warm-up and Warm-down**
Gentle stretching before exercising reduces the risk of injury and gradual progression decreases the probability of cardiac dysrhythmia. Circulatory adaptations during the recovery period are less effective in an elderly person than in a younger person, and the warm-down period should be slightly longer (10 minutes or more) in an older person than in a younger person.

- **Aerobic Activity Segment**
The main segment of the exercise should provide a period of moderate aerobic activity. Ideally this would be 20 minutes of activity sufficient to raise the heart rate to 75 to 85% of maximal attainable heart rate, or at least 110 to 120 beats per minute. Table 2 includes a list of age specific target heart rates.

For aerobic exercise to result in beneficial effects on the cardiovascular system, it should be performed at least three times a week. Many elderly patients are in such poor physical condition that they need to approach this target gradually. The exercise that is prescribed should leave the participant pleasantly tired the following day. It may be necessary to start training in two 10- to 15-minute sessions rather than a single session of 20 minutes.

Any large muscle exercise such as brisk walking, swimming, cycling, or cross-country skiing will theoretically develop aerobic fitness. In older persons, because of degenerate joints and limited support from surrounding muscles, the risk of injury may be high, particularly from vigorous activities, such as skiing or jogging. Older patients can develop just as large an oxygen consumption by fast walking as by jogging. Swimming is a good method of beginning the conditioning process, particularly for an obese or a disabled patient, but many elderly persons do not like to swim and dyspnea during swimming is a frequent complaint. Cycling may have a disadvantage, in that a major part of the effort is sustained by the quadriceps, and the exercise provokes a greater rise in blood pressure than an equivalent oxygen consumption developed by walking. Cycling can also be hard on persons with severe arthritis in the knees. Rhythmic calisthenics can provide the basis for useful warm-up; however, the exercises should be gentle and smooth to avoid causing injuries. Routines that involve the support of body weight, such as push-ups, are best avoided, since they induce an excessive rise in blood pressure and therefore cardiac work-load.

Exploit the exercise potential of normal daily living, both in the garden and in the home. Encourage the patient to use the stairs several times daily, to garden actively, or to pursue other pleasant walking activities, such as walking in shopping malls.

ADAPTING THE PROGRAM FOR PATIENTS WITH PHYSICAL PROBLEMS

Individual capabilities vary widely; some older adults lack the aerobic capacity to walk 2 miles/hour on level ground whereas others still participate in marathons. Many elderly persons have some type of medical abnormality that

TABLE 2.   Target Heart Rate*

Age (years)	Target Heart Rate (beats per minute)	Average Maximum Heart Rate (beats per minute)
40	108-135	180
45	105-131	175
50	102-127	170
55	99-123	165
60	96-120	160
65	93-116	155
70	90-113	150

* US Department of Health and Human Services. Public Health Service, National Institutes of Health. National Heart, Lung and Blood Institute. Exercise and Your Heart. NIH Publication No. 81-1677 Washington, D.C., U.S. Government Printing Office, 1981.

necessitates a more cautious approach to exercise prescription. A brief discussion of a few selected conditions follows.

Exercise-Induced Angina.   If there is a history of exercise-induced angina, the best response is to modify interval patterns of training. Shephard recommends interspersing 1 to 11/2 minutes of vigorous movement with equal periods of slow walking to allow oxidation of anaerobic metabolites.[20] If inhalation of cold air precipitates angina, the patient may arrange to exercise indoors. Patients with severe angina may take a anti-anginal medication before exercising. Patients with a history of angina or hypertension should avoid isometric contractions. Most authors recommend that at least in the beginning of the program those persons with angina should exercise in a monitored setting, such as a cardiac rehabilitation center or physical therapy clinic. These programs begin with an exercise stress test to identify the target level of exercise tolerated. Cardiac monitoring may need to be continued at subsequent exercise sessions, depending upon the severity of the disease.

Intermittent Claudication.   The appropriate pattern for training for vascular disease is an intermittent exercise schedule. Walking the patient to the point of symptoms several times a day is recommended unless the patient has ischemic rest pain and/or ulceration. There have been several reports that regular progressive activity extends the function of affected individuals, possibly by opening up alternative vascular pathways to muscles.[33]

Patients with peripheral vascular diseases should be advised to keep the extremities and body warm to avoid vasoconstriction. They should be instructed to wear good shoes, to take good care of their feet and to avoid trauma.

Chronic Obstructive Lung Disease.   In emphysema there is destruction of the alveolar structure, producing increased lung compliance and loss of elastic lung recoil. The lung retains larger volumes of gas, increasing thoracic diameter and preventing thoracic recoil that normally assists inspiration. The net result is a mechanically disadvantaged system performing the increased work of breathing with limited energy supply. This is superimposed on the decrease in pulmonary function normally seen with aging.

The implications for pulmonary rehabilitation in the geriatric population focus on the increased work of breathing and limited respiratory reserve capacities. Exercise training programs should respond to the patients' baseline status and their ability to exercise. The geriatric individual who is symptomatic may require medication, a bronchopulmonary hygiene program, and oxygen to participate in an exercise program. Respiratory therapists should help to train the patient about breathing exercises and methods to enhance secretory clearance. In general, the patient may be advised to practice deep nasal inspiration, hold the breath for 3 seconds and then relax and exhale before beginning the warm-up. The warm-up exercises might include walking in place 3–4 minutes while lifting the knees higher each time, then 3–4 minutes of stretching and inhaling while lifting the arms and exhaling as the arms are lowered. The final 3–4 minutes of warm-up could include trunk rotation and side bending.[34]

Aerobic exercise is going to allow for the greatest improvement in exercise capacity. The best time for an exercise session is late morning or afternoon. This allows time for the mucus to be cleared from the lungs. The best exercise mode, generally, is walking or stationary bicycling. The setting is also important. Humidity and pollution levels may affect exercise tolerance. If the ozone level is greater than .37 parts per million, exercising outdoors is not recommended. Bronchospasm precipitated by inhalation of very cold or dry air should be avoided. Indoor exercising with a humidifier may be necessary.

Frequently the initial exercise tolerance is extremely low in patients with COPD. It is desirable to start with several short exercise sessions during the day. These may be as short as 1–5 minutes in duration, with the time being increased progressively. Rather than setting a heart rate prescription, it may be more appropriate to set a level of dyspnea as the target for intensity.

Although most exercise programs have not demonstrated marked improvement in pulmonary function, one study reported that there was an average increase of 20% in the vital capacity after 42 weeks.[34] Exercise seems to help desensitize the patient to the sensation of dyspnea and may improve muscle function. Most programs have found that exercise allows patients with COPD to improve their functional capacity and abilities to perform ADL.

Degenerative Joint Disease, Orthopedic Problems, and Neurological Abnormalities. Patients will require adaptive exercise programs for joint diseases or neurological abnormalities. For arthritis patients, ideally activities should be chosen that are non-weight-bearing or do not involve the same joints on a continuous, daily basis. It is best to include an exercise physiologist or a physical therapist in the planning of exercise programs for this population.

Contraindications for Exercise. Relative contraindications in which exercise would generally be inadvisable include severe congestive heart failure, hypertophic cardiomyopathy, and moderate to severe aortic stenosis.

THE IMPORTANCE OF MOTIVATION IN EXERCISE

Motivation is a key component of a successful exercise program. Dropout rates from exercise programs for the elderly are frequently high, approaching 40–50%, even in relatively short programs. Slowly building intensity should be prescribed so as not to overstress the elderly in the beginning of a program. Otherwise the older participant may find that exercising is so unpleasant that he or she will not want to continue with it. A structured group program may be more effective. In a recent study, 22 postmenopausal women were divided into two groups matched for age, weight, current exercise habits and other variables.[25] One group was told to continue their current exercise program, and the other was enrolled in a formal exercise program. After 13 weeks, the women taking part in the structured program, unlike those who exercised independently, demonstrated objective improvement in cardiovascular fitness, strength, and flexibility.

In evaluating a program for your patients, remember that the person supervising group activities should have empathy for the needs and potential of an older person. An overly athletic youthful instructor can have a negative impact on both body image and motivation. Grouping classes by age and disability improves both real and perceived safety and helps to overcome some of the self-consciousness and embarrassment that some older people find in the early stages of renewed activity. Some older people will find companionship in social interchange, but in most cases the prime motivation will be to improve health. In consultations, therefore, stress the gains in health and fitness that can be realized in the program.

It is important to demonstrate progress, whether this be a gain of aerobic capacity or an improvement in body composition. One measure of cardiovascular fitness is when the exercise heart rate decreases by 30 beats per minute after 1 minute of cessation of maximum exercise sustained for 2 minutes or longer. Patients should be encouraged to keep a log or diary of their program, including information on pulse rates and duration of each exercise session. Although the extent of weekly gains diminishes as the individual approaches the standard for a fit person of his or her age, the program can be explained as a campaign of maintenance, and exercise should be commended as the basis of a happier life rather than just as a guarantee of longevity.

PROGRAM ACTIVITIES AND SOURCES

A wide range of activities similar to those of younger people may be undertaken by older adults with adaptation to suit their preferences and capabilities. Activities are categorized as conditioning programs, sports, or dance, and may be done individually or in groups. Table 3 summarizes the benefits of various exercise programs along with fitness components, needs, and interests to be considered in choosing the program.

Today a variety of innovative programs are available for older adults. Resources include local colleges, universities, and community colleges whose physical education or gerontology programs can often be of service. YMCAs and community centers, particularly senior citizen centers, often have very good programs. For those who cannot take part in an organized group (because of limited transportation, health, or funds), many programs are available in booklet form for home use. For example, the National Association for Human Development has exercise materials that older adults may obtain for use at home. Also most local and state divisions of aging and area agencies on aging have materials available or can help in locating them. Exercise booklets for the elderly have been also published by the American Physical Therapy Association and the American Association of Retired Persons.

SUMMARY

Physical fitness is a multifaceted concept that is an integral part of overall personal wellness. Health-related fitness is very important to the older adult

TABLE 3. Benefits of Exercise Activities*

Activity	Stamina	Muscular strength	Muscular endurance	Weight control	Flexibility	Skill Improvement	Individual	Group	Both	Comments**
Aerobic dance	XX	X	XX	XX	X	X			X	Very popular; widely available
Bicycling	XX	X	XX	XX	—	X			X	
Boating (rowing and canoeing)	XX	X	XX	XX	—	—			X	Stationary rowing machine can provide similar benefits
Bowling	—	—	—	—	—	X			X	A major participation activity in the U.S.
Circuit training	X	X	XX	X	X	—			X	Can be adapted to emphasize any fitness components
Dancing	X	—	X	X	—	X		X		Varied opportunities exist for participants
Fitness trail or par course	XX	X	XX	XX	X	—			X	Requires more space and precautions
Golf (walking)	X	—	X	X	X	X			X	
Handball/ racquetball	X	—	X	X	X	X			X	
Hiking	X	—	X	X	—	X			X	
Interval training	XX	X	X	XX	—	—			X	
Rhythmical endurance	XX	X	XX	XX	—	—			X	
Rope skipping	XX	—	X	XX	—	—	X			Fairly strenuous even at moderate pace; space/equipment efficient
Skating (ice & roller)	XX	—	X	XX	—	X			X	Seasonal aspect may add variety
Skiing: cross country	XX	X	XX	XX	—	—			X	Seasonal
Skiing: downhill	X	X	X	X	—	X			X	Seasonal; somewhat costly
Swimming	XX	X	XX	XX	X	X	X			Facility availability is a concern
Swim exercise	XX	X	XX	XX	X	—			X	
Tennis	X	—	X	X	—	X			X	
Walking/ jogging	XX	—	XX	XX	—	—			X	Readily available
Weight training	—	XX	X	—	X	—	X			Equipment is needed
Yoga relaxation	—	—	—	—	X	—			X	Often a good addition to other programs

XX = Very good; X = Moderate; — = Limited.
** The extent of benefit will relate to the intensity, frequency, and duration of the activity undertaken. The fun factor is possible in all the activities and is dependent upon the individual's attitude and approach.
 * From Clark BA: Physical activity programming. In Lewis CB (ed): Topics in Geriatric Rehabilitation. 1985; #1(1):68, with permission.

because of its role in both health maintenance and mobility. The benefits of exercise are myriad. They include improved cardiorespiratory capacity, muscular strength, and endurance, as well as changes in body composition and flexibility, improved range of motion, and improved general functional capabilities. In addition, exercise programs are helpful for relaxation and emotional stability. Physical activity for older adults can be extremely rewarding, providing sound physiologic guidelines are understood and reasonably implemented. Effective exercise programming requires taking specific individual characteristics into account, adjusting for fitness level and health as well as the patient's own desires. Most older adults feel they have earned the right to choose what they do. Therefore, exercising must be a pleasant experience.

PRACTICE RECOMMENDATIONS

1. Assess the appropriateness of an exercise program for the individual patient:
- Take into account the patient's desires as well as what you think would be best.
- Assess functional status and prescribe exercises accordingly.
- Evaluate cardiac risk factors.
- During the physical examination, evaluate body weight, range of motion, and presence of arthritis as well as blood pressure, pulse, and the signs of congestive heart failure.
- Consider ordering an exercise stress test. Most authors recommend a stress test for anyone who is sedentary and/or someone who plans to progress to aerobic or vigorous exercise as well as for anyone with cardiac risk factors or known coronary artery disease.

2. Prescribe a pattern of exercise that fulfills the purpose of the exercise program:

The type of exercise that one recommends is based on the needs, interest, and medical status of the potential exercise participant.

3. To be most effective, a prescribed program should provide written instructions for the type, intensity, duration, and frequency of exercise.

4. Encourage the patient to capitalize on the exercise potential of normal daily living in the garden, at home, or while shopping.

5. Adapt the program for patients with physical problems.

6. Relative contraindications in which exercise would generally be inadvisable include severe congestive heart failure, hypertrophic cardiomyopathy, and moderate to severe aortic stenosis.

7. Keep the importance of motivation in mind.

REFERENCES

1. Physical Fitness and Exercise. Public Health Reports Supplement. September-October 1983; 155–157.
2. Paffenbarger RS, Wing AL, Hyde RT: Physical activity as an index of heart attack risk in college alumni. Am J Epidemiol September 1978; 161–175.
3. Bortz WM: Disuse and aging. JAMA 1982; 248:1203–1208.
4. Vallbona C, Baker SB: Physical fitness prospects in the elderly. Arch Phys Med Rehabil 1984; 65:194–200.
5. Council on Scientific Affairs, American Medical Association: Exercise programs for the elderly. JAMA 1984; 252:544–546.

6. Fuller E: Exercise: Getting the elderly going. Patient Care 1982; 16:67–114.
7. Posner JD, Gorman KM, Klein HS, Woldow A: Exercise capacity in the elderly. Am J Cardiol 1986; 57:52C–58C.
8. Schocken DD, Blumenthal JA, Port S, et al: Physical conditioning and left ventricular performance in the elderly: assessment by radionuclide angiocardiography. Am J Cardiol 1983; 52:359–364.
9. De Carlo TJ, Castiglione LV, Cavusoglu M: A program of balanced physical fitness in the preventive care of elderly ambulatory patients. J Am Geriatr Soc 1977; 25:331–334.
10. Price JH, Luther SL: Physical fitness: its role in health for the elderly. J Gerontol Nurs 1980; 6:517–523.
11. Cummings SR, Nevitt MC, Haber RJ: Prevention of osteoporosis and osteoporotic fractures. West J Med 1985; 143:684–687.
12. Taylor CB, Sallis JF, Needle R: The relationship between physical activity and exercise and mental health. Public Health Reports.
13. Shephard RJ: Sudden death—a significant hazard of exercise? Br J Sports Med 1974; 8:101–110.
14. Koplan JP, Siscovick DS, Goldbaum GM: The risks of exercise: a public health view of injuries and hazards. Public Health Reports.
15. Koplan JP: An epidemiological study of the benefits and risks of running. JAMA 1982; 248:3118–3121.
16. Holloszy JO: Exercise, health, and aging: a need for more information. Med Sci Sports Exerc 1983; 15:1–5.
17. Erickson DJ: Exercise for the older adult. Phys Sportsmed 1978; 6(10):99–107.
18. Russell LB: Is Prevention Better Than Cure? Washington, D.C., The Brookings Institution, 1986.
19. The American Heart Association Committee on Exercise, Exercise Testing and Training for Healthy Individuals: Handbook for Physicians. New York, The American Heart Association, 1972.
20. Shephard RJ: Physical fitness: exercise and aging. In Pathy MSJ: Principles and Practice of Geriatric Medicine. New York, John Wiley and Sons, 1985.
21. Cantwell JD: Stress testing indicated in a variety of complaints. Phys Sportsmed 1977; 5(2):70–74.
22. Larsen OA, Lassen NA: Effect of daily muscular exercise in patients with intermittent claudication. Lancet 1966; 2:1093–1096.
23. Froelichen VG, Brown P: Exercises and coronary heart diseases. J Cardiac Rehab 1981; 277–288.
24. Rigott NA, Thomas GS, Leaf A: Exercise and coronary heart disease. Ann Rev Med 1983; 34:391–412.
25. Bachman GA, Grill J: Exercise in the postmenopausal women. Geriatrics 1987; 42:75–85.
26. Sandler RB, Canley JA, Hom DL, et al: The effects of walking on the cross-sectional dimensions of the radius in postmenopausal women. Calcif Tissue Int 1987; 41:65–69.
27. American College of Sports Medicine Guidelines for Graded Exercise Testing and Prescriptions. Philadelphia, Lea & Febiger, 1980.
28. Serfass RC, Agre JC, Smith EL: Exercise testing for the elderly. Topics in Geriatric Rehabilitation 1985; 58–67.
29. Jette M, Campbell J, Mongeon J, et al: The Canadian Home Fitness Test as a predictor of aerobic capacity. Can Med J 1976; 114:680–682.
30. Balke B, Ware RW: An experimental study of physical fitness of Air Force personnel. US Armed Forces Med J 1959; 10:675–688.
31. Amundsen LR, Eliason ML, Ellingham CT, et al: Cardiac considerations and physical training. In Jackson O (ed): Physical Therapy of the Geriatric Patient. New York, Churchill Livingstone, 1983, pp 181–201.
32. Schwimmer J: A new geriatric application of electrocardiographic treadmill testing in an office setting. J Am Geriatr Soc 1979; 27:337–344.
33. Spittell J: Rehabilitative aspects of peripheral vascular disease in the elderly. In Williams TF (ed): Rehabilitation in the Aging. New York, Raven Press, 1984.
34. Zadai C: Pulmonary rehabilitation of the geriatric patient. In Lewis CB (ed): Aging: The Health Care Challenge. Philadelphia, F.A. Davis Co., 1985, pp 181–214.
35. Health Promotion and Disease Prevention, United States, 1985. Data from the National Health Survey, Series 10, No. 163, DHHS Publication No. (PHS) 88-1591.

8
NUTRITION, ALCOHOL AND
TOBACCO IN LATE LIFE

Mary Ann Forciea, MD

The link between unwise consumption and morbidity and mortality is at least as old as Biblical times: partaking of the apple led to the end of Eden. Philosopher/scientists and physicians from ancient through medieval times increasingly recognized the role of diet in the pathogenesis of disease (red wine and gout), and used dietary manipulations in efforts to treat disease. Progress in the use of foods in illness prevention can be traced to Victorian times in England where sailors were given regular rations of limes as scurvy prophylaxis. Work in our century has led to definitions of essential amino acids and of vitamins as well as to increased understanding of the relationship between biochemical structure and function of these required foodstuffs.

Nutritional requirements for humans change during the lifespan. The majority of studies of age-related alterations have focused on early life: childhood and development. Only recently have careful studies begun to address nutrition in later life. Ideal studies would encompass possible changes in requirements of individual cells or organ systems during aging, as well as alterations in metabolite absorption, activation and excretion. In addition, changes in nutrient metabolism caused by co-existing disease would need to be addressed. While we are awaiting these definitive data, a great deal of new information on nutritional requirements during healthy aging is appearing. This chapter briefly reviews the available information about not only nutrition and aging but also the effects on the elderly of consuming the known toxins, alcohol and tobacco. Recommendations appropriate to the ambulatory setting summarize suggested approaches to detecting problems and counseling for change.

NUTRITION

There are many reasons why nutritional assessment and counseling are important with elderly patients. Approximately 30% of elderly patients living in the community are consuming diets deficient in at least one major nutrient.[1] Furthermore, according to a national survey, 16% of whites and 18% of blacks over 60 years old consume under 1,000 calories per day.[2] At highest risk are alcoholics, women, the poor, and persons living alone, either in high-rise housing or in rural areas. Over one-third of elderly blacks live below the poverty line[2] and therefore are at increased risk for undernutrition. Thus malnutrition and disorders of nutrition (whether they are due to inadequate intake, undernutrition, imbalanced intake or, more rarely, the inability to utilize nutrients) are common among the elderly. Such malnutrition, if significant and prolonged, can lead to nutritional deficiency diseases such as megaloblastic anemia. In addition, illness may precipitate the appearance of a nutritional deficiency syndrome in patients with borderline adequate nutritional intake. Those who are malnourished may be vulnerable to developing complications from pre-existing disease. Thus, nutritional assessment is a crucial part of preventive care for the elderly.

Currently, dietary therapy is being pursued for several disorders. While certain dietary modifications are effective and safe in many circumstances, others—especially those related to weight loss-can lead to dietary restrictions that impair the consumption of a nutritionally adequate diet. Improvement in diabetes, hypertension, and the lipid disorders provide good examples of beneficial effects of dietary modification. The American Cancer Society, noting that the incidence of colon cancer is lower in populations with high dietary fiber content, has recommended increased dietary fiber as a cancer preventive.[3] Dietary fiber is also often recommended for the management of various gastrointestinal disorders such as constipation, diverticulitis, and irritable bowel syndromes. Recent studies have documented the benefits of cholesterol reduction on atherosclerotic heart disease even in patients over age 65[4] (see Chapter 6 for guidelines). Many experts advocate the use of supplemental dietary calcium for prevention or treatment of osteoporosis[1,5] (see Chapter 9).

Elderly consumers are the target of advertising campaigns for a variety of products and procedures with purported beneficial effects, with little or no scientific evidence supporting the claims (Table 1). Consumption of these questionably useful over-the-counter food supplements, such as zinc tablets, is seen in older patients and may be costly. High doses of these products may produce the toxicity syndromes described in Table 2, such as hypercalcemia with high dose Vitamin D. In addition, consumption of multiple products and drugs may lead to potential interactions. For example, increasing dietary fiber may reduce trace mineral absorption due to binding of minerals to the nonabsorbable fiber. Patients should be advised to take vitamin supplements at a different time of day than when taking fiber preparations.

Therapeutic regimens for a variety of disorders may cause nutritional deficiencies. Excessive zeal in dieting can be dangerous; in diets containing less than 1,200 calories, it is difficult to meet Recommended Daily Allowances (RDAs) without supplements. Drugs may interfere with nutrient absorption or metabolism. Diphenylhydantoin use may lead to Vitamin D deficiency and osteomalacia, especially in elderly seizure patients in long-term care settings. Isoniazid therapy can interfere with Vitamin B_{12} and niacin availability.

On the other hand, obesity itself can be associated with increased morbidity and mortality in older patients. Excessive adiposity (more than 40% above ideal body weight) is associated with increased risk for malignancies of colon, breast, gallbladder and uterus.[3] Excessive weight gain can aggravate diabetes, hypertension, osteoarthritis, and many of the hyperlipidemias. Obesity can limit functional recovery after illness due to difficulties with skin breakdown and mobility.

Physicians treating elderly patients should carefully assess each patient's nutritional status and counsel patients based on thorough evaluation of the costs and benefits associated with various dietary therapies. The logical benefits of early identification of nutritional deficiencies include cheap and safe restoration of physiologic reserve, avoidance of unnecessary morbidity, reduction of excess mortality, and the possible avoidance of side effects and interactions of "unsuspected" medications used by our elderly patients. Good advice on

TABLE 1. Products Advertised to Older Patients for Health Promotion

Product	Purported Usefulness	Scientific Evidence
Leicithin	Memory preservation	Leicithin is a precursor of choline and acetylcholine. Acetylcolinergic pathways are important in intellectual function. No study has shown that increased dietary leicithin or choline increases brain neurotransmitters.
Zinc tablets	Increased sexual potency	Zinc deficiency is associated with hypogonadism. Nonalcholic elderly patients consuming a balanced diet can maintain zinc reserves without supplements.
Bee pollen	"Energizer"–decrease apathy, fight infections, heal skin disorders	No controlled trials to verify claims.
RNA, DNA skin creams	Decrease cellular aging	Many age-associated changes in skin are the consequences of life-long sun exposure. No controlled trials have shown benefits of DNA/RNA creams.
Superoxide dismutase (SOD) tablets	Prevent aging changes	SOD is a naturally occurring anti-oxidant. No study has shown that natural levels fall to dangerous levels in healthy older people. No beneficial effects have been shown with oral ingestion.
Cellular injections	Rejuvenation	European clinics inject animal fetal cell suspensions into elderly humans. No controlled trials have demonstrated beneficial effects in patients receiving injections

nutrition may save patients money. Patients can often make better use of their food budget (since fresh fruit and vegetables are more nutritious and cheaper than processed foods), with a simultaneous moderation of their expenditures on nutritional supplements.

When assessing and counseling elderly patients, it is important to consider several factors that may, from their viewpoint, be obstacles to improving their nutrition. Upon retirement, income may drop. The elderly poor are least likely to consume a nutritionally adequate diet. But even when finances are adequate, the purchase of healthful foods may be difficult. Older patients may be immobile due to arthritis, emphysema, angina, or stroke. Grocery stores with home delivery services are rapidly disappearing from many urban and rural settings. Mass transit to supermarkets or malls may be limited. Taxis may be too expensive or inaccessible. Food preparation may be impaired. Kitchens may be inadequate to provide both a stove and refrigerator, or functional limitations may prevent adequate mobility and manual dexterity in the kitchen to prepare food. A Massachusetts Department of Public Health survey found the elderly's greatest unmet need to be assistance with food shopping and preparation.[6]

The consumption of food may also be problematic. Half of all Americans over age 60 have lost all or a substantial portion of their teeth,[7] so they have difficulty chewing more nutritious foods such as meats and fresh vegetables. Loneliness and depression also affect food consumption. Twenty-seven percent

TABLE 2. Toxicities or Complications Possible in Mega Vitamin Usage

Fat-Soluble Vitamins	Symptoms
Vitamin A	Fatigue, headache, arthralgia, alopecia, weight loss
Vitamin D	Hypercalcemia, generalized calcinosis
Water-Soluble Vitamins	
Vitamin C	Renal calculi, false (-) fecal occult blood
Niacin	Flushing pruritus (nicotinic acid); GI distress, hepatic dysfunction
Minerals	
Calcium	Renal calculi

of women over 75 in a health survey of community-living Americans said that they had no interest in cooking for a single person versus 8% of women 51–64.[1]

Even with adequate income, access, preparation and eating, there are many patients who may be unaware of natural sources of basic nutrients (Table 3), or who may have limited sensory pleasures available and be reluctant to limit consumption of enjoyed foods. Illness and medications can also alter appetite and taste. And finally, patients may be unwilling to confide in physicians about dietary habits, because they may have been rebuffed or given inaccurate information in the past. All of these variables should be considered in assessing an elderly patient's nutritional status.

A further obstacle to effective nutrition assessment and counseling is the fact that most physicians have been poorly educated in nutritional guidelines, especially with respect to the elderly. Education during medical training may be scanty on deficiency disease states. In one study, physicians failed to recognize

TABLE 3. Natural Sources of Basic Nutrients

Nutrient		Natural Sources
Fat-Soluble Vitamins		
Vitamin A	Retinol	Liver, dairy products
	Carotene	Vegetables, fruits
Vitamin D	Cholecalciferol	Sun exposure, fortified milk
Vitamin E	Tocopherol	Vegetable oils, fruits, vegetables
Water-Soluble Vitamins		
Vitamin C	Ascorbic acid	Citris fruits
B_1	Thiamine	Whole grain cereals, breads
B_2	Riboflavin	Dairy products, organ meats, eggs
--	Niacin	Vegetables, cereals, nuts, fish, meats
B_6	Pyridoxine	Liver, meats, fish, cereals
Folate		Leafy vegetables, liver, fruits, yeast
B_{12}	Cyanocobalamin	Eggs, meats
Minerals		
Calcium		Dairy products, leafy vegetables, sardines
Zinc		Meats, vegetables
Iron		Meats

TABLE 4.   Weight for Height for Medium-Framed Individuals Aged
65-74 Based on Life Insurance Data*

Height (inches)	Men (lbs)	Women (lbs)
60	—	119
62	133	125
64	137	131
66	143	137
68	149	143
70	155	149
72	169	—
74	169	—

* Adapted from Russell RM, Sahyoun NR, Whinston-Perry R: In Calkins E, Davis PF, Ford AB
(eds): The Practice of Geriatrics. Philadelphia. W.B. Saunders, 1986, pp 135-145.

moderate or severe malnutrition in 50% of hospitalized patients diagnosed by
biochemical and anthropomorphic measurements.[5]

At the simplest level, tables of ideal body weight have been extensively
revised only recently (Table 4). Andres has extensively re-evaluated the data
supporting the Metropolitan Life Tables and found that for the elderly the lowest
mortality was seen at above-average weights. This observation has been
confirmed in other studies, and it is now postulated that modest weight gain
throughout life and into old age is associated with reduced mortality.[8] Therefore,
clinicians should identify and assess elderly who are below ideal body weight or
have recently and unintentionally lost more than 10% of their body weight.

While protein calorie malnutrition is the common type of malnutrition,
vitamin deficiencies leading to the classic deficiency states listed in Table 5

TABLE 5.   Nutritional Deficiencies in the Elderly: Key Signs and Symptoms

Nutrient	Signs or Symptoms
Proteins & calories	Reduced appetite, muscle wasting, parotid enlargement, extremity edema, flaking dermatitis
Vitamin A	Night blindness, xerophthalmia
Vitamin C	Scurvy: perifollicular petechiae, bleeding gums, bruising
Vitamin D	Osteomalacia: bone tenderness, weakness
Vitamin B_{12}	Pernicious anemia: glossitis, loss of vibration and position sense
Folate	Glossitis, macrocytic anemia
Thiamine	Beriberi: muscle pain, paresthesia, foot drop, edemia; Wernicke's encephalopathy: opthalmoplegia and confusion; Korsakoff syndrome: peripheral neuritis and confusion
Iron	Anemia, spooning of nails, tongue atrophy
Zinc	Hypogeusia, flaking dermatitis
Niacin	*Pellagra:* dermatitis, glossitis, diarrhea, dementia
B_6	Depression, dermatitis, glossitis

* Adapted from Shank RE: In Andreas R, Bierman EL and Hazzard WR (eds): Principles of
Geriatric Medicine. New York, McGraw-Hill, 1985, pp 444-460, and Russell RM, Sahyoun
NR, Whinston-Perry R: In Calkins E, Davis PJ, Ford AB (eds): The Practice of Geriatrics.
Philadelphia. W.B. Saunders, 1986, pp 135-145.

TABLE 6.   Recommended Daily Dietary Allowances, Ages 51+ Years

Fat-Soluble Vitamins			
Vit. A, mg retinol	1000	800	Dark adaptation, mucous membrane and skin integrity
Vit. D, mg cholecalciferol	5	5	Calcium absorption, phosphate excretion
Vit. E, mg (-? -tocopherol)	10	8	Probable effects on membrane stability; anti-oxidant
Water-Soluble Vitamins			
Vit. C, mg	60	60	Collagen formation
Thiamine, mg	1.2	1.0	Co-enzyme in oxidative decarboxylation; pentose shunt
Riboflavin, mg.	1.4	1.2	Co-factor in biological oxidation
Niacin, mg	16	13	Co-enzyme in tissue respiration, glycolysis, fat synthesis
Vit. B$_6$, mg	2.2	2.0	Co-enzyme in protein metabolism
Folacin, mg	400	400	Co-enzyme in nucleic acid synthesis
Vit. B$_{12}$	3.0	3.0	Co-enzyme in amino acid and fat metabolism
Minerals			
Calcium, mg	800	1500*	Skeletal integrity, cellular metabolism
Iron, mg	10	10	Hemoglobin synthesis
Zinc, mg	15	15	Co-enzyme in a variety of metabolic processes

* Pre-menopausal   1000 mg
  Post-menopausal   1500 mg

Adapted from Shank RD: In Andreas R, Bierman EL, Hazzard WR (eds): Principles of Geriatric Mediciine. New York, McGraw-Hill, 1985, pp 444–460.

certainly exist among the elderly. Since it is difficult to get the necessary vitamins on a diet of less than 1,200 calories, vitamin and mineral deficiencies are often found in association with protein calorie malnutrition. It should be remembered that deficiencies rarely occur singly; complex presentations may arise due to multiple deficiencies. A recent study indicates that "subclinical" malnutrition plays a role in a significant number of elderly with cognitive dysfunction.[9] Thus, nutritional deficiency diseases should always be considered in elderly patients with multiple symptoms or atypical presentations, particularly if they involve skin, oral cavity, or cognitive function.

Unfortunately, little information is available on true requirements for essential nutrients in people over 50. Limited information is available on possible changes in absorption, metabolism and excretion of nutrients. The National Institute on Aging has designated nutrition a priority area for investigation. The most recent version of the RDAs for people in late life are summarized in Table 6. A complete nutritional assessment should include the types of questions included in Table 7, a review of dietary intake, and a directed physical exam and laboratory evaluation. A validated questionnaire for nutritional screening in the elderly appears in Appendix A.[26] Asking about weight change gives the broadest indicator of nutritional adequacy. Inquiring about problems with chewing, food preparation and shopping, as well as diarrhea, vomiting, or change in appetite

TABLE 7. Nutritional Assessment Questions*

---

1. Has weight changed?

2. Has appetite changed?

3. Can the patient smell and taste normally?

4. Are there problems with chewing (dentures) or swallowing?

5. Does the patient have persistent nausea and vomiting, or persistent diarrhea?

6. How does the patiient manage food shopping?
   - Finances
   - Access to stores
   - Carrying bundles

7. How does the patient prepare food?
   - Adequate kitchen (stove and refrigerator)
   - Manual dexterity

8. How much alcohol is consumed?

9. Is the patient following a dietary restriction?

10. Is the patient using vitamins or food supplements?

---

* Adapted from Russell RM, Sahyoun NR, Whinston-Perry: In Calkins E, Dairs PJ, Ford AB (eds): The Practice of Geriatrics. Philadelphia. W.B. Saunders, 1986, pp 135–145.

may yield early clues to the existence or potential for malnutrition. Finally, questions regarding alcohol consumption, dietary preferences, or dietary restrictions will yield information required for effective dietary counseling. If, on the basis of the dietary history, low body weight or weight loss, the clinician suspects malnutrition, the physical exam should be directed toward skin (pallor, pitting, edema, petechiae, dryness enythema, hyperpigmentation, xerosis); hair (alopecia, dryness); eyes (xerosis); mouth (cheilosis, dentition, gingivitis, glossitis); abdomen (hepatomegaly); neurologic factors (mental status changes, loss of vibratory sensation, decreased reflexes, peripheral neuropathy); and musculoskeletal system (muscle wasting, particularly deltoid, suprascapular and intercostal). The laboratory tests for malnutrition most commonly ordered, serum albumin ($\leq$ 3.5 g/d) and total leukocyte count ($\leq$ 1500/mm^3), are insensitive and are often normal until the malnutrition is quite severe. Retinol-binding protein and pre-albumin are the most sensitive indicators of malnutrition. Transferin and thyroxine-binding protein, which are more readily available than the most sensitive indicators, are still more sensitive than albumin.[2,10] Skin hypersensitivity testing provides a good "functional" test for malnutrition, since people with significant malnutrition are often anergic.[11]

If, because of time constraints, it is difficult in the routine history to evaluate the patient's nutritional state, enlist the help of office nurses in collecting dietary histories. Other members of the office staff can also monitor compliance with dietary recommendations; however, it is important that the physician actively reinforce dietary goals and guidelines directly with the patient.

Counseling should be tailored to individual patient needs. Some patients will need to be educated in proper nutritional guidelines and sources of nutritious food (see Table 3). Others may benefit from being made aware of community programs such as meals-on-wheels or eating programs at senior centers. Most of these programs are administered by the local Area Agency on Aging (AAA), which can be contacted for specific information. It is worthwhile developing a list

TABLE 8.   Recommended Energy Intakes for Older Adults

Sex	Age	Weight (kg)	Height (cm)	Needs (Kcal)
Men	51–75	70	178	2000–2800
	76+	70	178	1650–2450
Women	51–85	55	163	1400–2200
	76+	55	163	1200–2000

From Recommended Dietary Allowances, 9th Revised Edition. Washington, National Research Council, National Academy of Sciences, Food and Nutrition Board Committee on Dietary Allowances, 1980.

of professionals in your area interested in working with the elderly: dentists for cases where poor dentition is the obstacle to adequate nutrition; physical and occupational therapists, who can help develop strategies to redress or compensate for mobility and dexterity impairments that discourage the preparation of meals; registered dietitians, who can provide specialized counseling for patients with dietary restrictions or weight problems; and social workers, who can identify available community programs. All patients should be provided with specific nutritional guidelines and goals.

For those patients who are 20% above ideal body weight, as defined by the guidelines in Table 4, counseling should include the negotiation of a program for gradual weight reduction that combines a reduction in calorie intake (that complies with the guidelines for basic energy requirements for nonobese elderly in Table 8), with an increase in exercise (see Chapter 7 for exercise guidelines). Very-low-calorie diets (< 800 calories) have been associated with increased risk in all ages.[12] In addition, patients ingesting less than 1,200 calories should probably take a multivitamin.

Follow-up visits with the patient every 2 to 4 weeks are recommended during the period of the weight reduction. These visits provide the opportunity to make any needed adjustments in the program and to provide the patient with reinforcement and encouragement. Patients who are underweight or have protein calorie malnutrition should be advised to increase their calories to 35 Cal/kg of ideal body weight. For most elderly, this can be done most easily by increasing portions of a balanced diet. However, some patients with problems chewing or swallowing may find it difficult to increase their caloric intake substantially without supplements. The composition of some supplements is given in Figure 1. Supplements in the form of pudding might be particularly helpful for patients with swallowing difficulty. It should be noted that they vary widely in not only protein but also sodium and potassium content. This can be of obvious importance to patients with underlying cardiac, renal, or hepatic disease. Generally, these supplements are not covered by prescription plans.

Definitive or even preliminary studies on the cost benefit of nutritional assessment in the elderly do not exist. Nor have there been studies to help define the most cost-effective approach to nutritional assessment in the elderly. However, the prevalence of malnutrition among the elderly suggests that the kind of systematic yet parsimonious approach to nutritional assessment and counseling discussed in this chapter has the potential to improve the elderly's lot.

ALCOHOLISM IN THE ELDERLY

Physicians have traditionally viewed alcoholism as a problem of young and middle-aged patients. In fact, alcohol use does decline among older cohorts in

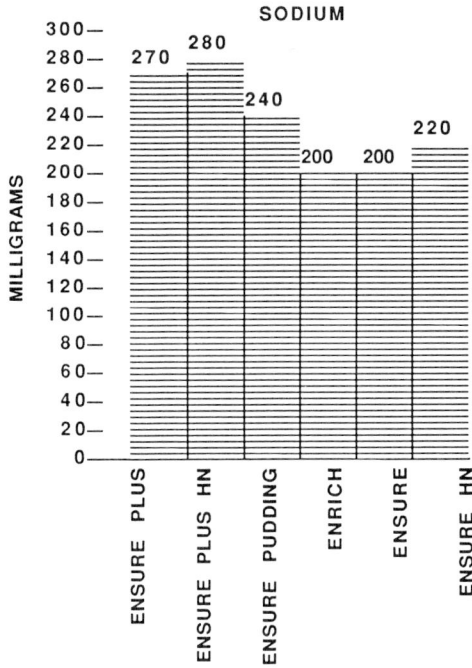

A

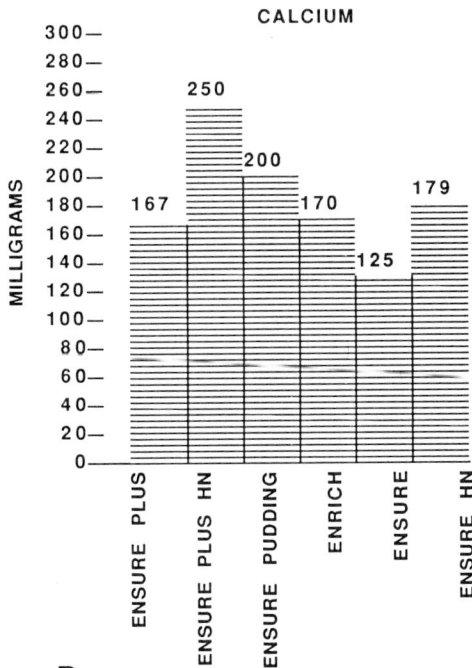

B

FIGURE 1. Composition of supplements: A. sodium,
B. calcium, C. iron, D., potassium, and E. magnesium.

IRON

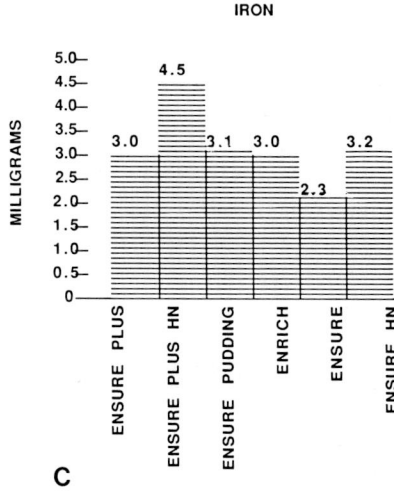

C

POTASSIUM

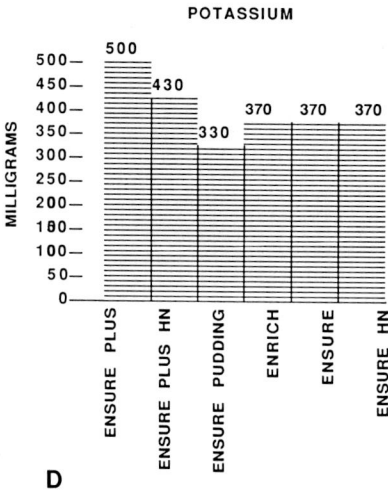

D

MAGNESIUM

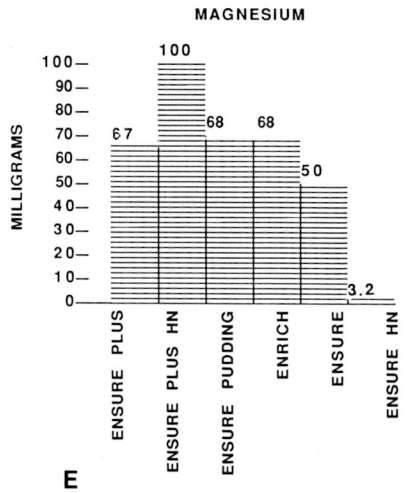

E

population surveys. For example, in one study 71% of subjects aged 30–49 drank alcohol, whereas only 45% of subjects over 65 consumed alcohol.[13] One explanation for the decline is substantial attrition of alcoholics in the population from deaths due to cancer, cardiovascular disease, accidents, and suicide.[14] However, problems of alcohol abuse are being increasingly recognized among elderly patients. Although a community study found significant alcohol abuse in only 1% of subjects over 75, the rate of alcoholism was 10% in elderly widowers.[15] Alcoholism is important in social disturbances among the elderly: 82% of 722 elderly subjects arrested were charged with public drunkenness.[16] Furthermore, alcohol abuse may have a late onset. In one study, approximately 30% of a group of elderly alcoholics began abusing alcohol after age 60.[17] Finally, the fact that the elderly are not usually employed where absenteeism, tardiness, or poor performance often prompt intervention may lead to delayed recognition.

Alcohol ingestion can result in serious metabolic consequences in the aged. Although consumption of alcohol by elderly subjects does decrease, blood levels after individual drinks may actually be higher in elderly subjects due to decreases in lean body mass and space distribution. Alcohol abuse is a frequent cause of malnutrition in elderly patients, as well as a risk factor for head and neck cancers, cancer of the esophagus, and hypertension. In addition, elderly drinkers are at increased risk for suicide.

Alcohol use may cause difficulties with drug interactions (Table 9). Ethanol is metabolized largely by the hepatic microsomal enzyme systems. Acute ingestion of alcohol competes with many drugs such as benzodiazepines and meprobamate for metabolism. The competition prolongs the efficacy of these drugs. With chronic alcohol ingestion, induction of microsomal enzymes occurs. This increases the degradation rate of various drugs such as tolbutamide, warfarin and diphenylhydantoin, and reduces the therapeutic effect of these medications. In addition, ethanol is a CNS depressant. Therefore, alcohol may potentiate the CNS effects of any sedative-hypnotic medication.

Finally, alcoholic patients show increased mental aging at every chronologic age. A study of admissions to psychiatric hospitals showed that, in patients with dementia, alcohol abusers were younger (mean age 67) than patients without a history of alcoholism (age 74). Families had significantly more negative attitudes toward alcoholic patients with dementia. Mortality at two years in the alcoholics with dementia was 37%, whereas nonalcoholic demented patients had a rate of 12%.[18]

Outcomes of therapy in elderly patients with alcohol abuse are at least as successful as therapy in younger patients and perhaps significantly more so.[19] In late-onset alcoholism, attention to precipitating social factors, such as social isolation and bereavement, will substantially improve outcomes. Education about potential alcohol/drug interactions may avoid toxicities even in patients who consume alcohol but are not abusers.

Increased time spent in screening for alcohol use, in education, and counseling is the main cost to the primary care practitioner. For the patient there is a range of costs. Some support groups are free or charge fees less than ethanol purchases would cost. Inpatient rehabilitation programs are expensive but have the highest success rates for alcoholic patients.

While many elderly patients will conceal their drinking habits, families may cooperate in minimizing alcohol intake. As discussed above, physicians may neglect alcohol screening in elderly subjects, believing this to be an uncommon disorder in older patients. A screening instrument, the Michigan Alcoholism

TABLE 9. Ethanol-Drug Interactions

Barbiturates	Insulin
Benzodiazepines	Meprobamate
Cephalosporins	Metoclopramide
Chloral hydrate	Metronidazole
Cimetidine	Phenformin
Disulfiram	Phenothiazines
Furazolidone	Salicylates
Glutethimide	Sulfonylureas

Screening Test, has been validated in the elderly and is short enough to be useful in an office setting (see Appendix A, p. 215).

Do not assume your older patients do not drink. Search for alcohol abuse in all patients, and be particularly attentive in those who may be socially isolated. Educate all your elderly patients concerning the changes in reaction to alcohol that occur with normal aging, and be sure to alert your patients to alcohol-drug interactions.

When you have identified problem drinking in an older individual, attempt to identify potential causes, such as depression, isolation or boredom, and seek out the patient resources for countering these problems, such as families, social centers, or possibly social work or psychiatry referrals. Community groups such as Alcoholics Anonymous or inpatient rehabilitation programs are appropriate for the elderly as in younger patients. Elderly alcoholics can be helped.

SMOKING AND THE ELDERLY PATIENT

Smoking remains prevalent among patients over 65. A large survey of community-living subjects disclosed prevalence rates of 17% for men over 65 and 12% for women of the same ages. Among urban poor elderly, the rates are much higher: 53% of respondents aged 65 to 75 were still smoking.[20]

Cigarette smoking remains the single most important risk factor for premature mortality in the United States. Life expectancy for a 65-year-old man in average health who has never smoked is 17 years (to age 82). An age-matched smoker has less life expectancy: if consumption is 2 packs per day, expectancy is 6 years less (to age 76). Even at 1/2 pack per day, expectancy is 3 years less (to age 79).[21] The associations between smoking and lung cancer have been well publicized. Smoking markedly increases the risks of coronary heart disease mortality; smokers' risk of death due to coronary disease is nearly doubled.[22] Smoking increases risk for stroke and multi-infarct dementia.[23] Smoking is highly associated with chronic bronchitis and emphysema. An accelerated rate of bone mineral loss is also seen in smokers of both sexes.[24] And, finally, elderly smokers may constitute fire hazards in their own homes or in congregate living situations.

As discussed above, elderly smokers who stop can expect moderate increases in life expectancy.[21] Decreased morbidity and mortality due to smoking-associated disease may still be seen. Smokers who were able to stop reduced their coronary heart disease mortality to nearly the levels of nonsmokers within 1 to 5 years of cessation.[22] Reduction in the lung cancer death rate is seen after smoking stops.[24] Improvement in cerebral blood flow with rises to baseline levels of nonsmokers is seen. Values of flow rise in a linear fashion throughout

TABLE 10.   Nicotine Withdrawal Symptoms

Symptoms:	Tobacco craving Increased restlessness and anxiety Difficulty concentrating Headache Gastrointestinal disorders
Duration:	Prominent in first 2–3 days after cessation • lessen over succeeding 1st week • worsen again for subsequent 2 weeks • then gradually abate
However,	individual symptoms may persist up to 3 months. Tobacco craving may persist longer

the first cigarette-free year.[23] Pulmonary function damage associated with smoking is at least partially reversible, with improvement measurable within 5 years.[21]

Physician advice and counseling on smoking cessation has documented effectiveness. Verbal advice for 60–120 seconds has been associated with a significant increase in the quit rate.[21] The rate improves further with educational material and nicotine gum. *Counseling is especially effective in the setting of an acute illness that is smoking-related.*[24]

Elderly patients may be unaware of possible physiologic improvements achieved with smoking cessation, or they may consider smoking one of their few remaining sensory pleasures. In addition, patients may be psychologically or physically addicted to nicotine and be intolerant of the withdrawal symptoms described in Table 10.

Physicians may also be unaware that physical benefits may accrue to elderly smokers who quit. Physicians may have doubts about the efficacy of programs to help elderly smokers quit, or they may have concerns about the potential side effects of nicotine gum. Nicotine gum is usually contraindicated in peripheral vascular disease, cerebrovascular disease or coronary disease. However, providers may assess the risk of continued smoking against ineffective counseling; switching patients to low tar/nicotine brands or to cigars and pipe does not usually lessen total nicotine exposure[21] since patients increase consumption to maintain nicotine levels.

The cost of nicotine gums compares favorably with the cost of continued smoking. Costs of increased physician office visits during the period of decreasing nicotine use are balanced by decreases in future smoking-related morbidity.

Figure 2 presents a suggested protocol for assisting patients in smoking cessation. After developing a clear picture of a patient's current smoking habits, spend at least 60–120 seconds firmly, but nonjudgmentally, advising the patient to stop smoking. This advice should consist of a review of the benefits to be derived from stopping rather than any emphasis on adverse consequences. Emphasize potential improvements in minor smoking-related symptoms such as reduced energy, coughing and wheezing. Describe to the patient the nicotine withdrawal symptoms in Table 10, stressing the fact that these symptoms are transient and controllable. Suggest that abrupt cessation is usually more successful than trying to taper cigarette use or changing to a lower-nicotine brand.[25]

Past unsuccessful quitting efforts should be praised, rather than used as examples of failure, and can be used as experiences in incremental learning by

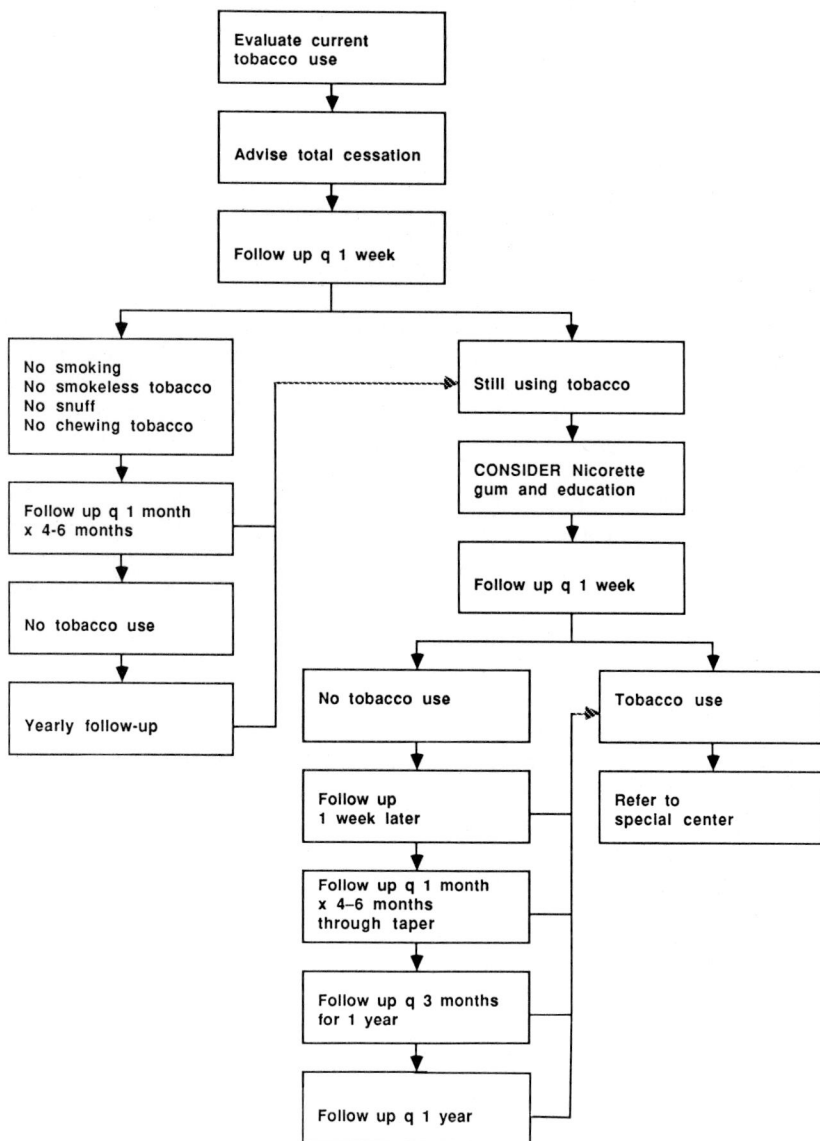

FIGURE 2.   Treatment protocol for smoking cessation.

reviewing the reasons for failure and identifying strategies to overcome past obstacles. Have on hand or suggest relevant literature from organizations such as the American Cancer Society (777 3rd Ave., New York, NY 10017) or the American Lung Association (1740 Broadway, New York, NY 10019). Local chapters of these organizations are listed in local telephone directories. It is also valuable to develop a list of local support groups and other smoking cessation programs so that you can pass this information on to patients.

For reinforcement, it is important to follow up on patients' progress at one week, then monthly intervals for 3 to 6 months, then according to routine intervals. If advice alone is not successful, consider recommending nicotine polarilex (Nicorette gum). Whenever the patient craves a cigarette, he or she should chew a 2 mg piece, up to an absolute maximum of 30 pieces daily. Be sure to instruct the patient in proper chewing techniques in your office and advise that the usual cost of Nicorette gum is $20 per box. A telephone prescription without office follow-up is no more effective than a placebo.[21] Follow-up at 1 week for effective chewing, side effects and abstention from all tobacco-containing products. Continue to follow the patient at 1-month intervals for 3 to 6 months during gum taper, then every 3 months for the remainder of the first cigarette-free year, then yearly. If smoking continues, consider referring the patient to a major smoking control center for behavior modification or other techniques to aid smoking cessation.

PRACTICE RECOMMENDATIONS

NUTRITION

1. Include time in the history for questions related to the adequacy of the diet and to the use of food supplements in use (Table 7).

2. In patients who are under 80% of ideal body weight, or who lose more than 10% of their baseline weight in 6 months, consider malnutrition evaluation.

3. Include careful examination of the skin, hair, tongue, and mucous membranes in the examination. Also evaluate muscle wasting, especially in the deltoid and intercostal muscles. This is especially important in high-risk patients: alcoholics, the poor, and patients in isolated living conditions.

4. When malnutrition is identified, make the patient aware of special community programs such as meals-on-wheels and congregate dining at senior centers or churches. Enlist the aid of a social worker or dietitian in providing access to such programs.

5. If functional obstacles such as poor dentition or impaired manual dexterity are contributing to malnutrition, refer to dentists, physical and occupational therapists.

6. Counsel patients who are obese (20% above ideal body weight) (Table 5) in a gradual program of weight reduction.
   - An appropriate reduction in calories should be suggested that complies with guidelines for basic energy requirements for non-obese elderly (Table 8).
   - Increase in exercise should be recommended as tolerated (see Chapter 7).
   - Follow the patient at regular intervals (every 2–4 weeks) during the period of weight loss for reinforcement.

7. Consider the use of office nurses as assistants in obtaining complete dietary histories and in monitoring dietary therapy. Retain an active and vocal interest in the problem with the patient yourself.

8. Consult with registered dietitians for education and counseling of patients, especially dieters and those with special diets (hypertensives, diabetics, etc.).

ALCOHOL

1. Screen for alcohol use in all patients. Be especially attentive in older patients who live alone and have few social contact.

2. Educate all patients in the accentuation of immediate alcohol effects during normal aging. Warn all patients about alcohol-drug interactions. **Do not assume that your older patients do not drink.**

3. When problem drinking is identified, consider root causes such as depression, isolation, boredom. Mobilize resources such as social centers, families, etc. Consider referral to psychiatry and social work.

4. Refer to community groups such as Alcoholics Anonymous. Consider inpatient rehabilitation programs. **Elderly alcoholics can be helped.**

SMOKING

1. Carefully ascertain current smoking habits.

2. Spend at least 60–120 seconds firmly, but nonjudgmentally, advising the patient to stop smoking.

3. Review benefits to be gained rather than dwelling on adverse consequences.

4. Review nicotine withdrawal symptoms, stressing that the symptoms are transient and controllable.

5. Praise unsuccessful quitting efforts. Review reasons for failures and suggest strategies to overcome past obstacles.

6. Suggest (or distribute) useful literature available from organizations such as the American Cancer Society or the American Lung Association.

7. Provide information on local support groups and other cessation programs.

8. Follow up at 1 week then monthly for 3–6 months, then per routine intervals.

9. If advice alone is not successful, consider nicotine polarilex (Nicorette gum). *Instruct the patient* in proper chewing techniques in your office.

10. Follow up at 1 week for effective chewing, side effects, and abstention from all tobacco-containing products.

11. Follow at 1-month intervals for 3–6 months during gum taper; follow every 3 months for the remainder of the first cigarette-free year, then yearly.

12. If smoking continues, consider referral to a major smoking control center for behavior modification or other techniques to aid smoking cessation.

REFERENCES

1. Shank RE: In Andres R, Bierman, EL, Hazzard WR (eds): Principles of Geriatric Medicine. New York, McGraw-Hill, 1985, pp 444–460.
2. Morley JE, Silver AJ, Fiatarone M, Mooradian AD: Geriatric Grand Rounds: Nutrition and the elderly. University of California, Los Angeles. J Am Geriatr Soc 1986; 34:823–832.
3. Holleb AI, et al: Nutrition and Cancer: Cause and Prevention. New York, American Cancer Society (Professional Education Publication), 1984.
4. Cummings SR, et al: Is hypercholesterolemia still important after age 65? Clin Res 1987; 35:736A.

5. Russel RM, Sahyoun NR, Whinston-Perry R: In Calkins E, Davis PJ, Ford AB (eds): The Practice of Geriatrics. Philadelphia, W.B. Saunders, 1986, pp 135–145.
6. Massachusetts Department of Public Health: Determining the needs of the elderly and chronically disabled. N Engl J Med 1976; 294:110–111.
7. Pritikin N, Asney N: In Dychtwald K, MacLean J (eds): Wellness and Health Promotion for the Elderly. Rockville, MD, Aspen Press, 1986, pp 179–200.
8. Andres R: In Andres R, Bierman EL, Hazzard WR (eds): Principles of Geriatric Medicine. New York, McGraw-Hill, 1985, pp 311–318.
9. Goodwin JS, Goodwin JM, Garry PJ: Association between nutritional status and cognitive functioning in a healthy elderly population. JAMA 1983; 249(21):2917–2921.
10. Morley JE: Nutritional status of the elderly. Am J Med 1986; 81:679–695.
11. Gordon S, Kelly S, Sybyl J, et al: Relationship in very elderly veterans of nutritional status, self-perceived chewing ability, dental status and social isolation. J Am Geriatr Soc 1985; 33:334.
12. Moss AJ: Caution: very-low-calorie diets can be deadly. Ann Intern Med 1985; 120(1):121–123.
13. Stotsky BA: Social and clinical issues in geriatric psychiatry. Am J Psychiat 1972; 129:117–126.
14. Schuckit MA, Miller PA: Alcoholism in elderly men: A survey of a general medical ward. Ann NY Acad Sci 1976; 273:558–571.
15. Bailey MB, et al: The epidemiology of alcoholism in an urban residential area. Q J Stud Alcohol 1965; 26:19–40.
16. Epstein LJ, et al: Antisocial behavior of the elderly. Compr Psych 1970; 11:36–42.
17. Pascarelli EF: Drug dependence. Geriatrics 1974; 29:109–115.
18. Gaitz CM, Baer PE: Characteristics of elderly patients with alcoholism. Arch Gen Psychiat 1971; 24:372–378.
19. Stultz BM: Preventive care for the elderly. West J Med 1984; 141(6):832–845.
20. Remington PL, et al: Current smoking trends in the United States. JAMA 1985; 253:2975–2978.
21. Sachs DPL: Cigarette smoking: Health effects and cessation strategies. Clin Geriatr Med 1986; 2:337–362.
22. Jajich CL, Ostfeld AM, Freeman DH: Smoking and coronary heart disease mortality in the elderly. JAMA 1984; 252:2831–2834.
23. Rogers RL, Meyer JS, Judd BW, et al: Abstention from cigarette smoking improves cerebral perfusion among elderly chronic smokers. JAMA 1985; 2970–2974.
24. Mellstrom D, et al: Tobacco smoking, aging and health among the elderly. Age Aging 1982; 11:45–58.
25. Orleans CT: Understanding and promoting smoking cessation: Overview and guidelines for physician intervention. Ann Rev Med 1985; 36:51–61.
26. Wolinsky FD, et al: Further assessment of the reliability and validity of a nutritional risk index: Analysis of a three-wave panel study of elderly adults. Health Serv Res 1986; 20:977–990.
27. Willenbring ML, et al: Alcoholism screening in the elderly. J Am Geriatr Soc 1987; 35:864–869.

9
PREVENTION OF OSTEOPOROTIC FRACTURES

Jeane Ann Grisso, MD, MSc
Maurice Attie, MD

Osteoporotic fractures result in substantial costs and personal morbidity. Since osteoporosis is the most important determinant of the risk of fracture in older age, the primary emphasis of this chapter will be on the prevention of osteoporosis. However, fracture pathogenesis is complex, and low bone density (osteoporosis) is a necessary but not a sufficient cause for a fracture to occur. The propensity of the elderly to fall is an independent risk factor for fractures, particularly for fractures of the hip and wrist. Since most of those over 65 will have already lost a significant amount of bone and be at risk for osteoporotic fractures, it is crucial to stress the prevention of falls in this population. Therefore, the chapter also includes a discussion of risk factors and preventive measures for falls.

THE SIGNIFICANCE OF OSTEOPOROSIS

Osteoporosis-associated fractures are a major public health problem in the United States. The total cost of osteoporosis and osteoporotic fractures may be as high as 10 billion dollars.[1] Osteoporosis predisposes to fractures of the hip, vertebrae, distal forearm (Colles'), humerus, and pelvis, as well as other less common types of fractures. It is predicted that over 50% of women in the Western world will develop a fracture in later life as a result of osteoporosis.[2]

Although the prevalence of vertebral fractures is difficult to ascertain, it is estimated that between 5% to 10% of white women aged 65 to 75 will have a vertebral fracture.[3] The amount of back pain and disability attributed to vertebral fractures is unknown. Colles' fractures are the most common fracture among white women in the United States until age 75. At age 50, a white woman has about a 15% lifetime risk of fracturing her forearm.[4]

Fractures of the hip are associated with more deaths, disability, and medical costs than all other osteoporotic fractures combined. In 1985, about 247,000 hip fractures occurred among persons over the age of 45 in the United States.[5] Of those who live to the age of 90, an estimated one-third of women and one-sixth of men will have a hip fracture.[4] The consequences of hip fractures are often severe. Of those who were functionally independent and living at home at the time of the fracture, 15-20% remain in long-term care institutions, and another 25-35% must depend on other people or mechanical aids for mobility.[4] Because of the increasing number of elderly persons in the population, the frequency of hip fractures can be expected to double or triple by the middle of the next century.

107

WHAT IS OSTEOPOROSIS?

Loss of skeletal mass is a normal consequence of aging. Bone mass in both men and women reaches a peak in the fourth decade of life and thereafter begins a slow decline at a rate of about 0.5% per year through at least the eighth decade.[6] To a large degree this is related to progressive age-related bone loss. In women, the annual rate of bone loss accelerates to approximately 2% per year through the first five to seven peri- and postmenopausal years.[6] The strength of the skeleton and the ability of bone to withstand trauma without fracture is related to the amount of bone in the skeleton. Osteoporosis is defined as a reduction in the amount of bone so that fractures occur after minimal trauma. In general, a reduction of approximately 30% of total bone mass in women from its peak is associated with an increase in the risk of osteoporosis related fractures.[6] In the absence of severe trauma, fractures are rare unless the bone density falls to 1.0 g/cm^2 for both vertebrae and femur. This level of bone density is often referred to as the fracture threshold.

Involutional bone loss affects the entire skeleton; however, bone loss is not always uniform. The more metabolically active trabecular or spongy bone in the spine is lost more rapidly than cortical bone in the first few years of menopause and in disorders such as hypercortisolism. Vertebral fractures may indicate osteoporosis occurring at an earlier age in postmenopausal women.

Osteoporosis cannot be approached as a single disease entity with a specific etiology. Rather, as discussed below it represents the accumulated effects of several factors on the skeleton throughout an individual's lifespan. The need for screening and diagnosis must therefore be considered in light of the almost universal occurrence of involutional bone loss and the high prevalence of this disorder in the older population. Rather than approach it as a single disorder, osteoporosis should be considered a composite of several risk factors, some of which can be altered later in life. Furthermore, a major focus of any program should be aimed at reducing injury in the older population where osteoporosis is highly prevalent.

RISK FACTORS FOR OSTEOPOROSIS AND OSTEOPOROTIC FRACTURES

There are many factors that increase the risk of osteoporosis. These causal factors can be traced in investigations by identifying risk factors associated with an increased incidence of either low bone density or of fractures. A discussion of the important established risk factors follows.

DEMOGRAPHIC RISK FACTORS

Age is the most important determinant of bone density and accurately reflects the slow bone loss that occurs over life in both sexes. Since the frequency of falling also increases markedly with age, and 90% of hip fractures result from a fall, age is the most important single risk factor for hip fractures. After age 50, the incidence of hip fractures rises dramatically with age, doubling every 5 to 10 years in both men and women.[7] Almost 50% of hip fractures occur in persons who are 80 years of age or older.[7-10]

Although in the United States all osteoporotic fractures occur more frequently in women than in men, the difference in risk varies markedly by type of fracture. While the incidence rate for hip fractures in white women is only about twice as high as for white men, that of Colles' fractures and fractures of the proximal humerus and pelvis are *six to eight times higher* in women than in men.[7-9,11,12] The reasons for the varying sex ratios in different skeletal sites are uncertain.

Blacks in the United States have higher bone mass, and fewer vertebral and hip fractures than whites.[13-15] Age-specific incidence rates of hip fractures are about twice as high in white women as in black women.[16-18] The incidence rate of hip fractures and vertebral fractures also appears to be less in Hispanic populations in the United States than in white populations.[19,20] Although bone density is less in Asians than in Caucasians, no data are available about the risk of fracture among Asians in the United States.

PRIMARY FACTORS AFFECTING BONE MASS

Bone mass in the elderly is a function of peak bone mass achieved earlier in life and subsequent rates of bone loss. The major cause of age-related bone loss is not known; however, several factors are known to be associated with a greater risk of osteoporosis, either because they reduce the peak bone mass achieved or because they accelerate the rate of bone loss (Table 1). Knowledge of these factors can be used to identify individuals who may be at risk of developing osteoporosis. Moreover, some of these factors can be modified to prevent osteoporosis.

Persons who accumulate a low peak bone mass may be more susceptible to fractures at an early age. Peak bone mass is determined by several factors, including racial and other genetic influences. Blacks amass more bone than whites and Orientals. Men also accumulate a larger peak bone mass than women. Body habitus is also an important determinant; underweight individuals have a lower bone mass than those who are overweight. Other factors that may reduce peak bone mass include lack of physical activity, amenorrhea, hypogonadism and low calcium intake.

In contrast to factors affecting peak bone mass, factors that increase the rate of bone loss can potentially be modified in an older population to prevent further bone loss. Menopause is one of the major factors contributing to bone loss in women. The accelerated bone loss in the peri- and postmenopausal years causes an excess of 15–20% loss from the spine and 10–15% loss from long bones.[21,22] Women who have had a premature surgical menopause have a lower bone density than their peers in later life.[22]

Levels of endogenous estrogen appear to be positively associated with bone mass at least in the years immediately after menopause. Heavy women have a lower risk of fractures at various sites and have a higher bone mass than thin women. This protection is conferred at least in part by the higher levels of circulating estrogen in obese than in thin postmenopausal women. Estrogen replacement therapy begun soon after menopause reduces the rate of bone loss[23,24] and the risk of spine, hip and wrist fractures.[25-28] In men, overt hypogonadism as a result of testicular or pituitary disease is associated with osteoporosis and vertebral fractures. However, aside from these disorders, men undergo a gradual and less drastic decline in gonadal function than women and osteoporotic fractures are less frequent and occur at an older age.[29]

The role of calcium intake in osteoporosis is controversial. Because of a decline in intestinal calcium absorption, the dietary requirement for calcium rises

TABLE 1.   Risk Factors for Osteoporosis

Factors That Reduce Initial Bone Mass
  Female sex
  White or Asian
  Family history of osteoporosis
  ? Low calcium intake
  Short stature and small bones

Factors That Increase Age-related Bone Loss
  Premature surgical menopause
  Hypogonadism (in men)
  Inactivity
  ? Low calcium intate
  Gastric or small bowel disease
  Long-term glucocorticoid therapy
  Hyperparathyroidism
  Smoking
  Heavy alcohol use
  Thyrotoxicosis

with age. Heaney et al. showed with calcium balance studies that perimenopausal women need 1000 mg and postmenopausal women 1500 mg to be in balance. This contrasts with the average estimated daily consumption of calcium of 550 mg in middle-age and elderly women in the United States.

It has long been recognized that prolonged immobility results in osteoporosis.[30-32] Tennis players, weight lifters, ballet dancers, and other athletes appear to have wider bones and more cortical bone in limbs that are involved in the particular activity.[33-35] However, the limited number of prospective studies of the effects of various exercise programs on bone mass have yielded conflicting findings.[36-40] This may occur because of different effects of exercise on different skeletal sites. A randomized trial of weight-bearing exercise did not result in a protective effect on bone density in the radius.[78] However, a recent non-randomized trial of weight-bearing exercise reported a marked improvement in bone density in the lumbar vertebrae.[77]

Heavy alcohol use in both men and women may be associated with an increased prevalence of osteoporosis. Also, cigarette smoking can accelerate the rate of bone loss in both men and women.[29,41] In women the mechanism of increased bone loss with smoking may be related to an increase in the catabolism of estrogens and lower body weight.[42]

A number of medical conditions listed in Table 2 may contribute to bone loss and are often categorized as causes of secondary osteoporosis. In as many as 20% of women and 40% of men presenting with spontaneous vertebral fractures, a secondary cause of osteoporosis can be identified.[43] The most common causes are hypogonadism (in men), early oophorectomy (in women), subtotal gastrectomy, and pharmacologic doses of glucocorticoid or thyroid hormones.[6]

THE RISK OF FALLING

Although osteoporosis or a reduction in bone mass is thought to be the main determinant of the risk of fracture, other factors are important as well. The

TABLE 2. Causes of Secondary Osteoporosis

Endocrine Diseases	Bone Marrow Disorders
Hypogonadism	Multiple myeloma and
Ovarian agenesis	related disorders
Hyperadrenocorticism	Systemic mastocytosis
Hyperthyroidism	Disseminated carcinoma
Hyperparathyroidism	
Diabetes mellitus	Connective Tissue Diseases
Acromegaly	
	Osteogenesis imperfecta
Gastrointestinal Diseases	Homocystinuria
	Ehlers-Danlos syndrome
Subtotal gastrectomy	Marfan's syndrome
Malabsorption syndromes	
Chronic obstructive jaundice	Miscellaneous Causes
Primary biliary cirrhosis	Chronic obstructive pulmonary disease
Severe malnutrition	Chronic heparin administration
Anorexia nervosa	Rheumatoid arthritis

dramatic increase in incidence of hip fractures with age cannot be explained solely by decreased bone mass with age. It is likely that decreased bone mass and an increased frequency of trauma due to falls combine to produce the pattern of increased risk of hip fractures with age.

About 90% of fractures of the hip, forearm and pelvis result from a fall. Generally, the frequency of falls increases markedly with age and is higher for women than for men.[44-46] Each year, almost one third of persons 65 or older fall.[47] Risk factors for falls include both environmental and personal factors.

The best documented personal risk factors for falls include cognitive impairment, problems with gait and/or balance, diminished hearing or vision, and decreased functional status.[48-50] In addition, several studies have found that certain medications predispose to falls and hip fractures.[49,51] Hypnotics, sedatives, and anti-psychotic medications, particularly doses excessively high for the elderly, have been implicated.[51-53]

Environmental factors have been less consistently identified but include loose rugs, inadequate lighting, slippery footwear, and trailing electrical cords.[53,54]

Risk factors for falls are discussed in more detail in Chapter 10. However, it is important to remember that for older persons, the prevention of falls may be the most promising way to prevent osteoporotic fractures. For the elderly, efforts should be directed at preventing falls by removing environmental hazards and by improving neuromuscular protective responses to trauma.

SHOULD PERIMENOPAUSAL AND POSTMENOPAUSAL WOMEN BE SCREENED FOR OSTEOPOROSIS?

Osteoporosis is sometimes compared to hypertension; in both conditions irreversible damage is likely to have occurred if the clinician waits until symptoms have developed before starting treatment. Given the morbidity and mortality of osteoporotic fractures and the availability of treatments that may be effective in preventing fractures, osteoporosis is a condition that fulfills many of the criteria that are used to judge the merits of screening programs. Some preventive measures, such as exercise and increasing dietary calcium, are relatively safe and inexpensive and therefore may be recommended without screening measurements. Estrogen therapy, on the other hand, has potential risks and, ideally, should be reserved for women at greatest risk for future fractures. The important question that remains controversial is whether there are screening tests that can predict those at increased risk for osteoporotic fractures.

The increasing availability of noninvasive methods for measuring bone mass raises the issue of whether postmenopausal women should routinely have such measurements or other tests to identify those at highest risk for osteoporotic fractures. A recent book on osteoporosis recommends screening for osteoporosis in all women,[55] and a number of clinics have sprung up which offer measurements of bone mass to screen women for osteoporosis. The new techniques are much more sensitive than standard x-rays (which may not detect bone loss unless 30% of the bone is gone) and include single-photon absorptiometry, dual-photon absorptiometry, and quantitative computed tomography. Table 3 includes summary information about each method.

Cummings and Black have published a thoughtful assessment of the merit of screening asymptomatic women with bone mass measurements.[56] They do not support the routine use of noninvasive measurements of bone mass because: (1) bone density measurements have not been shown to predict who is at risk for fractures of the hip or wrist; (2) bone mass assessments of the wrist (those used most frequently in screening clinics) correlate poorly with that of other skeletal sites and with total body calcium; (3) studies have generally found that, on average, women with hip fractures have only slightly less bone mass than normal women of similar age and therefore bone mass measurement does not even differentiate persons who already have fractures from those who do not; and (4) currently available methods to measure bone mass are not precise enough to accurately assess bone loss rates.

The problem with measuring bone loss is that rates of bone loss are relatively small compared with the reproducibility of the measurement. Most existing noninvasive techniques are reported to have a 1% to 5% reproducibility (or precision)[57-59] and even during the perimenopausal years bone loss rates rarely exceed 2% per year. For example, Heaney[60] has demonstrated that if 100 women who are not losing *any* bone have two measurements of bone density using a method with 2% precision, about 15 of the women will falsely appear to have lost at least 3% of their bone. Thus, measurement of the rate of bone loss based on two measurements of bone mass over a period of time leaves considerable uncertainty about the rate of loss.

Even if we could accurately assess the rate of bone loss, a clinician cannot assume that a woman who appears to have lost bone density at 2% per year will continue to lose bone at that rate and therefore be at increased risk of fracture. Unfortunately, there are poor data about how well past rates of loss predict future rates of loss. In addition, studies have found no correlation between short-term rates of change in bone density at various sites.[61,62] Thus, a change in bone density observed at one location may not reflect changes in other parts of the skeleton.

Although it is not recommended to use bone mass assessments as routine screening tools, there are other important indications for their use. It may be important for some patients to learn whether they have established osteoporosis or not. For many women the decision about whether to take postmenopausal estrogens might be influenced by information about their current level of bone mass. In addition, multiple measurements of bone density may be valuable for

TABLE 3. Methods to Assess Bone Mass

Methods	Skeletal Site(s)	Precision	Radiation Exposure
Quantitative CT	Vertebrae	1–3% in normal 3–5% in osteoporosis	150–250 mrem
Dual-photon absorptiometry	Vertebrae Hip Total body	2–4%	5–10 mrem
Single-photon absorptiometry	Radius	1–3%	5–10 mrem

assessing responses to experimental therapies, such as sodium fluoride or calcitonin, which produce variable but sometimes quite marked responses.

If the clinician and patient decide that the patient should undergo an assessment of bone mass, it is important to decide which methods and skeletal site(s) to select. It is beyond the scope of this chapter to review the various methods to assess bone density. (See the ACP Health and Public Policy Committee review in Annals of Internal Medicine, 1984, for more information.[57]) The most precise methods having predictive value (for vertebral fractures) are CT scanning or dual-photon absorptiometry of the lumbar spine. Single photon densitometry of the wrist has not been shown to predict fracture risk or to correlate well with other skeletal sites. See Table 3 for summary information on each method. When deciding where to refer a patient, it is important to remember that most reports of reproducibility (or precision) have come from specialized referral centers, and the accuracy of results may not be as great for scans obtained in other clinical settings.

Whether other laboratory measurements can predict those at highest risk of future fractures is similarly unknown. One recent study suggested that a single determination of body fat mass, urinary calcium and hydroxyproline, and serum alkaline phosphatase early in the postmenopausal period could identify women who were "fast bone losers," i.e., those who lost 4% or more per year over 2 years.[2] However, predicting those who lose bone rapidly over a short time may not predict those who will continue to lose bone rapidly and ultimately are at greater risk of fracture.

The most cost-effective approach to select those at increased risk is to use historical risk factors (Table 1). Although it is not yet possible to weigh these factors according to their relative importance, and the ability of risk factor profiles to predict future fractures has not been tested by a prospective study, individually these risk factors have been well established and constitute the best information currently available for selecting high risk patients. It is recommended that clinicians consider advocating estrogen therapy to perimenopausal women who have one or more of the following risk factors for osteoporotic fractures: thin body build, Caucasian of Northern European ancestry, premature surgical menopause, and/or cigarette smoking.

PREVENTION OF OSTEOPOROSIS IN PERIMENOPAUSAL AND POSTMENOPAUSAL WOMEN

ESTROGEN REPLACEMENT THERAPY

For the Perimenopausal Woman. Estrogen replacement therapy (ERT) is the most effective therapeutic measure available to prevent bone loss in the first

TABLE 4. Beneficial and Harmful Effects of Estrogen Replacement Therapy in Postmenopausal Women

Beneficial Effects
   Reduction in rate of bone loss
   Reduction in menopausal symptoms
   ? Reduced incidence of ischemic heart disease

Harmful Effects
   Increased risk of endometrial cancer
   ? Increased risk of breast cancer
   ? Thromboembolic disease
   Increased incidence of cholelithiasis

five to seven postmenopausal years.[23,24,27] It has been well established that estrogen replacement therapy protects against osteoporotic fractures.[25-28] However, estrogens have other potentially beneficial and harmful effects (Table 4) and these should be weighed when deciding whether to use estrogen replacement therapy.[63,64] When used without a cyclic progestational agent, estrogens increase the risk of endometrial cancer. The use of a cyclic progesterone reduces the risk of endometrial cancer but results in a return of menses which is a bothersome concern for many women. Cyclic progesterone may have a similar effect to estrogen on preventing bone loss and is usually recommended in combination with estrogen to reduce the risk of endometrial cancer.[79] However, progestational agents may counteract the beneficial effect of estrogen on HDL levels, and it is not known what impact progestives have on the risk of cardiovascular disease. Estrogens may slightly increase the risk of developing breast cancer. Therefore estrogens may be relatively contraindicated in a woman with a high risk of developing breast cancer (e.g., a woman with a positive family history of breast cancer). Since estrogens can enhance the growth of breast cancers, they are contraindicated in a woman who has or has had breast cancer. In a small proportion of women, estrogens may cause an increase in blood pressure and therefore blood pressure should be monitored. There may also be a slight increase in risk of thrombophlebitis and cholelithiasis (these risks appear to be considerably less than with oral contraceptives and other premenopausal estrogen use). Estrogen replacement therapy is very effective in reducing symptoms of estrogen deficiency such as hot flashes and vaginal dryness.[65]

   One of the major concerns of clinicians deciding whether to start ERT is the question of possible cardiac risk. Several large studies have shown that the incidence of ischemic heart disease is reduced in women taking estrogen replacement therapy. However, some studies have shown no effect or even an increase in risk.[64] At present, the weight of evidence suggests that ERT reduces this risk. Because of the high incidence of ischemic heart disease in women in the United States, even small protective effects on this risk may outweigh other potential harmful effects.[63] Prevention of ischemic heart disease rather than the risk of osteoporosis may eventually be the most important factor in the decision on the use of ERT.

   How does prevention of osteoporosis fit into the decision of using ERT? For one, prevention of osteoporosis is only one of the potential effects of ERT. Second, if ERT is going to be used for prevention of osteoporosis, it should ideally be provided to women who are at greatest risk of developing osteoporosis. Recommendations for whom ERT should be used are included at the end of this section.

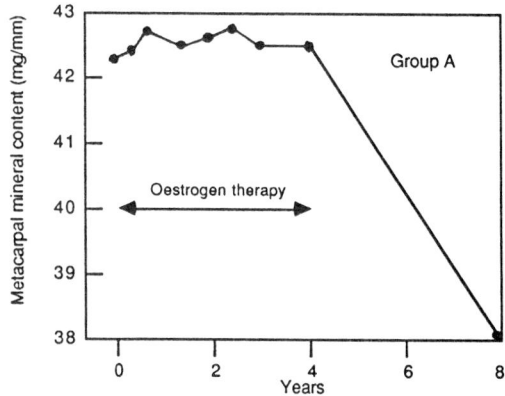

FIGURE 1. Effects of withdrawal of estrogen therapy on bone mineral content after 4 years of active treatment. Reprinted with permission from Lindsay R, Hart DM, MacLean A, et al: Bone response to termination of estrogen treatment. Lancet 1978; #1:1325–1327.

For the Older Woman. The efficacy of ERT in women who are 5 to 10 years past menopause is not known. Christiansen et al. found that ERT begun two years after menopause in women who were previously untreated was effective in halting further bone loss.[66] Initiation of estrogen therapy for older women would presumably have less benefit since the accelerated phase of perimenopausal bone loss slows from 2 to 3% bone loss per year immediately after menopause to only .3 to .6% per year 8 to 10 years after menopause.[67] Since ERT can only slow or halt further bone loss and most white women over 65 years of age have bone densities below the fracture threshold, starting estrogens in older women is unlikely to confer marked protection. Yet a recent analysis of ERT in women from the Framingham study suggested the ERT was protective in women between 65 and 74 years of age.[68] Whether women of this age who took estrogens were less likely for other reasons to be at risk for fractures is not known. The authors suggest that we should be cautious in interpreting the results to mean that ERT is protective in this age group.

Another important question that needs to be answered is how long to continue estrogens in women who started them around the time of menopause. Two studies have found that accelerated bone loss (similar to that observed in perimenopausal women) occurs after stopping ERT (Fig. 1).[66,69] Retrospective studies of osteoporotic fractures have reported that the longer the duration of ERT, the greater the protective effect.[25–27] We do not know whether stopping ERT after 4 to 6 years will confer the same protective effect as continuing ERT for life. Most experts recommend continuing ERT for at least 10 years.[70]

RECOMMENDATIONS FOR ERT

The decision to use ERT must evolve from thorough discussion with the patient of its potential advantages and disadvantages. ERT should be initiated in high-risk women as soon after the onset of menopause as possible, with a view to continuing therapy for 10 years. Women who are more than 10 to 16 years postmenopausal may not benefit from ERT, since they already experienced the period of accelerated bone loss that accompanies and follows the menopause; it is this period during which ERT is maximally effective. ERT should be considered for women who are at particular risk for the development of osteoporosis, or who have existing osteoporosis at a relatively young age, in whom prevention of

TABLE 5.   Guidelines for Estrogen Therapy

- Consider ERT to prevent osteoporosis in women who are at high risk, who have no contraindications, and who understand the benefits and complications.

- Prescribe low-dose ERT (e.g., 0.625 mg) for 25 or 26 days monthly, and a progestin (e.g., 10 mg medroxyprogesterone) on days 12-15 to days 25 or 26.

- Insure that the patient undergoes frequent manual breast examinations, yearly mammography, and thorough investigation of abnormal vaginal bleeding.

- Initiate ERT as soon as possible after the menopause, and plan to continuue it for at least 10 years. Women who have had hysterectomies need not receive concomitant progestin replacement.

- ERT may also be considered for older women within 5 to 15 years postmenopause who have fractures (e.g., have clinically evident osteoporosis).

Adapted from National Osteoporosis Foundation: A Physician's Resource Manual on Osteoporosis. Washington, D.C., 1987.

additional losses can be achieved. Guidelines (discussed below) for use of ERT are also summarized in Table 5.

Contraindications to ERT include the possibility or known presence of an estrogen-dependent malignancy (including history of breast cancer), history of previous complications of estrogen use, thrombophlebitis or other evidence of increased coagulability, evidence that the patient is likely to be noncompliant, and unexplained vaginal bleeding. Endometriosis and uterine myoma should also deter estrogen use. ERT is not recommended for women who have significant benign breast disease of the dysplastic type or who have a family history of breast cancer.

The only estrogens shown to preserve bone density or reduce fracture frequency are orally active, short-acting preparations. Transdermal patch preparations, though effective in preventing menopausal symptoms, are currently being evaluated for preventing bone loss and their efficacy in this area has not yet been established. Depot estrogen preparations may not be effective and may expose the patient to inappropriate concentrations, increasing the risk of complications that cannot be treated by withdrawing the hormone. High doses of oral estrogen are no more effective than low doses in limiting bone loss. The optimal dose is 0.625 mg of conjugated estrogen daily or its equivalent in other oral, short-acting preparations.

CALCIUM THERAPY

For the Perimenopausal Woman.   Although several controlled clinical trials have found lower rates of bone loss for perimenopausal women who received calcium supplementation compared to controls, the effect on bone loss has been modest. However, it seems unlikely that bone loss can be prevented without an adequate intake of calcium to maintain a positive calcium balance. In addition, there may be subpopulations with low calcium intake or inefficient calcium absorption in whom calcium deficiency may be adversely affecting bone mass. It is recommended that perimenopausal women consume at least the recommended dietary allowance for calcium (800 mg) and that high-risk perimenopausal women consume 1000 mg daily. If this cannot be achieved because of dietary habits or intolerance of dairy products, calcium supplements should be given to raise calcium intake.

TABLE 6. Major Dietary Sources of Calcium

Food	Serving Size	Calcium Content (mg)
Parmesan, grated	1 ounce	390
Vanilla shake	averagee	361
Sardines, canned in oil with bones	8 medium	354
Yogurt (lowfat, fruit-flavored)	1 cup	345
Gruyere cheese	1 ounce	308
Milk, skim	1 cup	303
Milk, whole (3.5% fat)	1 cup	288
Tofu	8 ounces	280
Cheddar cheese (American)	1 ounce	211
Creamed cottage cheese	1 cup	211
Muenster cheese	1 ounce	203
American cheese (processed)	1 ounce	195
Chocolate fudge	3½ ounces	100

Adapted from National Osteoporosis Foundation: A Physician's Manual on Osteoporosis. Washington, D.C. 1987.

Prescribing vitamin D with calcium is not recommended. For most adults, cutaneous vitamin D generation by sun exposure and a balanced diet assures adequate vitamin D nutrition. Clinical trials of calcium with and without vitamin D have not shown an added effect with vitamin D and high levels of vitamin D supplementation increase the risk of vitamin D intoxication, a dangerous, potentially fatal disorder.

For the Older Woman. The efficacy of calcium supplementation among older persons is not known. However, because of the decrease in calcium absorption with aging in both sexes, especially after age 70, most experts recommend *at least* increasing dietary consumption of calcium to the recommended daily allowance of 800 mg per day for adults. The recent National Institutes of Health Consensus Conference on Osteoporosis recommended a calcium intake of 1000 to 1500 mg per day for all postmenopausal women.[72] In postmenopausal women with established osteoporosis and women at high risk of fracture it is prudent for clinicians to recommend a calcium intake of about 1500 mg a day. Table 6 includes a list of foods that are relatively high in calcium.

One of the problems with increasing dietary calcium is that the major dietary sources are dairy products that are high in cholesterol and calories. In addition, dairy products can be a problem for those who have lactose intolerance, which is especially common among Asians and blacks. Lactose intolerance, however, need not be a problem since yoghurt, a rich source of calcium, is tolerated by many who are lactose intolerant. Lactose-free milk preparations are also available.

Table 7 includes a list of the strengths of selected calcium supplements. There is currently a great deal of discussion about which calcium supplements are best absorbed. A recent study in normal young people found no difference in absorption among any of the calcium products.[73,74] Calcium carbonate may be absorbed less well in persons with gastric achlorhydria and achlorhydria may exist in about 10% of elderly women; therefore, calcium carbonate should be administered with meals which improves calcium absorption.[75]

Side Effects of Calcium Supplements. Adverse effects of calcium supplementation are few and generally not severe. An increased frequency of

TABLE 7. Calcium Supplements*

Product (manufacturer)	Calcium per tablet	Cost of 1000 mg
Calcium carbonate tablets		
Tums Antacid (Norcliff-Thayer)	200 mg	$0.12
Caltrate 600 (Lederle)	600 mg	$0.18
Biocal (Miles)	500 mg	$0.21
Calcium Carbonate (Lilly)	260 mg	$0.23
Alka-2 Chewable Antacid (Miles)	200 mg	$0.27
Os-Cal (Marlon)	500 mg	$0.27
Biocal (Miles)	250 mg	$0.34
Calcium lactate tablets		
Calcium Lactate (General Nutrition Corp.)	100 mg	$0.26
Natural Calcium Lactate (Schiff)	100 mg	$0.28
Formula 81 (Plus)	83 mg	$0.40
Calcium Lactate (Lilly)	84 mg	$0.55
Calcium gluconate tablets		
Calcium Gluconate	62 mg	$0.56
Calcium Gluconate (Lilly)	47mg	$1.51
"Chelated" calcium tablets		
Chelated Calcium (Solgar)	167 mg	$0.35
Calcium Orotate 2000 (Nature's Plus)	100 mg	$1.70
Calcium Orotate (Kal)	50 mg	$2.33

* Listed by types; within types, listed in order of increasing cost.
From Consumer Reports, October, 1984, pp 576–580, with permission.

kidney stones in those who have a personal or family history of kidney stones is a possible concern. Twenty-four hour urinary calcium determinations should be obtained in those persons and calcium intake should probably not be increased without further evaluation if the 24-hour urinary calcium is above 300 mg/ml. Constipation is frequently associated with the use of calcium carbonate. Elderly individuals who are susceptible to constipation should be encouraged to maintain adequate fluid intake and to follow a program of regular exercise. Some persons report increased bloating or gas with calcium carbonate. Taking the calcium in divided doses or changing the preparation can eliminate this effect.

EXERCISE

Although the effect of exercise programs on bone density is probably not dramatic, there may be another reason to prescribe an exercise regimen for older persons. Regaining physical fitness may help to prevent falls among the elderly. The aging process is associated with slower reflex reaction time and, frequently, impaired gait. Studies have found that impaired mobility and gait are risk factors for falls in the elderly.[48] Preliminary results of a randomized trial to prevent falls that includes both home environmental modification and physical therapy show a significant reduction in falls among community-dwelling elderly persons.[76] The physical therapy part of the intervention includes training in the proper use of exercises for strength, balance, flexibility, posture, and general physical conditioning. Unless there are contraindications to exercise (see Chapter 7 on

Exercise), clinicians should advise a program of moderate weight-bearing exercise for older persons similar to that described in Chapter 7.

PREVENTION OF FALLS

Several overall strategies are important for preventing falls (see Chapter 10 for more detailed discussion): optimal management of balance-disturbing disorders and sensory impairment; limitation of the patient's use of balance-disturbing drugs, including alcohol; appropriate education for the patient and/or family concerning the dangers of falling, including information about who is at greatest risk, and awareness and reduction of home hazards. Patients should be cautioned about rising too quickly after eating or resting and should use a support aid if they tend to experience dizziness. An exercise program, in conjunction with physical therapy, may do much to restore balance and confidence.

Increasing home safety includes a compendium of approaches that includes provision of optimal lighting, elimination of slippery or otherwise hazardous floor surfaces, and ensuring adequate hand supports in key home areas. A knowledgeable visiting health nurse or other health professional is the most efficient way of identifying areas for improvement in home safety.

CONCLUSIONS

Fractures due to osteoporosis are a major public health problem in the United States. At present there are no reliable laboratory screening methods for identifying women at high risk for osteoporotic fractures. Historical factors listed in Table 1 have been well documented individually as predictive of increased risk for both osteoporosis (decreased bone mass) and the risk of fracture. The clinician should consider a person as being at increased risk if one or more of these factors are present.

Various strategies are available for primary prevention of osteoporosis; that is, intervention before substantial bone loss has occurred. These include estrogen replacement therapy, applicable to women at high risk for osteoporosis; adequate calcium nutrition and/or calcium supplementation; and weight-bearing exercise. Similar approaches may be used for secondary prevention; that is, intervention among older women in whom significant bone loss has already occurred, although estrogen replacement therapy is most effective when used during the first 5 to 10 years following menopause.

PRACTICE RECOMMENDATIONS

FOR MEN

The risk of osteoporotic fracture is low in men and therefore no special preventive measures are advised. It is reasonable to advocate an intake of calcium of 800 mg daily and a moderate weight-bearing exercise program. Smoking and excessive alcohol intake should be discouraged.

FOR PERIMENOPAUSAL WOMEN

A. Screening with Bone Mass Assessment
1. Routine noninvasive bone mass measurements are not recommended for asymptomatic women. They may be helpful in the decision of whether to use

ERT and in monitoring response to experimental therapies, such as fluoride or calcitonin.

B. Estrogen Replacement Therapy

1. Clinicians should consider advocating estrogen replacement therapy for women who are at increased risk by one or more the following factors: thin body build, Caucasian of Northern European ancestry, premature surgical menopause, and/or cigarette smoking.

2. The decision to use estrogen replacement therapy should evolve through discussion with the patient of its potential advantages and disadvantages (Table 4).

3. Prescribe low-dose estrogen replacement therapy (e.g., 0.625 mg) for 25 or 26 days monthly and add a progestin (10 mg medroxyprogesterone) on days 12–15 to day 25 or 26 in women who have not had hysterectomies.

4. Insure that the patient undergoes yearly breast examinations and mammography and thorough investigation of abnormal vaginal bleeding.

5. Initiate estrogen replacement therapy as soon as possible after the menopause, and plan to continue it for 10 years.

C. Calcium Intake

1. Take a dietary history for calcium by asking about consumption of foods listed in Table 6. It is recommended that perimenopausal women consume at least the recommended dietary allowance for calcium (800 mg daily) and that high risk perimenopausal women consume 1000 mg daily.

2. If adequate dietary intake of calcium cannot be achieved either because of dietary habits or intolerance of dairy products, calcium supplements should be given to raise calcium intake. Calcium carbonate is the least expensive calcium product and is generally well tolerated. Vitamin D supplementation is not recommended.

3. If the patient has a history of kidney stones in the past or a family history of kidney stones, obtain a 24-hour urine for urinary calcium. If it is greater than 300 mg, further evaluation is necessary before advising calcium supplementation.

4. Bloating and constipation can be alleviated by taking calcium divided doses, drinking adequate fluids, and/or by changing the calcium preparation.

D. Exercise

1. Moderate weight-bearing exercise is recommended according to the guidelines listed in Chapter 7.

FOR POSTMENOPAUSAL WOMEN

A. Screening

Routine noninvasive bone mass assessments are not recommended for asymptomatic women.

B. Estrogen Replacement Therapy

1. Initiating ERT for women 65 and older is of questionable benefit and is not generally recommended. It may be considered for women within 5 to 15 years postmenopause who have osteoporotic fractures (e.g., have clinically evident osteoporosis).

2. Women who began ERT around the time of menopause should be advised to continue ERT for around 10 years.

C. Calcium

1. Adequate calcium intake is especially important for the elderly because of decreased calcium absorption with aging.

2. For high risk postmenopausal women (those with one or more risk factors listed in Table 1) 1500 mg of calcium a day is recommended. Others should take 800 to 1000 mg daily.

3. If adequate calcium intake cannot be achieved through dietary sources, calcium supplementation is recommended. Calcium carbonate preparations are the least expensive and have the highest amount of elemental calcium per tablet. However, calcium carbonate is not well absorbed between meals in subjects with low gastric acid secretion. Advising patients to take calcium carbonate with meals insures adequate absorption. Constipation and bloating can be eliminated by taking the calcium in divided doses, drinking plenty of fluids and/or by changing the preparation. Vitamin D supplementation is not recommended.

D. Exercise

1. Although the effect of exercise programs on bone density is probably not great, regaining physical fitness may help to prevent falls among the elderly.

REFERENCES

1. Holbrook TL, Grazier K, Kelsey JL, et al: The frequency of occurrence, impact, and cost of musculoskeletal conditions in the United States. Chicago: American Academy of Orthopedic Surgeons, 1985.
2. Christiansen C, Riis BJ, Rodbro P: Prediction of rapid bone loss in postmenopausal women. Lancet 1987; 5:16.
3. Mellon TJ III, Riggs BL: Epidemiology of age-relate fractures. In Avioli LV (ed): The Osteoporosis Syndrome. New York, Grune & Stratton, 1983, pp 45–72.
4. Cummings SR, Kelsey JL, Nevitt MC, O'Dowd KJ: Epidemiology of osteoporosis and osteoporotic fractures. Epidemiol Rev 1985; 7:178–208.
5. National Center for Health Statistics: Advance data from vital and health statistics 1985 summary national hospital discharge survey. Hyattsville, Md. Public Health Service, 1986. U.S. Public Health Service Publication no. (PHS) 86-1250.
6. Riggs BL, Melton LJ: Involutional osteoporosis. N Engl J Med 1986; 3:1676–1684.
7. Gallagher JC, Melton LJ, Riggs BL, et al: Epidemiology of fractures of proximal femur in Rochester, Minnesota. Clin Orthop 1980; 150:163–171.
8. Alffram P: An epidemiological study of cervical and trochanteric fractures of the femur in an urban population. Acta Orthop Scand (Suppl) 1964; 65:1–109.
9. Knowelden J, Buhr AJ, Dunbar O: Incidences of fractures in persons over 35 years of age: a report to the MRC working party on fractures in the elderly. Br J Prev Soc Med 1964; 18:130–141.
10. Lewinnek G, Kelsey J, White A, et al: The significance and comparative analysis of the epidemiology of hip fractures. Clin Orthop 1980; 152:35–43.
11. Owen RA, Melton LJ, Johnson KA, et al: Incidence of Colles' fracture in a North American community. Am J Public Health 1982; 72:604–607.
12. Rose SH, Melton LJ, Morrey BF, et al: Epidemiologic features of humeral fractures. Clin Orthop 1982; 168:24–30.
13. Trotter M, Broman GE, Peterson RR. Densities of bones of white and Negro skeletons. J Bone Joint Surg (Am) 1960; 42A:50–58.
14. Cohn SH, Abesamis C, Yasumura S, et al: Comparative skeletal mass and radial bone mineral content in black and white women. Metabolism 1977; 26:171–178.
15. Garn SM, Sandusky ST, Magy JM, et al: Advanced skeletal development in low income Negro children. J Pediatr 1972; 80:965–969.
16. Nordin BEC: International patterns of osteoporosis. Clin Orthop 1966; 45:17–30.
17. Farmer ME, White LR, Brody JA, et al: Race and sex differences in hip fractures incidence. Am J Public Health 1984; 74:1374–1380.
18. Bollett AJ, Engh G, Parson W: Epidemiology of osteoporosis. Arch Intern Med 1965; 16:191–194.
19. Bauer RL, Deyo RA: Low risk of vertebral fracture in Mexican American women. Arch Intern Med 1987; 147:1437–1439.
20. Bauer RL, Diehl AK, Barton SA, Brender J, Deyo RA: Risk of postmenopausal hip fracture in Mexican American women. Am J Public Health 1986; 76(8):1020–1021.

21. Hillner BE, Hollenberg JP, Pauker SG: Postmenopausal estrogens in prevention of osteoporosis. Benefit virtually without risk if cardiovascular effects are considered. Am J Med 1986; 80(6):1115–1127.

22. Richelson LS, Wahner HW, Melton LJ, Riggs BL: Relative contributions of aging and estrogen deficiency to postmenopausal bone loss. N Engl J Med 1984; 311(20):1273–1275.

23. Lindsay R, Aitken J, Anderson J, et al: Long term prevention of postmenopausal osteoporosis by estrogen. Lancet 1976; 1:1038–1041.

24. Riis B, Thomsen K, Christiansen C: Does calcium supplementation prevent postmenopausal bone loss? A double-blind, controlled clinical study. N Engl J Med 1987; 316(4):173–177.

25. Kreiger N, Kelsey JL, Helford TR, et al: An epidemiologic study of hip fracture in postmenopausal women. Am J Epidemiol 1982; 116:141–148.

26. Hutchinson TA, Polansky SM, Feinstein AR: Postmenopausal oestrogens protect against fractures of hip and distal radius: case-control study. Lancet 1979; 2:705–709.

27. Weiss NS, Ure CL, Ballard JH, et al: Decreased risk of fractures of the hip and lower forearm with postmenopausal use of estrogen. N Engl J Med 1980; 303:1195–1198.

28. Ettinger B, Genant HK, Cann CE: Long-term estrogen therapy prevents bone loss and fractures. Ann Intern Med 1985; 102:319–324.

29. Seeman E, Melton LJ III, Fallon WM, Riggs BL: Risk factors for spinal osteoporosis in men. Am J Med 1983; 75(6):977–983.

30. Kelsey J, Hoffman S: Editorial. N Engl J Med 1987; 316:404–406.

31. Dietrick JE, Whedon GD, Shorr E: Effects of immobilization upon various metabolic and physiologic functions of normal men. Am J Med 1948; 4:3–36.

32. Donaldson CL, Hulley SB, Vogel JM, et al: Effect of prolonged bed rest on bone mineral. Metabolism 1970; 19:1071–1084.

33. Nilsson BE, Westlin NE: Bone density in athletes. Clin Orthop 1971; 77:179–182.

34. Jones HH, Priest JD, Hayes WC, et al: Humeral hypertrophy in response to exercise. J Bone Joint Surg (Am) 1977; 59A:204–208.

35. Aloia JF, Cohn SH, Bab T, et al: Skeletal mass and body composition in marathon runners. Metabolism 1978; 27:1793–1796.

36. Smith EL, Reddan W, Smith PE. Physical activity and calcium modalities for bone mineral increase in aged women. Med Sci Sports Exerc 1981; 13:60–64.

37. Smith EL, Reddan W: Physical activity: a modality for bone accretion in the aged. AJR 1976; 126:1297.

38. Aloia JF, Cohn SH, Ostuni JA, et al: Prevention of involutional bone loss by exercise. Ann Intern Med 1978; 89:356–358.

39. Smith EL, Smith PE, Ensign CJ, et al: Bone involution decrease in exercising middle-aged women. Calcif Tissue Int 1984; 36(S):129–138.

40. Krolner B, Toft B, Pors Nielson S, Tondevold E: Physical exercise as prophylaxis against involutional vertebral bone loss: A controlled trial. Clin Sci 1983; 64:541–546.

41. Aloia JF, Cohn SH, Vaswani A, et al: Risk factors for postmenopausal osteoporosis. Am J Med 1986; 78:95–100.

42. MacMahon B, Trichopoulos D, Cole P, et al: Cigarette smoking and urinary estrogens. N Engl J Med 1982; 307:1062–1065.

43. Peck WA, Riggs BL, Bell NH: Physician's Resource Manual on Osteoporosis. National Osteoporosis Foundation, 1987.

44. Melton LJ, Illstrup DM, Beckenbaugh RD, et al: Hip fracture recurrence: a population-based study. Clin Orthop 1982; 167:131–138.

45. Campbell A, Reinken J, Alan B, et al: Falls in older age: a study of frequency and related clinical factors. Age Aging 1981; 10:264–270.

45a. Cooper C, Barker DJP, Morris J, Briggs RSJ: Osteoporosis, falls, and age in fracture of the proximal femur. Br Med J 1987; 295:13–15.

46. Prudham D, Evans J: Factors associated with falls in the elderly: a community study. Age Aging 1981; 10:141–146.

47. Gryfe CL, Amles A, Ashley MJ: A longitudinal study of falls in an elderly population: I. Incidence and morbidity. Age Aging 1977; 6:201–210.

48. Tinetti ME, Williams TR, Mayewski R: Fall risk index for elderly patients based on number of chronic disabilities. Am J Med 1986; 80:429–434.

49. Wild D, Nayak USL, Isaacs B: Characteristics of old people who fell at home. J Clin Exp Gerontol 1980; 2:271–287.

50. Morris, Runbin EH, Morris EJ, Mandel SA: Senile dementia of the Alzheimer's type: an important risk factor for serious falls. J Gerontol 1987; 42:4:412–417.

51. Ray WA, Griffin MR, Schaffner W, et al: Psychotropic drug use and the risk of hip fracture. N Engl J Med 1987; 9:316–363.
52. MacDonald J: The role of drugs in falls in the elderly. In Biological and Behavioral Aspects of Falls in the Elderly. Proceedings of a conference sponsored by the National Institute on Aging, Sept. 17–18, 1984.
53. Wild D, Nayak U, Isaacs B: Descriptions, classification and prevention of falls in old people at home. Rheumatol Rehabil 1981; 20:153–159.
54. Waller J: Falls among the elderly: human and environmental factors. Accident Anal Prev 1978; 10:21–33.
55. Notelovitz M, Ware M: Stand Tall!: The Informed Woman's Guide to Preventing Osteoporosis. Gainesville, FL, Triad Publishing Company, 1982.
56. Cummings SR, Black D: Should perimenopausal women be screened for osteoporosis? Ann Intern Med 1986; 104:817–823.
57. Health and Public Policy Committee, American College of Physicians: Radiologic methods to evaluate bone mineral content. Ann Intern Med 1984; 100:908–911.
58. Johnston CC: Noninvasive methods for quantitating appendicular bone mass. In Avioli LV (ed): The Osteoporotic Detection Prevention, and Treatment. New York, Grune & Stratton, 1983, pp 73–84.
59. Riggs BL, Wahner HW, Seeman E, et al: Changes in bone mineral density of the proximal femur and spine with aging: differences between the postmenopausal and senile osteoporosis syndromes. J Clin Invest 1982; 70:716–723.
60. Heaney RP: Enrechercha de la difference (P < .05). Bone Mineral 1986; 1:99–114.
61. Riggs BL, Wahner HW, Melton LJ, et al: Rates of bone loss in the appendicular and axial skeletons of women: Evidence of substantial vertebral bone loss before menopause. J Clin Invest 1986; 77:1487–1491.
62. Ott SM, Kilcoyne RF, Chestnut CH: Longitudinal changes in bone mass after one year as measured by different techniques in patients with osteoporosis. Calcif Tiss Int 1986; 39:133–138.
63. Hillner BE, Hollenberg JP, Pauker SG: Postmenopausal estrogens in prevention of osteoporosis. Benefit virtually without risk if cardiovascular effects are considered. Am J Med 1986; 80:1115–1127.
64. Bush TL, Barrett-Connor E: Noncontraceptive estrogen use and cardiovascular disease. Epidemiol Rev 1985; 7:80–103
65. Judd GL, Cleary RE, Creasman WT, et al: Estrogen replacement therapy. J Obstet Gynecol 1983; 58:267–275.
66. Christiansen C, Christiansen MS, Transbol I: Bone mass in postmenopausal women after withdrawal of estrogen/gestagen replacement therapy. Lancet 1981; 1:459–461.
67. Krolner B, Nielsen SP: Bone mineral content of the lumbar spine in normal and osteoporotic women: cross-sectional and longitudinal studies. Clin Sci 1982; 62:329–336.
68. Kiel DP, Felson DT, Anderson JJ, et al: Hip fracture and the use of estrogens in postmenopausal women. N Engl J Med 1987; 317:1169–1174.
69. Lindsay R, Hart DM, MacLean A, et al: Bone response to termination of estrogen treatment. Lancet 1978; 1:1325–1327
70. Consensus development conference: prophylaxis and treatment of osteoporosis. Br Med J 1987; 295:914.
71. Ettinger BR, Genant HK, Cann CE: Postmenopausal bone loss is prevented by treatment with low-dosage estrogen with calcium. Ann Intern Med 1987; 106:40–45.
72. Consensus Conference: Osteoporosis. JAMA 1984; 252(6):799–802.
73. Nicar MJ, Pak CYC: Calcium bioavailability from calcium carbonate and calcium citrate. J Clin Endocrinol Metab 1985; 61:391–393.
74. Sheikh MS, Santa Ana CA, Nicar MJ, et al: Gastrointestinal absorption of calcium from milk and calcium salts. N Engl J Med 1987; 317:532–536.
75. Rodysill KJ: Postmenopausal osteoporosis—intervention and prophylaxis. A review. J Chron Dis 1987; 40:743–760.
76. Personal communication. Darlene Wingfield, CDC Injury Meeting, February 1987.
77. Dalsky GP, Stocke KS, Ehsani AA, et al: Weight-bearing exercise training and lumbar bone mineral content in postmenopausal women. Ann Intern Med 1988; 108:824–828.
78. Sandler RB, Cauley JA, Hom DL, et al: The effects of walking on the cross-sectional dimensions of the radius in postmenopausal women. Calcified Tissue International 1987, 41:65–69.
79. Abdulla HI, Hart DM, Lindsay R, et al: Prevention of bone loss in postmenopausal women by norethisterone. Obst Gynecol 1985; 66:789–792.

10
PREVENTING DEPENDENCE AND INJURY: AN APPROACH TO SENSORY CHANGES

Mathy D. Mezey, RN, EdD
Jeane Ann Grisso, MD, MSc

Irrespective of age, one's environment can mean the difference between relative independence and total dependence. Someone confined to bed or chair, for whatever reason, is totally dependent on others for all items that are out of reach. Similarly, an elderly person with limitations of vision, hearing or mobility can be made more independent if the deficits are properly assessed and the environment appropriately designed. Arranging an environment so an activity or a group of activities can be carried out safely, effectively, and efficiently is common in everyday life. Any camper can appreciate the ways a kitchen facilitates food preparation or a wood-worker how a workshop facilitates using simple tools. Furthermore, pediatricians have long recognized the need to structure environments in order to maximize a child's safety and development. A toddler who walks on unsteady feet, or whose judgment is questionable at best and who does not always accurately interpret sensory input, should move about in a different world than a sure-footed confident 12-year-old. The same argument holds for the elderly whose sensory function and sense of balance are in a state of flux. Just as parents have come to turn to pediatricians for guidance in making their children's environment safe, increasingly family care-givers of the elderly will turn to primary care physicians for guidance in this area. Therefore, this chapter will describe the sensory changes that often accompany aging, recommend environmental adaptations that might reduce injuries and improve independence and, finally, discuss the role of assessment and reassessment in this dynamic process.

The prevalence of sensory changes and injuries among the elderly dictates the importance of addressing them in primary care settings. The elderly individual's perception of the environment changes subtly as the senses age. Changes in vision, hearing, taste, and smell are almost universal. Only 5% of persons over 80 have 20/20 vision, and nearly 60% of those aged 65 to 70 show evidence of cataracts or glaucoma.[15,13,15] Twenty-five percent of those over 65 have some type of hearing problem, and among persons over 75 the incidence increases to over 40%.[16,14] Sixteen percent of the elderly report they hear only shouted speech.[5,16,14] Similarly, the thresholds for taste and smell increase with age.[5]

The incidence of sensory losses is greatest among the very old and the institutionalized. The Framingham Eye Study reports the percentage of persons with good visual acuity (20/25 or better) is 98% of those 62 to 64, 92% of those aged 65 to 74, but only 69% of those aged 75 to 85.[13] Moreover, the incidence and prevalence of sensory changes are higher in the institutionalized elderly population when compared to the elderly residing in the community. For example, 12% of community-dwelling older people have been reported as having visual impairments, while 51% of institutionalized elderly report similar impairments.[13]

Sensory losses are of major importance to the elderly in that they limit self-care and activities of daily living, and significantly alter communication and interaction patterns. Impairment of the senses can, therefore, make an important contribution to a decline in functional state and lead to an increasing isolation of the elderly individual. Losses in hearing, in particular, may contribute to psychological disturbances, such as paranoia, depression, and hallucinations.

Perhaps the greatest impact of the sensory changes described above is their contribution to the high incidence of injuries in the elderly. Injuries are the fifth leading cause of death in persons older than 65.[18] The elderly have twice as many deaths from injury and three times as many days of restricted activity and bed confinement as any other age group.[12] Each year almost 5 million elderly persons sustain nonfatal injuries, about three-fourths of them at home.[2] Falls, motor vehicle collisions, and fires account for most injury deaths among the aged.

Three-fourths of all fatal falls occur to persons 65 years and older.[18] The frequency of falls increases dramatically with age, as does the risk of sustaining a significant injury. A third of community-dwelling elderly persons fall each year; two-thirds of those who fall once will fall again.[17] In all, 90% of the 200,000 elderly Americans who break a hip each year do so as a result of a fall; of these, 15% die from complications and many others suffer prolonged or permanent disability. Although the etiology of falls in the elderly is multifactorial, sensory loss is more often than not contributory.

Elderly persons have a higher rate of motor vehicle injuries than any age group except those aged 25 and younger.[12] In addition to having high injury rates, the elderly are more likely to die from motor vehicle injuries. Baker et al. found that people over 70 suffering moderately severe trauma were nine times as likely to die as those under 50 years of age.[1] The elderly are also particularly at risk for pedestrian injuries. Of all pedestrian deaths, 20% occur in persons aged 65 and older even thought this age group only represents 11% of the population.[12]

In general, the economic cost of injuries to society is huge and includes both direct (e.g., surgery and hospitalization) and indirect (e.g., lost time from work) medical costs.[23] Few studies have assessed injury costs for the elderly. However, given that the elderly have disproportionately high rates of significant injuries, the costs of direct medical care and institutionalization for the elderly are likely to be particularly great. The estimated cost per year due to hip fractures alone in those age 65 and older is 6.1 billion dollars.[6] Reducing the incidence of injuries would, therefore, be expected to have a positive financial benefit for society. In part, this goal might be achieved by preventing sensory loss in the elderly.

AGE-RELATED SENSORY CHANGES AND THE ROLE OF THE PRIMARY CARE PROVIDER

Sensory deficits and injuries are often evaluated and treated by a variety of subspecialists: the ophthalmologist, the otorhinolaryngologist, the orthopedist, and the emergency room physician. However, the primary care provider plays a crucial role in prevention, early identification, and management of sensory losses and injury prevention.

VISION

The eye's susceptibility to trauma, infection, and inflammatory conditions is increased in the elderly individual due to a number of factors that affect the eye's external protective mechanisms. Senile entropion (in-turning) and ectropion (eversion) of the eyelid are common. Although there is decreased lacrimation, tear overflow is common due to impaired drainage of the ductal system. In addition, there is conjunctival thinning and fragility.

Other age-related changes affect the individual's vision itself. Presbyopia (farsightedness) is caused by degenerative changes in the lens that decrease its ability to focus on nearby objects. These changes first lead to difficulty reading and performing close work beginning in the fourth decade.

Older people need more light to see clearly and a longer time to adapt to light changes. This increase in absolute threshold is due to two major factors. The first is related to the degenerative process in the lens just noted. With age, the lens yellows, increases in density, and decreases in transparency. The net effect is that between the ages of 25 and 60 the efficiency of light transmission through the lens drops about 66%. Another factor affecting absolute threshold in vision is senile miosis—decrease in pupillary size—which further limits the amount of light reaching the retina. Older people require 30 to 40 minutes to achieve full dark adaptation and never achieve the same degree of adaptation as younger people.

The lens changes noted above also result in decreasing color discrimination. As the lens yellows, the shorter-wavelength blue-green rays tend to be filtered out. As the yellowing progresses, all wavelengths are eventually affected, and the person's ability to discriminate between shades is lessened. The elderly individual can best distinguish between the colors red and white.

Formal vision testing reveals changes in visual fields and visual perception. Peripheral field deficits are common among the elderly, particularly during upward gaze. In addition, the ability to gaze upward decreases with age. While peripheral field defects may be related to age alone, it is important to remember that central field deficits (scotoma) are always abnormal and require further evaluation. As with other organ systems, changes in function are often the result of the interaction between aging and disease. Several diseases of the eye— cataracts, glaucoma and senile macular degeneration are very common among the elderly.[9]

Cataracts. Cataracts involve the gradual opacification of the cortex or nucleus of the crystalline lens; the opacification may be partial or complete. Paradoxically, the patient may experience an improvement in near vision during the early stages of cataract development because of increased lens density. The most common symptom of the disease is progressive unilateral or bilateral painless loss of vision. Diagnosis can be made using the number 10 lens of the ophthalmoscope and observing the opacity against the red reflex. The amount of difficulty that the observer has in seeing the macula is an indication of the size and density of the cataract. In some instances the swelling of the lens may cause a reduction in the depth of the anterior chamber. Pupillary response to light normally is preserved. Cataract removal with or without the use of a contact lens or an intraocular lens implant can restore vision if retinal function posterior to the cataract remains intact.[11] Thus, anyone with a cataract *and* decreased vision should be referred to an ophthalmologist for further evaluation. Even with the new surgical techniques now available, the probability of success is dependent on the amount of vision loss due to the cataract as opposed to that due to retinal damage from disease. This is best assessed by an ophthalmologist. If such an assessment shows that cataract extraction is likely to improve vision, surgery is indicated when the patient's functioning is being hampered.[11] This will obviously vary greatly among patients.

Glaucoma. Glaucoma is largely a disease of the elderly and is the second most common cause of legal blindness among those over 65. The evaluation of glaucoma involves assessment of the intraocular pressure by tonometry, visual field testing, and fundoscopic examination. Measuring intraocular pressure alone is associated with a large number of false negatives, and therefore false reassurance. In addition, the poor correlation between intraocular pressure and the glaucoma-related visual limitations, the existence of normal pressure glaucoma, and the diurnal variation in intraocular pressure are all reasons for the insensitivity of the test. While peripheral field testing may be most accurate, it is difficult to perform in the elderly. Other tests including gonioscopy, tonography, and provocative testing are necessary to confirm a suspected diagnosis or to distinguish narrow-angle from open-angle glaucoma.

While open-angle glaucoma is more common, narrow-angle glaucoma can present more acutely. An elderly person with narrow-angle glaucoma may give a history of headache and visual symptoms associated with being in a darkened room. In advanced stages either type of glaucoma may be associated with symptoms that may include abrupt or prolonged onset of blurred vision, halos around lights, pain in the eye, nausea and vomiting, and abdominal pain. Treatment includes medications and peripheral iridectomy. A complete discussion of therapy is beyond the scope of this chapter; however, the potential for glaucoma medications to cause adverse reactions when used in association with other commonly prescribed drugs should be kept in mind. Medications placed in the eye are absorbed systemically; therefore, an anticholinergic agent or β blocker instilled in the eye is the same double edge sword as it is when given orally or parenterally.[8]

Senile Macular Degeneration. About 165,000 new cases of senile macular degeneration are identified annually.[7] Clinical features of the disorder include slow, progressive, painless onset of loss of central vision over many months or years, with loss of fine discrimination such as is involved in close reading. Peripheral vision discrimination, which is coarser, remains unaffected. The condition rarely causes total blindness. Assessment is difficult, because the degree of macular degeneration does not always correlate with the level of visual acuity reported by the patient. A finding that the patient continues to perceive glare for a prolonged period after gazing at a bright light for a fixed time or that straight lines or edges appear wavy may be indicative of macular degeneration. Treatment involves maximizing vision through the use of magnifying lenses and correcting concomitant cataracts. There is evidence of some success with laser photocoagulation in preventing further degeneration.[2,10]

ROLE OF THE PRIMARY CARE PROVIDER

The primary care provider creates an important link among the elderly patient, ophthalmologic follow-up and services that help the individual with visual impairment to cope. The primary care physician may be the first to detect

TABLE 1. Agencies Serving the Blind and Patients with Low Vision*

American Foundation for the Blind 15 West 16th Street New York, NY 10011 (212) 620-2000	American Council of the Blind, Inc. 1010 Vermont Avenue Suite 1100 Washington, DC 20005 (202) 393-3666
Association for Education and Rehabilitation of the Blind and Visually Impaired (AERBVI) 206 North Washington Street, Suite 320 Alexandria, VA 22314 (703) 548-1884	National Federation of the Blind 1800 Johnson Street Baltimore, MD 21230 (301) 659-9314

American Association of Retired Persons (AARP)
1909 K Street, NW
Washington, DC 20049
(202)872-4700

* A full listing of all local and national agencies serving the visually impaired is available in Directory of Services for Blind and Visually Impaired Persons in the United States, New York, American Foundation for the Blind, 1988.

a subtle history of visual changes, which may seem insignificant to the patient but provide an indication for intervention by the ophthalmologist. The history may be supplemented by in-office tonometry and visual field testing. However it should be remembered that tonometry alone is an inadequate screen for glaucoma. Furthermore, it may be unreliable in inexperienced hands. Current recommendations are that all patients over the age of 60 should undergo ophthalmologic evaluation every two years. The primary care provider can play an important role insuring that such screening does take place.

Once a visual impairment has developed, the primary care physician may facilitate the coordination of available community services. Caring for an elderly person with vision defects entails an interdisciplinary approach. Training of this kind is available through agencies serving the blind and visually impaired (Table 1). Characteristically, in such programs an instructor accompanies the patient through a typical day, provides instructions about the use of what sight the patient has, coaches in techniques of memory retrieval and cuing for simple tasks, and provides mobility training.

Careful attention to the design of products and the surrounding environment can enhance the mobility and function of those with all degrees of visual impairment. One of the most available visual aids is light. Age-related changes in the lens, cataract, and macular degeneration substantially increase the amount of light required to produce an image on the retina. Elderly patients should be made aware of this and encoraged to use large wattage light bulbs for their activities that require macular vision, such as reading or sewing. The inability to accommodate quickly to darkness can be compensated by encouraging the use of 5 to 10 watt night lights; even better one should encourage the patient to always turn on the light when moving about the house at night. Similarly, dark spots in the house should be eliminated. Many older homes have poorly lit hallways or stairways, and the transition from a well-lit to a poorly-lit area is particularly dangerous for the elderly because of the slow accommodation to darkness. Contrasts using color and light should be used to provide meaningful edges and to emphasize important object features.

While good lighting is essential, suggestions should be given on ways to minimize glare, particularly for those elderly with cataracts. Polished, shiny surfaces and direct light can produce blinding glare for elderly patients with cataracts. By instructing individuals with cataracts and their families to seek a position in the room such that the light will be behind rather than directly in front of them, the disability associated with cataracts may be minimized. In addition, highly polished floors should be avoided. In summary, bright light that is properly positioned is probably the most important visual aid.

It is also important for clinicians to be mindful of changes in color perception. As the lens yellows, it can become very difficult for elderly to perceive differences between colors. This is especially important in distinguishing medications. Therefore, the elderly should be cautioned not to rely solely on color cues in differentiating substances, particularly medications. Patients with macular degeneration can be greatly helped by the use of magnifying glasses. By magnifying an image, they can rely on a larger portion of the retina. These aids are relatively inexpensive, thereby allowing a person with macular degeneration to keep several on hand and to distribute them throughout the house. As the visual loss progresses, large print newspapers and books, as well as talking books, can be obtained by contacting local agencies for the blind. Such agencies are often able to provide information regarding self-help groups and instruction on household tasks such as cooking.

HEARING

As persons age, their voices change, becoming lower in frequency, pitch and tone. This coincides with a number of characteristic age-related changes in hearing. With age there is also an increase in sound threshold, especially for high-pitched sounds. These changes mean that the elderly may be unable to hear such sounds as a clock ticking or some female voices. Speech discrimination and auditory judgment decrease; the consonants *s, z, t, f* and *g* are especially problematic. Yet consonants are the sounds that allow words to be distinguished one from another.

While most speech is in the range of 500 to 2,000 Hz, sounds such as *s, th, j, k,* and *f* are heard at higher frequencies. Older people lose the ability to perceive pitch above 4,000 Hz and have difficulty in hearing these sounds and distinguishing speech.[4] For example, the platitude, "When the going gets tough, the tough get going." would be reduced to the unintelligible "When e oin e ough e ough e oin" if one has difficulty hearing consonants. The ability to filter out extraneous noise declines. Thus, it can be extremely difficult for an elderly person to follow a conversation in a noisy room, whether the setting is a cocktail party or a waiting room.

Other changes in the ear such as decreased bone conduction and proprioception occur as well. Bone conduction diminishes because of bone reabsorption and damage. Proprioception decreases owing to a decline in the excitability of hair cells in the semi-circular canals, which may well contribute to the elderly's tendency to fall.

Hearing loss falls into three general categories: conductive or bone loss, loss through changes in air and auditory nerve conduction, and mixed hearing loss. Ninety percent of presbycusis in the elderly is due to *sensory nerve hearing loss* caused by diseases or changes in the inner ear, trauma, drugs, infectious diseases, damage to the cranial nerve, and degeneration of the organ of Corti. It is important to remember that a very common and reversible problem, impacted cerumen, may contribute to or augment presbycusis by decreasing air conduction. Similarly, iatrogenic factors may play a role; ototoxic drugs, including antibiotics, aminoglycosides, diuretics, and salicylates, can cause temporary or permanent hearing damage. Combined hearing losses can occur when sensory neural losses are combined with conductive losses from such diseases as otosclerosis or Paget's disease.

ROLE OF THE PRIMARY CARE PHYSICIAN

The primary care physician plays an important role in identifying patients with hearing impairment.[19] High-risk patients, who may require more frequent evaluation for hearing loss, include those patients with a history of recurrent otitis media or other ear problems and those individuals who worked in a noisy environment, experiencing barotrauma. In all patients, certain clues to hearing impairment can be obtained during a routine history. First and foremost is the question whether the patient is aware of any difficulty hearing. If the patient or family reports any of the following behaviors, there is a high likelihood that a hearing loss exists:

- Excessive amplification of radios and television
- Inability to hear people on the telephone
- Turning the head to the "better" ear or to face a person who is speaking
- Frequent request to repeat information
- Withdrawal from conversations or lack of recollection of discussion
- Unwillingness to participate in activities that involve more than one person

An occupational and recreational history should be obtained, and elderly with a history of trauma or repeated episodes of otitis media as well as those that show signs of hearing loss should be referred to an audiologist.

Examples of specific questions to assess hearing deficits are shown in Table 3. Complete assessment includes physical examination of the ears, nose, and throat, a review of past and current medication, and referral for an audiometric examination. Complete office testing should include otoscopic exam and removal of impacted cerumen, and the evaluation of air and bone conduction using a low and a high frequency tuning fork. The question of when it is appropriate to perform a formal audiologic evaluation in asymptomatic individuals is controversial. If the patient is truly asymptomatic and has a normal exam audiologic testing will probably have a low yield.

The benefits from early detection relate mainly to early intervention with hearing aids and environmental modifications that may reduce the subtle but disturbing difficulties with communication often encountered by mildly impaired individuals. Some experts recommend formal screening every 5 years.[5]

STRUCTURING THE ENVIRONMENT TO PREVENT DYSFUNCTION

Since the majority of the elderly with hearing loss have difficulty with word discrimination as a result of their inability to discriminate among high frequency sounds, attempts to structure the environment should focus on this deficit. Instruct the elderly on the kinds of consonant sounds that are most difficult for them to hear, so that they can educate those with whom they are trying to converse. Suggest that elderly patients in a noisy room position themselves near a wall, so that the wall can act as a sounding board. If an elderly person has difficulty understanding a particular work or phrase, the phrase should be repeated once, and if still not understood, rephrased preferably using lower frequency sounds. For example "You *seem to* be *feeling fine*," can be rephrased to "Are you okay?" Instructing the elderly and their families on this strategy can be extraordinarily helpful.

In addition, there are a number of assistive listening devices. FM and infrared assistive devices consist of a microphone that is worn on the clothing of the hearing-impaired person and an amplifier that is worn in the ear. These devices allow conversations to be picked up by the microphone and amplified, so that the elderly person can filter out extraneous noises more easily. Similarly, hard-wired amplifiers for television, radio and telephone are available. The home environment can be made more safe for the hearing-impaired person by using signaling devices that use vibration or light. Telephones, doorbells, and smoke detectors can be adapted to generate a flashing light rather than a sound when activated.

Of course hearing aids can be very helpful in situations where there is not a lot of background or extraneous noise. The in-the-ear type of hearing aid is currently the most popular type. This hearing aid, like other types, requires a motivated patient who is willing to learn how to adjust the hearing aid in different settings, as well as a patient who has the hand and finger dexterity to adjust the controls on a hearing aid.

While there have been additional advances in hearing aid technology, including the cochlear implant, most elderly do not have hearing loss severe enough to warrant this kind of hearing aid. Hearing aids are not covered by Medicare or third-party payers, and are quite expensive—ranging from $300 to $500. Therefore, for many elderly, learning to structure the environment is the only viable method of coping with presbycusis.

Most important in ensuring the success of these therapies is that the physician anticipate negative attitudes toward interventions that compensate for sensory losses (such as hearing aids), and that he or she work with the patient to overcome these feelings. Acknowledging and seeking treatment for difficulty operating in the local environment requires that the elderly recognize and accept permanent changes in themselves—that they recognize clear evidence of aging and deal with their own and other's attitudes toward dependence.

Once identified, management of hearing impairments involves both environmental modifications and use of hearing aids. Communication strategies for talking with a hearing-impaired older person, for environmental modification, and for the use of assistive devices are outlined in Tables 2, 3, and 4. Information about hearing deficits can be obtained from the National Information Center for Deafness and the American Speech, Language and Hearing Association, the National Association for the Deaf, and Self-Help for Hard of Hearing People, Inc.[15,19]

TASTE AND SMELL

With age the decline in ability to taste sweet substances is especially pronounced, and older people may consume increasing amounts of sugar to compensate for this deficit. The threshold for salt is also increased; that is, more salt is necessary to achieve baseline taste sensations.

These age-related changes in taste correlate with a gradual decrease both in the number of fungiform papillae and in the number of taste buds per papilla; as many as two-thirds of the papillae become atrophic in old age.[2] There is also a

TABLE 2. Communication Strategies for Talking with the Hearing Impaired

RULES TO REMEMBER WHEN SPEAKING TO SOMEONE WITH A HEARING LOSS

- DO NOT SHOUT
- SPEAK CLEARLY AND SLOWLY
- REPHRASE A MISUNDERSTOOD SENTENCE
- MOVE AWAY FROM BACKGROUND NOISE
- STAND IN CLEAR LIGHT FACING THE PERSON WITH WHOM YOU ARE SPEAKING
- DO NOT OBSCURE YOUR MOUTH WITH A CIGARETTE OR HANDS AND DO NOT CHEW FOOD WHILE SPEAKING
- ASK THE PERSON WHAT YOU MIGHT DO TO MAKE CONVERSATION EASIER

To increase awareness of hearing impairment, the Suzanne Pathy Speak-Up Institute has developed this large sign to place above the bed of the hearing-impaired patient. Smaller gummed stickers are also available to mark the medical chart of each hearing-impaired patient. Also, a gummed card is available for the medical chart to remind hospital staff of rules for communicating with the hearing impaired.

Source: U.S. Congress, Office of Technology Assessment, Hearing Impairment and Elderly People. A background paper. OTA-BP-BA-30 (Washington, D.C.: U.S. Government Printing Office, May 1986) p. 53.

decrease in the flow of saliva, which contributes to xerostomia, or dry mouth. These changes are increased by the wearing of dentures as well as with cigarette and pipe smoking. Taste loss is also thought to be exacerbated by certain medications.[9,13] The age-related decline in the ability to smell (anosmia) is probably due to a combination of decrease in factory bulb size and in some cases nerve damage, nasal polyps, or mucous membrane changes exacerbated by smoking.

Changes in taste and smell have major implications not only for nutritional status but also for injury prevention, such as in the areas of detection of smoke or gas and ingestion of noxious substances. The elderly may appreciate educational efforts that reveal the normal changes in taste and smell. Smokers may be motivated to decrease use of cigarettes by increased awareness of the effect on both taste and smell.

INJURY PREVENTION

Sensory deficits, particularly multiple sensory deficits, contribute to the elderly's increased risk for injuries. The high incidence and high costs associated with injuries make it crucial for the provider to become involved in injury prevention. The three most common causes of injuries are falls, motor vehicle accidents, and burns.

Falls. Assessing the risk of falling involves identifying the high-risk patient. A simple balance maneuver can be conducted quickly in the physician's office and is described in Appendix A. This test can be incorporated into the

TABLE 3.   Strategies for the Use of Hearing-Assisted Devices

To the newly aided person:

1. Begin with a comfortable volume level.
2. Begin with easy listening challenges.
3. Don't overtire yourself.
4. Relearn the trick of concentration.
5. When in church or group meetings, sit up close.
6. Experiment with difficult listening environments or situations (noisy places, TV or stereo listening, telephone use). Try different volume settings on the aid or tone controls on the stereo. Use the telephone with and without the aid. Parttime hearing aid use may be a solution.
7. Listen with your eyes. Be visually observant.
8. Be patient and keep trying.

When an aid is nonfunctional or weak or is not performing well in other ways, there are a few simple remedies that may be tried. **If the aid is giving a weak signal or none at all:**

1. Place a new battery in the aid, taking care to put it in properly and completely. Check the battery contacts and clean them with a sharpened pencil eraser if they show corrosion.
2. Check the telephone switch to make sure it is in the (M) position.
3. Turn the volume control of the aid up and down, listening for scratchiness or "cutting on and off."
4. Check the cord of a body aid to see if it is intact and firmly connected to its sockets. Roll it in the fingers to see if this causes intermittency.

If the aid is producing inappropriate feedback:

1. Try reseating or adjusting the earmold.
2. Check the tubing to see if there are any cracks or looseness in the tubing or receiver.
3. If the feedback persists when the sound outlet is plugged, the mold or tubing or receiver is probably faulty and will need replacement or repair.

---

physical examination and provides a visual measure of the risk for falling for both patient and physician. In addition, all elderly should be assessed for postural changes in blood pressure, disturbances of gait, and changes in proprioception, as well as for adverse reactions to medications or alcohol use, which may also increase the risk of falling. The risk factors reported most frequently in studies of falls are as follows:

- Postural blood pressure decline (20 mmHg postural drop in mean blood pressure)

TABLE 4.   Examples of Communication Devices for the Hearing Impaired

Telephone Aids:

Amplified public telephones
Telephone handset amplifiers
Portable amplifiers
Telephone adapters for hearing aids
Speaker phones
Telecommunication devices for the deaf

Altering Devices:

Flashing-light alarm system
Wrist-worn vibrator
Tactile paging devices

Assisting Listening Systems:

Communication access systems
Infrared systems
AM/FM loop systems

Television and Film Access:

Telecaption adapters
Captioned

TABLE 5.   Hazards

Home:

Inadequate lighting, especially in bathroom and stairs. Light switches should be easily accessible at door of room and near bed.

Low-lying objects, such as foot stools, tables, toddlers, and pets.

Slippery surfaces.

Loose rugs.

Faulty flooring.

Rickety stairs with loose banisters.

Personal:

Improper shoes, especially worn slippers.

Nighttime trips to bathroom; if frequent, consider bedside commode.

- Medication (number and types including tranquilizers, diuretics, antipsychotic and antidepressant medications, and antihypertensives)
- Abnormal vision and hearing
- Decreased mobility; gait disturbances, such as those seen in Parkinson's disease or after a stroke
- Decreased mental status; psychiatric illnesses
- Previous history of a fall
- Decreased ability to perform activities of daily living (needs help with more than two of six activities of daily living—see Appendix A)
- Serious cardiovascular and neurological diseases
- Alcohol use

Some community nursing services have professionals trained in home assessments and can be called upon to make home visits. Patients and their families should be made aware of the home hazards listed in Table 5 and be reminded that most falls occur during usual daily activities in the rooms at home where the patients spend the most time.

Motor Vehicle Accidents.   The second area to focus on for injury prevention is motor vehicle injuries. The risk of crashes for elderly drivers is probably increased in those who suffer from dementia or cardiovascular diseases associated with fluctuation in mental status, or who are unstable.[12] Such patients should be advised not to drive or to restrict driving. Decreased visual threshold and peripheral vision as well as decreased hearing may also contribute to increased risk of injuries and should be brought to the patient's attention.

With regard to motor vehicle injuries, patients should be instructed to follow the recommendations in Table 6; specifically, they should avoid driving on high-speed and unfamiliar roads and driving at night. The elderly should be warned that their ability to drive may be impaired by small amounts of alcohol and by drugs that would not have affected them when they were younger.

A physician who feels a patient is not safe to drive for any of those or other reasons has several options:

1. Counsel the patient on the risks to him or herself as well as to others. Enlist the help of a social worker at the Area Agency on Aging in finding alternate types of transportation. Work with family members to develop a strategy for limiting or eliminating the patient's driving while minimizing the loss

TABLE 6.   Measures to Prevent Auto Accidents

- See your physician if you suspect you have a hearing problem
- Leave your car window partially open to let you hear warning signals. Set the air conditioner or heater and the radio low so that their noise does not mask outside sounds. Place mirrors on both sides of the car and use them and a wide rear-view mirror when you change lanes or pass other vehicles
- Stop frequently to stretch your muscles and rest your eyes.
- Schedule regular eye examinations to check for vision changes or health problems that may affect your vision
- Follow the physician's recommendations, if any, about limiting when and where you drive
- Before driving, give yourself time to adjust to new lenses, especially bifocals or trifocals.
- Wear good quality sunglasses (gray or green are usually best) to reduce glare. Wear them only in the daytime.
- Keep windshield and all windows clean inside and out. Replace worn wiper blades. Keep headlights, tail lights, and turn signals clean to maintain maximum lighting.
- If you take medication, know its long-term and short-term effects on your driving ability
- Do not smoke while driving at night. Smoking impairs vision.
- Do not drive when you have been drinking
- Enroll in a driver-training course through your state motor vehicle department

From AARP: Your Retirement Driving Guide. Pub. #1260 (1079), 1979, pp. 12–13, with permission.

of independence. Beware, for there is a real potential for straining family relationships as well as the doctor-patient relationship.

2. Recommend that the patient be retested (by both a written and a road test) before the driver's license is renewed. This recommendation should be made directly to the Department of Motor Vehicles.

3. Notify the Department of Motor Vehicles that the patient has medical problems that might interfere with driving. This will probably lead to the suspension of the patient's license and should be considered only if the patient represents a significant hazard to himself or herself on the road.

Ambulatory individuals are also at increased risk for injury from a motor vehicle. Patients should be told that the risk of pedestrian injuries is greatest at night. They should be reminded to stand on the sidewalks and not on the street when waiting to cross. Since many elderly are unable to cross intersections during the time alloted by the traffic light, the elderly should ask for assistance when crossing busy streets where traffic lights only allow a short duration for crossing.

Burns.   Finally, it should be appreciated that in the elderly multiple sensory deficits might contribute to their risk for burns. Diminutions in smell may decrease the ability to detect smoke. Therefore, electronic smoke detectors with a loud siren should be purchased and maintained. Similarly, decreased sensitivity to hot and cold coupled with a high temperature setting on a hot-water heater frequently lead to scalds among the elderly. Most hot-water heaters are set at or above 150° F (55° C). Turning the temperature down to 110–120° F will reduce the risk of scalding old, fragile skin.

TABLE 7. Reimbursement Considerations

Reimbursable Items	Items Not Covered
wheelchairs	raised toilet seats
walkers	bath tub seats
hospital beds	safety grab bars
eye glasses	stairway elevators
prosthetic devices	

SUMMARY

The data collected in the history and physical may help identify specific areas for intervention by the physician: cardiovascular and neurologic problems can be treated; medications can be adjusted; and appropriate referrals can be made for vision and hearing evaluations. Other professionals, such as physical therapists, can help stabilize decline and reverse some functional impairments.

The primary care provider is in a position not only to recognize early sensory changes and risk factors for injury, but also to suggest modifications in the environment that will prevent disability. While major renovations or structural changes in an elderly person's environment may be both costly and difficult to accomplish, there are many self-help aids and simple tips that are likely to promote independence. It should be noted that many if not most of these items are not reimbursed by Medicare or Medicaid (Table 7).

PRACTICE RECOMMENDATIONS

1. Incorporate sensory evaluation into routine review of systems.
2. Maintain a flow-sheet of sensory evaluations.
3. Review medications for possible iatrogenic causes of sensory loss (see Table 8).
4. Assess nutritional status for causes of sensory loss such as B_{12} or folate deficiency.
5. Develop a referral network of specialists interested in sensory deficits in the elderly.
6. Routinely screen elderly patients for visual acuity, color perception, and visual fields.
7. Refer all patients with evidence of visual impairment to an ophthalmologist and suggest to a symptomatic patient that routine exams be obtained every two years.
8. Discuss with visually impaired patients the importance of adequate glare-free lighting.
9. Prescribe magnifying glasses for patients with macular degeneration that is still at an early stage.
10. Obtain information on large-print books and newspapers to give to visually impaired patients.
11. Routinely ask all patients questions that will uncover hearing loss.
12. Perform an office hearing evaluation at least once a year and refer all patients with abnormalities to an audiologist.
13. Suggest routine screening by an audiologist every five years.

TABLE 8. Medications Potentially Causing Iatrogenic Sensory Problems*

Health Problem	Medication		Side effects			
	Generic name	Trade name	Eye	Ear	Nose	Mouth
Anxiety	Chlordiazepoxide	Librium	Blurred vision			
	Diazepam	Valium	Blurred vision			
	Meprobamate	Equanil				Dry mouth
Arthritis	Salicylates	Aspirin	Visual disturbances	Tinnitus		
	Phenylbutazone	Butazolidin	Optic neuritis; retinal hemorrhage	Hearing loss		Stomatitis Salivary gland enlargement
	Chloroquine		Retinopathy; blindness			
	Corticosteroids		Cataracts; glaucoma			
	Indomethacin	Indocin	Corneal deposits; retinal disturbances			
Heart disease	Digitalis		Visual disturbances			Anorexia
	Nitroglycerin			Vertigo		Anorexia
Glaucoma	Cholinergics		Miosis; diminished light adaptation; increased tearing		Rhinorrhea	Increased salivation
Hyperlipidemia	Clofibrate	Atromid				Sweet taste to food
Hypertension	Thiazides	Diuril Hydrodiuril		Tinnitus Decreased hearing		Dry mouth
	Furosemide	Lasix		Tinnitus; decreased hearing		Dry mouth
	Triamterene	Dyrenium				Dry mouth
	Reserpine				Nasal stuffiness	
	Methyldopa	Aldomet			Epistaxis	Dry mouth
Infections	Streptomycin Neomycin Kanamycin Gentamiciin			Tinnitus; decreased hearing; Meniere's syndrome		
	Nitrofurantoin	Furandantin		Vertigo		
Muscle cramps	Quinine		Visual disturbances	Tinnitus; vertigo		

* From Mezey M, Rauckhorst L, Stokes S: Health Assessment of the Older Individual. New York, Springer Publishing Company, 1980, pp 52–53, with permission.

14. Teach elderly patients how to position themselves in a room in order to minimize visual and hearing deficits.

15. Advise patients that taste and smell diminish with age and that smoking will further decrease these senses.

16. Inquire about the safety of the home. If there are questions or concerns about the safety of the home environment, make a referral to the physical therapist of a home health-care agency, who can make an in-home assessment.

17. Identify patients with risk factors for falling and orthostatic blood pressure changes. Check proprioception and balance at least once a year.

18. Identify and advise patients who are at increased risk for motor vehicle accidents.

REFERENCES

1. Baker SP, O'Neill B, Haddon W Jr, et al: The injury severity score: A method of describing patients with multiple injuries and evaluating emergency care. J Trauma 1974; 14:187.
2. Bartoshuk LM, Refkin B, Markes LE, et al: Taste and aging. J Gerontol 1986; 41:51.
3. Breslow L, Somers AR: The Lifetime Health-Monitoring Program. N Engl J Med 1977; 22:269–273.
4. Cooper S: Accidents and older adults. Geriatr Nurs July/Aug 1981; 287–290.
5. Corse J: Sensory processes and age effects in normal adults. J Gerontol 1971; 26:90–105.
6. Cummings SR, Kelsey JL, Nevitt MC, O'Dowd KJ: Epidemiology of osteoporosis and osteoporotic fractures. Epidemiol Rev 1985; 7:178–208.
7. Ferris FL: Senile macular degeneration: Review of epidemiologic features. Am J Epidemiol 1983; 118:132–149.
8. Fraunfelder FT, Meyer SM: Safe use of ocular drugs in the elderly. Geriatrics 1984; 39:97–102.
9. Ghafour M, Allan D, Foulds W: Common causes of blindness and visual handicap in the west of Scotland. Br J Ophthal 1983; 67:209–213.
10. Hiatt L: Technology and chronically impaired elderly: Interpretations leading to performance demands and products in institution and community care systems. Paper presented at National Research Conference on Technology and Aging, 1981.
11. Hoffer J: Preoperative evaluation of the cataract patient. Surv Ophthalmol 1984; 29:55–69.
12. Hogue CC: Injury in late life: Epidemiology and prevention. J Am Geriatr Soc 1982; 30:183–190, 276–280.
13. Kahn H, Leebowitz H, Ganley J, et al: The Framingham Eye Study outline and major prevalence findings. Am J Public Health 1977; 106:17–32.
14. Koopmann C: Symposium of geriatric otolaryngology. Otolaryn Clin North Am 1982; 15(2).
15. Mezey M, Rauckhorst L, Stokes S: Health Assessment of the Older Individual. New York, Springer Publishing Co., 1980.
16. Hearing impairment and elderly people: Background paper. Office of Technology Assessment. Congress of the United States. OTA-BP-BA-30. Washington, D.C., U.S. Government Printing Office. May, 1986.
17. Perry BC: Falls among the elderly: A review of the methods and conclusions of epidemiologic studies. J Am Geriatr Soc 1982; 30:367–371.
18. Rubenstein LZ: Falls in the elderly: A clinical approach (Topics in Primary Care Medicine). West J Med 1983; 138:273–275.
19. Rupp RR, Jackson PD: Primary care for the hearing impaired: A changing picture. Geriatrics 1986; 41:75–84.
20. Rupp RR, Vaugh GR, Lightfoot RK: Nontraditional "aids" to hearing: Assistive listening devices. Geriatrics 1984; 39:55–73.
21. Tinetti ME: Performance-oriented assessment of mobility problems in elderly patients. J Am Geriatr Soc 1986; 34:119–126.
22. Tinetti ME, Williams TF, Mayewski R: Fall risk index for elderly patients based on number of chronic disabilities. Am J Med 1986; 80:429–434.
23. U.S. National Center for Health Statistics: Episodes of Persons Injured: United States, 1975. Advance date No. 18. DHEW Publication No. (PHS) 78-1250. Hyattsville, MD, U.S. Dept. of Health, Education and Welfare, 1978.

11
FUNCTIONAL STATUS ASSESSMENT: AN APPROACH TO TERTIARY PREVENTION

Jerry C. Johnson, MD
Mathy D. Mezey, RN, EdD

CLINICAL RELEVANCE

Functional status assessment is a major part of the multi-dimensional process of evaluating elderly patients, and it is essential for effective tertiary prevention.[20,23] Physicians and elderly patients appreciate the importance of functional status, though for different reasons. To patients, loss of function threatens independence. Geriatricians recognize that change in function in a healthy elderly patient is sometimes the earliest manifestation of an acute illness. In addition, routine assessment of functional status can provide the clinician with an indication of a progressing chronic illness and help direct changes in management, particularly in the frail elderly.

Functional status assessment complements disease-specific clinical and physiological data.[10] In some cases, elderly patients with multiple diseases function independently. In other cases, individuals with one disease are seriously disabled and unable to function independently. The clinician cannot assume that among several co-existing chronic diseases, a single acute disease is responsible for existing functional deficits. For example, although congestive heart failure may be the acute presenting diagnosis, the combination of congestive heart failure plus osteoarthritis, mild dementia, and multiple medications may better explain a patient's current functional status than does congestive heart failure alone.

Because of the therapeutic and prognostic implications and the decreased physiological reserve seen in the elderly, accurate identification of disease states is especially important, but the complementary importance of functional status assessment cannot be overstated. A functional status assessment expands the clinician's data base, so that therapeutic emphasis shifts from curing diseases to improving function in some instances and preventing further dysfunction in others. This change in focus can decrease the clinician's sense of frustration and therapeutic impotence often associated with the care of patients with multiple chronic, slowly progressive diseases. Particularly for the frail elderly, functional status assessment provides the clinician one of the most common and important opportunities for tertiary preventive health care. By identifying and addressing existing but unreported functional impairments, the clinician can significantly contribute to improving an elderly individual's daily quality of life.

141

Alterations in functional status threaten independence, suggest the presence of illness, and therefore often prompt elderly patients to seek medical care. Even small deficits may severely impair ability to manage day-to-day activities and independent living. For example, ordinary daily activities for 80-year-olds may require close to maximal energy expenditure.[9] For those individuals close to the thresholds of performance or nonperformance, small improvements or decrements in exercise tolerance can make great differences in functional independence. Severe functional deficits, particularly loss of toileting skills (leading to urinary incontinence) and complete loss of mobility, present the most difficult management problems for caregivers and often lead to frustration and sometimes unnecessary institutionalization.[4] When identified functional deficits cannot be reversed, clinicians in collaboration with other health professionals can obtain assistance for patients in the home, in senior centers or, if necessary, in a nursing home. Caregivers and patients can be counselled, resulting in more appropriate expectations and improved coping skills.

Accurate functional assessment not only benefits patients but also has important health policy implications. Denson and Jones point out the use of functional assessment in regional planning, in monitoring the quality of care, and in policy making.[5,6] Comprehensive assessment, of which functional assessment was a major component, followed by efforts to restore function, resulted in decreased hospitalization rates and mortality in one randomized clinical trial.[19] In addition, functional status has been found to be a better indicator of need for nursing home care than either medical diagnosis or number of chronic diseases.[22,23]

EPIDEMIOLOGY AND COST-EFFECTIVENESS

While the foregoing clinical observations highlight the importance of functional status to patients and clinicians, a greater appreciation is derived from a review of epidemiologic data.[23,24] Most studies suggest that while one of five of the over-65 population reports a mild degree of disability, only a small proportion are severely disabled. Nineteen percent of the elderly have some limitations in their ability to meet such basic self-care needs as eating, dressing, toileting, grooming, physical ambulation, and bathing, or in their ability to carry out activities necessary to maintain themselves independently in the community, such as shopping, food preparation, house cleaning, laundering, and use of transportation. However, only 4% report major disabilities (for example, limitations in performing five or six activities of daily living) and 5% of the elderly are housebound.[24]

In a Swedish study, noteworthy because of its population-based, longitudinal design, 112 women and 93 men aged 79 were randomly selected from the community. No subjects could, without exertion, achieve the recommended walking speed necessary to safely cross a busy intersection between changes in traffic signals.[14] Whereas almost all were able to stand in front of a wash basin when washing, 20% had great difficulty climbing in, sitting down, and getting out of a bathtub, although they preferred using the bathtub to showering.[15] When sitting down and rising from a toilet seat, 38% of the women and 21% of the men used a support such as the wall or bathtub. Other disabilities seen in this same population were difficulty in removing items from shelves, opening jars, and picking up items from the floor.

The rates of functional disability increase with age. Those over 85 are four times more likely to be disabled than those aged 65 to 74. While only 4% of people 65 to 74 need help with dressing, 18% of people over 85 report such a need. Fifteen percent of people over 75 are housebound, whereas this number rises to 20% for people over 80 years of age.

Unfortunately, there is only limited data available at this time concerning the cost-effectiveness of functional assessment. Geriatric assessment units, employing extensive functional assessments, have demonstrated a reduction in acute hospital and total health care costs by reducing re-hospitalization rates and preventing or delaying nursing home placement.[20,21] The cost of maintaining a patient in a nursing home averages $16,000 to $26,000 per year, and studies have suggested that use of functional assessment could prevent inappropriate placement of nursing home residents.[23] Cost-effectiveness solely within out-patient settings has not been studied, although studies are in progress within health maintenance organizations.[8]

FUNCTIONAL ASSESSMENT

Functional assessment measures should meet specific clinical objectives. Usually these are to define the patients baseline function and, on subsequent visits, to determine whether the individual is better, worse or unchanged. To accomplish these objectives, lengthy multidimensional tools used in research are unnecessary and may provide irrelevant information.[7,11] Nevertheless, clinicians should carry out an assessment of function fully analogous and complementary to a careful disease-oriented diagnostic work-up.[23] The types and degree of functional capabilities must be carefully assessed, as well as the extent of family and other resources available for assistance.

Terminology. A discussion of terminology related to functional status measures is necessary before discussing the specific data to be obtained. The domains of functional status include two elements of physical function: self-care activities, such as hygiene and mobility, and the more complex activities required to maintain the person in the community, such as shopping and food preparation. Additionally, mental, emotional and social function, and life satisfaction are sometimes described under functional status.[6,13,20,23] Since another chapter in this book discusses mental and emotional function, this chapter will discuss functional status as defined by physical and social function. Physical self-care activities will be referred to as activities of daily living (ADL), and more complex self-maintenance functions will be called instrumental activities of daily living (IADL).[13] Social competence will refer to the individual's abilities to carry on usual activities at home, at work, if appropriate, and in his or her social and recreational pursuits.

ASSESSMENT PROCESS

Functional assessment data can be obtained by several collaborating health professionals. However, in outpatient settings, such a team often does not exist, and the physician must learn to elicit efficiently as much of the important data as possible. Collaborating health professionals can obtain additional data through visiting nurse associations, home visits, enrollment in day hospitals, or admission to a rehabilitation hospital.

Patients can be observed performing functional status tasks or they can report on their performance, that is, what they have done or what they can do.

Self-reported data may be obtained by interview or by asking the patient to complete a questionnaire. Actual observation of performance is most accurate but can be used only for activities that can be reasonably assessed in a clinical setting and in a reasonable amount of time.[1] Mobility and the ability to transfer from a chair and from an examining table should be directly observed. However, other important activities—social function, self-care and the IADL activities— cannot be rated feasibly by direct observation in an outpatient or acute general medicine setting. Often these data must be obtained by self-report from the patient, or from friends or family. In obtaining self-reported data, an attempt should be made to determine what the patient has actually performed. If a task has not been performed—for example, cooking—this may be a function of personal choice or culture rather than a reflection of health status. Whenever feasible and appropriate—for example, during a hospitalization or home visit— patients should be observed directly.

The clinician should select short, established functional status questionnaires containing questions related to ADL, IADL and social function. The Physical Self-Maintenance Scale and the IADL Scale developed by Lawton are recommended for physical function (Tables 1 and 2). The ADL component assesses six skills: toileting, feeding, dressing, grooming, physical ambulation, and bathing. The IADL scale assesses eight skills: telephone use, shopping, food preparation, housekeeping, laundering, use of transportation, responsibility for taking medications, and ability to manage finances. To assess social competence, questions developed by Benoliel and colleagues are suggested.[2] These questions assess social and recreation activities, usual activities around the home, and work role (Table 3).

Although reliable and valid in discriminating those who function from those who don't, often the ADL and IADL scales are not sensitive to change in condition, particularly among the healthiest patients. Since clinicians are concerned with assessing change over time, it is useful to complement the measures of functional status, which reflect a single state or point in time, with other questions that directly assess change or transition.[17] Using this approach, the clinician first asks each patient his or her own maximal level of function related to a specific activity, thereby establishing a baseline. For example, regarding bathing, the clinician asks the patient to describe how he or she goes about bathing. On subsequent visits, the clinician should ask whether the patient, has more, less or the same level of difficulty in performing this activity. Mobility is readily assessed using this approach. The patient is asked to describe his or her ambulation in terms of maximal performance and need for any assistive device. The clinician then asks the patient at a subsequent visit to state whether his or her best performance is better, worse, or the same as at the baseline visit.

In obtaining functional status data, details are important. Hearing that a patient dresses herself is insufficient. What does "dress herself" mean? Who selects the clothing? Can buttons, zippers and laces be fastened? Often patients take assistance for granted and do not mention some of the assistance required. Washing is an example where patients may claim independence but not indicate that a caretaker is necessary to assist the patient in and out of the bathtub or shower. Additional questions can determine whether patients are satisfied with their performance of an activity and how much effort is required. An activity may be neglected not because of health status but because of lack of interest or motivation. In other instances, functional status may be maintained but require greater effort.

TABLE 1. Physical Self-maintenance Scale (ADL)*

A. Toilet
   1. Cares for self at toilet completely; no incontinence.
   2. Needs to be reminded, or needs help in cleaning self, or has rare (weekly at most) accidents
   3. Soiling or wetting while asleep, more than once a week.
   4. No control of bowels or bladder.

B. Feeding

   1. Eats without assistance.
   2. Eats with minor assistance at meal times, with help in preparing food or with help in cleaning up after meals.
   3. Feeds self with moderate assistance and is untidy.
   4. Needs major assistance in dressing but cooperates with efforts of others to help.
   5. Completely unable to dress self and resists effort of others to help.

C. Dressing

   1. Dresses, undresses and selects clothes from own wardrobe.
   2. Dresses and undresses self, with minor assistance.
   3. Needs moderate assistance in dressing or selection of clothes.
   4. Needs major assistance in dressing but cooperates with efforts of others to help.
   5. Completely unable to dress self and resists effort of others to help.

D. Grooming (neatness, hair, nails, hands, face, clothing)

   1. Always neatly dressed and well-groomed, without assistance.
   2. Grooms self adequately, with occasional minor assistance (e.g., in shaving).
   3. Needs moderate and regular assistance or supervision in grooming.
   4. Needs total grooming care, but can remain well-groomed after help from others.
   5. Actively negates all efforts of others to maintain grooming.

E. Physical Ambulation

   1. Goes about grounds or city.
   2. Ambulates within residence or about one block distance.
   3. Ambulates with assistance of (check one):

      (a)_____ wheelchair, (b)_____ railing, (c)_____ cane, or (d)_____walker;

      1. _____ gets in and out without help; 2. _____ needs help in getting in and out.

   4. Sits unsupported in chair or wheelchair, but cannot propel self without help.
   5. Bedridden more than half the time.

F. Bathing

   1. Bathes self (tub, shower, sponge bath) without help.
   2. Bathes self, with help in getting in and out of tub.
   3. Washes face and hands only, but cannot bathe rest of body.
   4. Does not wash self, but is cooperative with those who bathe him.
   5. Does not try to wash self, and resists efforts to keep him clean.

Start by asking the patient to describe her/his ability to perform a given activity, e.g. feeding. Then ask specific questions as needed.

* Reprinted with permission from Lawton MP: The functional assessment of elderly people. J Am Geriatr Soc, 1971; #19(6):465–481.

TABLE 2.   Scale for Instrumental Activities of Daily Living (IADL)*

A. Ability to Telephone

   1. Operates telephone on own initiative: looks up and dials numbers, etc.
   2. Dials a few well-known numbers.
   3. Answers telephone but does not dial.
   4. Does not use telephone at all.

B. Shopping

   1. Takes care of all shopping needs independently.
   2. Shops independently for small purchases.
   3. Needs to be accompanied on any shopping trip.
   4. Completely unable to shop.

C. Food Preparation

   1. Plans, prepares and serves adequate meals independently.
   2. Prepares adequate meals if supplied with ingredients.
   3. Heats and serves prepared meals, or prepares meals but does not maintain
      adequate diet.
   4. Needs to have meals prepared and served.

D. Housekeeping

   1. Maintains house alone or with occasional assistance (e.g., heavy work
      done by domestic help).
   2. Performs light daily tasks such as dishwashing and bedmaking.
   3. Performs light daily tasks but cannot maintain acceptable level of cleanliness.
   4. Needs help with all home maintenance tasks.
   5. Does not participate in any housekeeping tasks.

E. Laundry

   1. Does personal laundry completely.
   2. Launders small items: rinses socks, stockings, etc.
   3. All laundry must be done by others.

F. Mode of Transportation

   1. Travels independently on public transportation or drives own car.
   2. Arranges own travel via taxi but does not otherwise use public transportation.
   3. Travels on public transportation when assisted or accompanied by another.
   4. Travel limited to taxi or automobile, with assistance of another.
   5. Does not travel at all.

G. Responsibility for Own Medication

   1. Is responsible for taking medication in correct dosages at correct time.
   2. Takes responsibility if medication is prepared in advance in separate dosages.
   3. Is not capable of dispensing own medication.

H. Ability to Handle Finances

   1. Manages financial matters independently (budgets, writes checks, pays rent
      and bills, goes to bank); collects and keeps track of income.
   2. Manages day-to-day purchases but needs help with banking, major purchases, etc.
   3. Incapable of handling money.

Start by asking the patient to describe his/her functioning in each category;
then complement with specific questions as needed.

---

* Reprinted with permission from Lawton MP: The functional assessment of elderly people.
JAGS. 1971; #19(6):465–481.

TABLE 3. Social Competence Activities *

Activities in the Home

Can you describe what your primary responsibilities have been in your home? Has this changed in recent weeks? If yes, in what ways? For example:

> Who prepares the meals?
>> If the patient does, ask if his health has affected this activity.
>
> Who does the shopping?
>> If the patient does, ask if his health has affected this activity.
>
> Who does the laundry?
>> If the patient does, ask if his health has affected this activity.
>
> Who cleans the house?
>> If the patient does, ask if his health has affected this activity.
>
> Who does repairs around the house?
>> If the patient does, ask if his health has affected this activity.
>
> Who does the yard work?
>> If the patient does, ask if his health has affected this activity.
>
> Who runs errands?
>> If the patient does, ask if his health has affected this activity.

Work Questions

A. Do you work? That is, do you receive pay for the work you do? If yes:

1. What kind of work are you presently doing?

2. Are there some things at work you used to do that you aren't doing now?

B. If you don't work, did you stop working for pay because of illness? If yes:

1. What kind of things do you do now that you think of as work? That is, things you are responsible for such as chores around the house, volunteer club duties?

2. Are there some things you used to do that you aren't doing now?

C. If you have never worked for pay or have not worked for pay for a considerable period of time unrelated to current illness:

1. What kind of things have you done that you consider work? That is, things you are responsible for such as chores—yard work, repairs, cooking, cleaning, shopping—or volunteer work?

2. Are there some things you used to do that you aren't doing now?

Recreational and Social Activities

A. What kind of things do you do for recreation or just for fun? What about TV?

B. Has this changed in any way since your illness?

C. How much contact do you have with people not a part of your family, and where does this occur?

D. Do you keep in touch with your friends like you used to?

E. Are there things you'd like to do in the way of recreation or entertainment that you aren't doing right now?

F. What did you do (do you plan to do) on the most recent (upcoming) major holiday?

* Adapted from Benoliel JQ, McCorkle R, Young K: Development of a Social Dependency Scale. Res Nurs Health 1980; #3:3–10.

As with other clinical and physiological measures, the variability of functional status among the elderly is great.[3] The clinician will encounter many elderly who are fully independent and others who are totally dependent. It is with those between the extremes, who are partially disabled or have a chronic disease known to be progressive, where the measures described here are most useful. Screening questions in each category of ADL and IADL should be asked of all patients, but the full ADL, IADL and social battery described in Tables 1, 2 and 3 need not be asked of all patients. A comprehensive clinical examination will help determine who should be asked all questions. For example, a healthy 76-year-old woman with high blood pressure who walks into your office unaccompanied and indicates that she plays golf, drives an automobile, and does volunteer work three days a week need not be asked about feeding and toileting skills. However, an 81-year-old man with a history of gait imbalance and early signs of Parkinson's disease should be asked detailed questions. In all cases, mental status screening as described in Chapter 12 of this book is important to determine the reliability of the patient's responses. If the patient gives evidence of cognitive impairment, a family member should be asked to verify the patient's responses. Definitely impaired individuals should be asked questions about ADL first, then IADL and social function. In contrast, the obviously healthy elderly individual should be questioned about social function first, followed by IADL. If no limitations of IADL and social function exist, questions of ADL are probably unnecessary.

Newly found functional deficits should prompt a thorough evaluation for potential disease processes, either physical or mental. Remediable causes should be treated and the social support system modified to adapt to the patient's level of disability. Medication may have to be adjusted. For example, diuretics in patients with urinary incontinence and immobility may have to be changed for another antihypertensive. Physical therapy may delay deterioration of patients with chronic neurological conditions. Once a pattern of progressive disability is clear, the family should be informed of community and nursing home resources so that adequate planning and intervention can occur.

BARRIERS TO ASSESSING FUNCTIONAL STATUS

Aside from lack of physician appreciation of the importance of obtaining functional status data, the greatest barrier to obtaining these data are time constraints of both the physician and patient. All the data need not be obtained in one visit nor does all the functional status data have to be obtained by the physician. Patients will be fatigued by long questionnaires of 30–60 minutes, but the data asked in Tables 1, 2 and 3 can be obtained in 5–15 minutes. The use of standardized instruments in the tables as guidelines in history-taking will assure that all items are assessed but carries the disadvantage of additional paperwork. Therefore, some clinicians may prefer to incorporate the functional assessment data in the standard clinical record.

When in the encounter should these data be obtained? Frequently, another practitioner, nurse or social worker can obtain data before the physician encounter. The physician will then want to repeat some of the questions and observe the patient directly perform other activities to get his or her own impression of the patient's responses. The timing of specific questions should be individualized. Those patients who are apparently healthy can be questioned as part of the review of systems. With patients known to have chronic disease, functional status questions can be asked along with clinical questions during the history of present illness. For example, in a patient with a stroke, questions of mobility and other ADL naturally follow questions of weakness and balance.

Answers to functional status questions may vary even when the same tool is used.[21] Patients often describe a higher level of performance than is real, and caregivers describe a lower level. Determination of the consistency of responses is helpful. For example, a person who cannot walk with good balance on level ground is unlikely to be able to climb into a bathtub, sit down, and get out unassisted. One who cannot eat without assistance is unlikely to be able to dress independently. When questions remain after discussion with all parties, a home visit is the best way to clarify discrepancies and can be arranged through a visiting nurse association.

Case Example.   An 81-year-old woman presented because of weakness of her legs and increasingly frequent falling episodes of two years' duration. She had no known illnesses and was on no medications. She denied urinary incontinence, syncopal episodes, a past stroke, transient ischemic attacks, or joint pain. On examination, she appeared weak but in no acute distress. There was decreased distal strength in both lower extremities with bilateral foot drops, right greater than left. The upper extremities were also weak and showed marked thenar atrophy bilaterally. The deep-tendon reflexes were normal in the upper extremities but absent at the knees and ankles. There was no Babinski sign and the rectal sphincter tone was normal. She could stand unassisted and walk 3–4 steps, after which she tended to fall because of loss of balance. Her verbal responses were short, often vague and tangential though sensible, and her affect was constricted. Both long- and short-term memory were impaired and she scored 17 out of 30 points on the Mini-Mental State Examination suggesting cognitive impairment.

She lived alone and described complete independence in transferring, eating, dressing, toileting and washing at a basin but could not bathe or shower. A friend visited the patient at least 2–3 hours each day, assisting her with IADL activities. The patient, over the past 12 months, had not left her home, and her only recreational outlet was talking to her friend.

Further evaluation was directed at (1) elucidating the cause of the gait disturbance and cognitive impairment; (2) verifying the patient's competence in ADL; (3) defining the social support system; and (4) improving her mobility. Her physical and mental state contradicted her stated level of function. After multiple hematological and metabolic studies; plain films of the cervical and lumbar spine, and a CT scan of the head and lumbar spine, it was determined that the patient had severe lumbar stenosis with lumbosacral radiculopathies, bilateral carpal tunnel syndrome, and dementia, probably of the Alzheimer's type. Consultation from neurology and psychiatry uncovered no other diagnoses.

The physician contacted the patient's friend and primary care-giver, who consented to a meeting with a geriatric nurse practitioner and social worker; they elicited additional pertinent details. The memory impairment was progressive of 1–2 years in duration. The patient through young adulthood had been fiercely independent, relying on no one for help. Even at the time of the initial evaluation, she was refusing assistance from her friend in some ADL except when absolutely necessary. However, she could not perform any ADL unassisted except transferring from bed to chair and eating. The friend, a neighbor, spent 2–3 hours each day with the patient assisting in ADL as well as shopping. She was becoming increasingly over-burdened and felt over-stressed by the patient's increasing disability. The patient's only relative living in the city, a nephew, had limited power of attorney and managed the finances.

The principal goal of management was to improve ambulation, if possible, and to decrease the frequency of falling. Therefore, the following team effort was organized:

1. The physician explained the nature of the illness to the patient, and to the friend and nephew, and explained the therapeutic options. The patient would not consider any surgical intervention, even minor procedures, to ameliorate the carpal tunnel syndrome, and she wanted to remain in her home.

2. A physical therapy consultation resulted in a brace for the right foot and wrist splints.

3. A nurse specialist counselled the friend on a diet plan that would increase the patient's caloric intake and reviewed safety measures in the home.

4. A social worker counselled the nephew on options for home care and arranged it, and, along with the nurse practitioner, provided three counselling sessions for the friend, advising her on coping skills and community resources to alleviate her burden.

Subsequently the falling episodes stopped. In this case, the diagnostic evaluation was important but insufficient by itself to indicate the patient's needs. First of all, the patient's own report of her ADL performance was inaccurate, underscoring the importance of a concurrent cognitive assessment when evaluating functional status reports of elderly patients. Had the subsequent interview of the care-giver/friend not taken place, the extent of the patient's disability would not have been known. Secondly, the identification of the increasing care-giver burden and stress in caring for the patient led to consultations that benefited not only the patient but also those around her, improving the quality of life of all involved. It was imperative that the physician know the details of the patient's functional abilities in order to develop a comprehensive management and present a baseline for subsequent evaluations. Some of the details were obtained by the physician and others were gleaned through the collaborative effort with nursing and social work. The collaboration both expedited the evaluation and relieved the physician of several hours of work.

SUMMARY

Functional status assessment of elderly patients provides the clinician with important information that complements the regular diagnostic and therapeutic aspects of care. It can offer early indications of the onset of an acute illness in healthy elderly patients and it can provide direction for management of those with multiple chronic illnesses. Even when a disease cannot be eliminated, functional status information offers the clinician the opportunity to prevent unnecessary reductions in a patient's independence and activity by highlighting and translating illness into terms that express its impact and meaning in a patient's daily life. Tertiary prevention, the identification and subsequent minimization of existing disability, is a hallmark of high-quality care for elderly patients. The functional status assessment is a centerpiece of tertiary prevention.

PRACTICE RECOMMENDATIONS

1. Screen all patients for functional status abilities assessing activities of daily living (ADL), instrumental activities of daily living (IADL) and social function (Tables 1, 2 and 3).

2. If functional deficits are obvious—for example, in the case of advanced dementia, Parkinsonism or stroke—then proceed from ADL to IADL to social function.

3. If there are no obvious functional deficits, proceed from social function to IADL. If no deficits are found, then ADL questions need not be asked.

4. New outpatients should be assessed during the first 2–3 visits, and general medical or surgical inpatients should be assessed when clinically stable before discharge.

5. During revisits, changes in functional status should be obtained at a frequency determined by degree of disability and occurrence of important changes in medical conditions or social supports. A person with a chronic progressive disorder should be reassessed every 4–6 months, whereas a generally healthy person need be reassessed only after an acute illness or hospitalization.

6. During revisits, to elicit directly evidence of change in condition for each type of activity, inquire as to whether the patient has more or less difficulty, requires more or less assistance, or is unchanged from some prior time point.

7. Verify the reliability of self-reported data by a screening mental status examination and, in some cases, asking a second person for verification.

8. Ask whether the patient is satisfied with his or her performance of specific activities.

9. Maintain a uniform data base, using the items in Tables 1, 2 and 3 to create a functional status flow chart. Update every 6–12 months.

10. Attempt to determine the medical reason(s) for any identified functional deficits.

11. Enlist the service of social workers, geriatric nurse specialists, rehabilitation therapists and other professionals when necessary. When the physician encounters patients who have a dementing illness and functional deficits or care-givers who are expressing frustration or stress, a social-work consultation is almost always helpful to the patient, family and physician.

12. Modify medications to compensate for functional deficits: for example, diuretics in a patient with gait imbalance may result in urinary incontinence because of the immobility. Psychotropics can further impair all functional deficits.

13. Consider modifications in the social support system; home care programs and senior centers provide a respite for caregivers. A nursing home may be necessary.

REFERENCES

1. Applegate W: Use of assessment instruments in clinical settings. J Am Geriatr Soc 1987; 35:45–50.
2. Benoliel IQ, McCorkle R, Young K: Development of a social dependency scale. Research in Nursing and Health 1980; 3:3–10.
3. Becker P, Cohen H: The functional approach to the care of the elderly. J Am Geriatr Soc 1984; 32:923–929.
4. Brody E: Basic data requirements for geriatric institutions and services. Medical Care 1976; 14:60–70.
5. Densen PM, Jones EW: The patient classification for long-term care developed by four research groups in the United States. In Murnaghan JH (ed): Long Term Care Data: Report of the Conference on Long Term Health Care Data. NCHS, Johns Hopkins University. Philadelphia, PA, J.B. Lippincott, 1976, pp 126–133.
6. Falcone A: Comprehensive functional assessment as an administrative tool. J Amer Geriatr Soc 1983; 31:642–650.

7. Feinstein A: Scientific and clinical problems in indexes of functional disability. Ann Intern Med 1986; 105:413–420.
8. Fretwell MO, Cutler C, Epstein AM: Outpatient geriatric assessment in a health maintenance organization. Clin Geriatr Med 1987; 3:185–191.
9. Grimby G: Physical activity and muscle training in the elderly. Acta Med Scan (Suppl) 1986; 711:233–237.
10. Jette A: Functional disability and rehabilitation of the aged. Topics Geriatr Rehab 1986; 3:1–7.
11. Kane P, Kane R: Assessing the Elderly. Lexington, MA, D.C. Health & Co., 1981.
12. Kane R: Assessing social function in the elderly. Clin Geriatr Med 1987; 3:87–98.
13. Lawton MP: The functional assessment of elderly people. J Am Geriatr Soc 1971; 19:465–481.
14. Lundgren-Lindquist B, Aniansson A, Rundgren A: Functional studies in 79-year-olds: Walking performance and climbing capacity. Scan J Rehab Med 1983(a); 15:124–131.
15. Lundgren-Lindquist B, Grimbly G, Landahl S: Functional studies in 79-year olds: Performance in hygiene activities. Scan J Rehab Med 1983(b); 15:109–115.
16. Lundgren-Lindquist B, Sperling L: Functional studies in 79-year-olds: Upper extremity function. Scan J Rehab Med 1983(c); 15:117–123.
17. MacKenzie CR: A patient-specific measure of change in maximal function. Arch Intern Med 1986; 146:1325–1329.
18. Mezey M, Rauchhorst L, Stokes S: Health Assessment of the Older Individual. New York, Springer Publishing Co., 1980.
19. Rubenstein L: Effectiveness of a geriatrics evaluation unit: A randomized clinical trial. N Engl J Med 1984; 311:1664–1670.
20. Rubenstein LZ: Geriatric assessment: An overview of its impact. Clin Geriatr Med 1987; 3:1–15.
21. Rubenstein LZ, Schairer WS, Wieland GD, et al: Systematic biases in functional status assessment of elderly adults: Effects of different data sources. J Gerontol 1984; 39:686–691.
22. Williams ME: Assessment of the elderly for long term care. J Am Geriatr Soc 1982; 30(1):71–75.
23. Williams TF: Comprehensive functional assessment: An overview. J Am Geriatr Soc 1983; 31:637–641.
24. Aging America: Trends and Projections, 1985–86 Edition. Prepared by U.S. Senate Special Committee on Aging: AARP; FCDA; AOA. Printed USDHHS PF #3377 (1985).

12
OPTIMIZING MENTAL FUNCTION
OF THE ELDERLY

Gary L. Gottlieb, MD, MBA

The American people cautiously welcome increased life expectancy. As the population ages, we increasingly are concerned about the quality of life that can be attained. Middle-aged and elderly individuals concur that a long life is desirable provided that function and, especially, intellectual ability are maintained. Fears about loss of intellectual abilities have been heightened by increasing awareness of pathologic processes associated with aging. Many face the aging process with severe apprehension. They are concerned that they will lose basic human qualities and identity. The aging process may threaten capacities to think, love and communicate. Early recognition of disturbances of cognition and affect allows rapid treatment of reversible etiologies and exploitation of retained assets in chronic and deteriorating conditions. Additionally, optimization of mental ability will strongly influence prognosis, outcome and the need for long-term care.[1]

More than 18% of older adults are thought to suffer significant mental health problems at any given time.[2] However, almost universally, patients and their families depend upon primary care providers to recognize and address complaints related to intellectual and emotional function, specifically depression and dementia.[3] Inasmuch as the elderly consume a substantial proportion of general medical services, prevention and early detection of disorders of high prevalence in this population are essential to successful practice.[4,5] However, the subtlety of mental impairment in this population severely limits the ability of primary physicians to recognize, diagnose and appropriately treat these disorders.[6] This limitation is of great concern in light of an extreme preference among older adults to employ medical providers to care for identified psychiatric disorders.[7]

Mental function explicitly influences all other areas of individual function. The abilities to interact, communicate and autonomously manage personal affairs are concretely controlled by higher-order cortical functions, and virtually all activities of daily living are subject to limitation when cognitive or emotional status is disturbed.

Similarly, medical well-being and health promotion are severely undermined by psychiatric disorders. Compliance with complicated medical regimens is notoriously poor among older adults.[8] Individuals with minor impairments in memory and learning are less likely to be able to follow prescribed protocols. Additionally, older patients with even mild depressive symptoms express a negative perception of their own health status, have more physical complaints, and make significantly more physician visits than do normal elderly patients.[9]

Early recognition of mental disorders is important for a number of reasons. Older adults are extraordinarily vulnerable to central nervous system effects of somatic illnesses and their treatments. The common but unfortunate assumption that changes in mental well-being are part and parcel of the normal aging process may inhibit the practitioner's aggressiveness in determining the etiology of a change in cognition, affect or thought content.[6] One series found that close to 28% of 200 patients carefully evaluated for suspected dementia showed some improvement with appropriate medical or psychiatric intervention.[10] Numerous studies indicate that between 55 and 80% of elderly depressives will respond to psychotherapeutic or somatic treatments.[11–13] However, the reversibility of these disorders appears to be related to early recognition and treatment. Chronic deterioration appears to be a major risk of delayed intervention.[14,15] The cost ramifications of prompt intervention are clear. Improvement in symptoms may prolong productive and autonomous function and postpone or prevent the need for acute or long-term institutionalization. Mental disorders are the most frequently diagnosed problems in nursing homes.[16] Families report that difficulty in managing the behavior of an impaired older adult is of substantial importance in the decision to seek nursing home placement for the affected individual.[17] Early, accurate intervention by the primary care provider can potentially prolong an individual's ability to reside in the unrestricted environment of choice.

Mental disorders are highly prevalent in the elderly population. The exact prevalence of dementia is unknown. Community surveys estimate that severe forms of dementing illness affect more than 5% of people over 65 years of age. Another 10–15% of elderly adults are thought to suffer mild to moderate dementia.[18] Nearly 70% of primary care medical patients who present with evidence of significant cognitive impairment may have Senile Dementia of the Alzheimer's Type (SDAT).[10]

The prevalence of depressive symptoms among the elderly is similarly impressive. Two groups of investigators found a 13–18% point prevalence of depression in large samples of community-residing elderly.[19,20] Studies of elderly medical patients reveal even higher rates (approximately 20%).[6] Suicide rates among the elderly are disproportionately high. This population comprises only 11.9% of the population but accounts for nearly a quarter of all suicides. For example, whereas the suicide rate for the general population is approximately 13 per 100,000, the rate for men in their eighties is close to three times that level.[21] These patients have more somatic symptoms and visit primary care providers more frequently than their nondepressed counterparts, and they rarely are treated by mental health specialists.[8] Therefore, identification and treatment or referral of depression in older adults is within the purview of the skilled and enlightened primary physician.

Prevention and early recognition of these disorders are essential to appropriate holistic care of older adults. Although other mental disorders are common in this population, depression and dementia are probably the most subtle and the most demanding of the clinician's skills.

1. Identify psychosocial and environmental stressors in the patient's life.

Losses and life events have re-emerged as major determinants of psychiatric illness in the elderly.[22] The losses imposed upon individuals by the aging process are numerous. As friends and loved ones die, social isolation may replace firmly-established networks of support. Retirement (or loss of primary function in the home), especially when it is unplanned or forced by an employer or unforeseen circumstances, is strongly correlated with apathy, involution, and depression.[20]

TABLE 1.   Risk Factors for Depression and Depressive Symptoms[20-24]

Grief and Bereavement:

- Loss of child
- Loss/disability of spouse
- Death of siblings
- Death(s) of friends/extended family

Changes in Network of Support:

- Geographic isolation
- Loss of loved ones due to death/illness
- Unplanned retirement
- Lack of confiding relationships

Changes in Physical Function

- Medically imposed limitation
- Limitations in strength/ambulation
- Sensory losses

However, grief and bereavement are probably the most powerful external threats to emotional well-being.[21] Loss of a child or, more commonly, a spouse is an important risk factor for major depression, hypochondriasis, and severe decline in functional status (Table 1).[22]

Although these environmental and psychosocial stressors are unavoidable concomitants of normal aging, their identification by the primary physician can prevent extreme consequences.

2. **Encourage the bereaved or grieving patient to establish at least one intimate and confiding relationship.**

Grief and bereavement can be eased by the establishment of at least one intimate and confiding relationship. At least one researcher has shown that development or involvement in such a relationship can serve to protect against depression.[23] The primary care provider, aware of a recent or impending loss, is equipped to assist the grieving patient in strengthening a relationship with a friend or relative and encouraging its exploitation. The physician can educate family members about the need for this level of intimacy and support. Isolated elderly must be encouraged repeatedly to participate in senior adult programs and, if necessary, group therapies for the bereaved. If no network of support or relationship can be established, a referral for supportive psychotherapy during the period of acute loss may be necessary.

3. **Encourage the person about to retire to plan carefully.**

Retirement can induce depression. However, appropriate planning can mitigate the severity of the patient's response. Individuals who structure their retirement with activities that they value are least likely to suffer depressive symptoms. As soon as the physician is aware of retirement plans, a planning process should be initiated. Social workers, occupational therapists, and career counselors may be extraordinarily helpful in determining available sites for skilled volunteer work, part-time employment, and structured recreational activities.

4. **Assess the extent of loss in the functionally impaired patient.**

Disability resulting from multiple medical, orthopedic, and neurologic conditions must also be seen as a major loss. However, education about the severity of illness, prognosis, and the utility of medication regimens can allow the patient to maintain control and self-esteem when fears about complete dependency become dominant.[24] As disability becomes evident, assessment of patient function (see Chapter 11) is essential. The physician then has adequate data to help improve function while maintaining retained assets. Physical and occupational therapies should be prescribed when tolerable.

Sensory function must be evaluated and optimized. Auditory and visual impairments are common in elderly medical patients. These disabilities naturally heighten isolation and often masquerade as cognitive or emotional disorders. Additionally, sensory losses are associated with both paranoid disorders and depression. Paraphrenic (late life paranoia) disorders are highly correlated with hearing loss and, to a lesser extent, with blindness. Audiometric screening and appropriate use of a hearing aid have been shown to reverse some of these disorders. Additionally, deafness has been argued to "accentuate alienation and discrimination," which may be reversible with the use of an aid.[22] Similarly, cataracts and glaucoma commonly impair vision in the elderly. However, psychiatric symptoms—including confusion, anxiety, fearfulness, and depression—may antecede complaints of visual impairment. Improvement of sensory function may eradicate these symptoms without the need for psychiatric intervention.

SCREENING

All of the risk factors just mentioned can be identified in the process of routine medical history-taking. The description of medical symptoms and related systems review is the essential core of the patient interview. However, the same rapport required to obtain an accurate medical history will allow essential psychosocial data to be obtained.

1. **Include a brief examination of mental status with the primary care evaluation.**

Record appearance, affect, mood, psychomotor function (i.e., retardation or agitation), speech, and thought process and content (including suicidal and homicidal ideation) in the history. Doing so should add little to time requirements. Close attention to these functions will enhance sensitivity to affective disturbances, symptoms of anxiety and panic, paranoid thinking, hallucinosis and other elements of psychosis, and cognitive impairment. The review of systems should also include sleep function, appetite, concentration, memory, and sexual function.

2. **Use an established assessment tool in screening for depression.**

The *Beck Depression Inventory* (BDI) (see Appendix A),[25] has been used in several studies to screen for depression in inpatient and outpatient medical populations.[26] This self-report questionnaire has been validated in geriatric populations and has demonstrated ability to provide important information about patient affective status to primary care providers (a score of over 14 on this test is cause for concern).[26,27] *Zung's Self-Rating Depression Scale* has been used similarly (scores of over 60 are associated with at least mild to moderate depression) (see Appendix A).[28] While some elderly patients (especially those with cognitive impairment) may have difficulty in completing these instruments, they are relatively simple to use and score and require little added time of the practitioner. Data from these screens will heighten clinician awareness of ongoing disorders masked by a focus on medical problems or by the patient's behavior with the provider.[6,26] This information may allow earlier recognition of symptoms and lead to psychosocial or pharmacologic intervention or prompt referral for psychiatric care.

Screening for cognitive deterioration may be impeded by retained social skills, the subtlety of findings, and patient and family denial.[6] The lack of clear age-related norms for intellectual ability (and decline) also hampers efforts to distinguish normal aging from pathology. However, because many of the factors that may impair cognitive function are treatable, the primary care provider must be able to rapidly screen for dysfunction. Several short, structured examinations of cognitive ability are adequate to screen for impairment in memory, concentration and new learning ability. The *Mini-Mental State Examination* (Folstein, et al.) is widely used in clinical research and in clinical practice (see Appendix A).[29] Its correlation with sophisticated psychometric testing has been established, and cut-off scores for "normal" and impaired function have been determined. Orientation, registration, calculating ability (concentration), recall, naming, figure copying, graphic ability, and ability to follow complex commands are superficially screened in only a few minutes. The exam provides a simple method of determining the need for further evaluation and quickly reassessing cognitive status. Cognitive impairment can be documented even more quickly with *Kahn's 10-item Mental Status Questionnaire* (MSQ).[30] This questionnaire is quite limited in scope. (For a detailed description of numerous scales and questionnaires, see *Assessing the Elderly* by Kane and Kane.)

Geriatric depression is a subtle and peculiar entity. The disorder is easily confused with numerous medical conditions. Somatic complaints, disturbances of sleep and appetite, anxiety, and apathy often predominate. Subjectively depressed mood, guilt and suicidal ideation are rarely expressed. Patients insist that the disorder is physical in nature. Gastrointestinal discomfort is common. This complaint, in conjunction with fatigue and weight loss, should precipitate an extensive workup (Table 2). Unquestionably, there is a need for a workup to rule out an occult malignancy, an infectious process (like viral pneumonia or hepatitis), an endocrine disorder (including hypothyroidism, apathetic hyperthyroidism, Cushing's disease, Addison's disease, panhypopituitarism, etc.), CNS disease including Parkinson's disease, SDAT and intracranial mass lesions, and major systemic illnesses such as CHF, CRF and COPD. These disorders often affect mood and function and can impose symptoms resembling those of major depression. However, even completely negative exhaustive workups rarely convince patients that their symptoms are functional in origin.

Scrutiny of medication regimens may uncover an iatrogenic etiology for this change in function and perceived quality of life (Table 3). Many of the pharmaceuticals used by the elderly have adverse central nervous system side effects. Depression is not uncommonly associated with antihypertensives, including reserpine, methyldopa, beta blockers (with the possible exception of

TABLE 2. Medical Disorders Which May Cause Depressed Mood

Occult malignancy	Panhypopituitarism
Infectious process	Parkinson's disease
Hypothyroidism	Dementing illnesses
Apathetic hyperthyroidism	Congestive heart failure
Cushing's disease	Chronic renal failure
Addison's disease	Obstructive pulmonary disease

TABLE 3.   Medications Associated With Depressed Mood[31]

Antihypertensives:	CNS Depressants:
Reserpine	Barbiturates
Methyldopa	Neuroleptics
Beta Blockers (except possibly Atenolol)	Opiates
Hydralazine	Alcohol
Histamine Type II Receptor Blockers:	Other:
Cimetidine	Digoxin
Ranitidine	Oral hypoglycemics
	Steroids
	Cytotoxic agents

atenolol), and hydralazine. Additionally, H_2 antagonists (cimetidine and ranitidine), digoxin, oral hypoglycemics, steroids, and cytotoxic agents may cause depression.[31] Virtually any CNS depressant—including barbiturates, benzodiazepines, neuroleptics, and alcohol—may also precipitate the symptom complex mentioned above.[31]

Frequently, after extensive medical evaluation and reorganization of medications, somatic complaints, vegetative symptoms, apathy and lethargy persist. Despite the patient's argument to the contrary, major depression is a likely diagnosis. Similarly, a patient who has recently suffered an acute illness or trauma (e.g., myocardial infarction or hip fracture), and who is unable to recover premorbid function, should be examined closely. If depression screening and formal mental status examination reveal anorexia, insomnia, fatigue, hopelessness and apathy, consider treatment for depression. Many depressives have "a good reason" for becoming depressed. Support alone, however, is unlikely to remedy the situation or promote recovery from the primary medical or surgical illness.[32] Appropriate treatment of the depression will enhance rehabilitation and permit prompt return to previous functional level. Accurate diagnosis can prevent the need for supervised or skilled care.

Summary.   **Depression in older adults is often diagnosed in the absence of depressed mood.**[31,32] Nearly 20% of elderly depressives present with complaints of physical illness.[31] Appropriate diagnosis requires **appreciation of constricted affect, elicitation of vegetative symptoms, demonstration of pervasive and autonomous dissatisfaction and apathy.** Routine use of the screening instruments may be quite helpful.

Much has been written about cognitive impairment in the presentation of depression in the elderly. The so-called dementia of depression, or pseudodementia, can easily be confused with dementias of other etiologies. Most importantly, much of the memory impairment associated with major depression may be reversible.[33] Considerable controversy exists in regard to the complete remission of dementing symptoms in depressives with cognitive impairment. It is clear, however, that cognition will improve somewhat with improvement in depression, even in patients with mild-to-moderate dementia of organic etiology.[33,34] Discrimination of pseudodementia from a primary degenerative dementia can be quite difficult (Table 4). In the dementia of depression, onset of symptoms is usually more sudden and patients readily admit to awareness of impairment, classically responding with "I don't know" answers rather than confabulating.

TABLE 4. Classical Comparison of Dementia of Organic Etiology
and Dementia of Depression[35]

Organic Dementia	Dementia of Depression
Slow, insidious onset	Rapid onset (days-weeks)
Course: slow; worse at night	Course: rapid and uneven, little variation during evening
Often unaware of cognitive deficit; usually denies problem	Complains of memory loss; problem emphasized
Greater impairment of recent memory and orientation	Greater impairment of attention and concentration
Approximate, perseverative and confabulated responses	Apathetic "I don't know" responses
Emphasizes trivial accomplishments	Emphasizes failures
Inappropriate, shallow or labile affect	Constricted affect
No neurovegetative signs	Possible neurovegetative symptoms (sleep, appetite, bowel, sexual dysfunction)

Additionally, psychomotor retardation is prominent, as are constriction of affect and classic vegetative signs. On cognitive screening, a disorder of concentration and long-term memory are more prominent than the deficits in recall and registration associated with dementias like Alzheimer's disease and multi-infarct dementia (MID).[33]

Management of depression in older adults is a difficult but rewarding pursuit. As with all somatic interventions in the elderly, caution and conservatism are essential. Antidepressant pharmacotherapy is the mainstay of treatment for major depression in the primary care setting. While several psychotherapies have proven efficacy in the management of this disorder, they are not fully proven in geriatric settings, require substantial training, and are impractically time-consuming for primary providers.

Obtain psychiatric consultation for

1. patients with major depression with delusional or other psychotic features;
2. patients with suicidal or homicidal ideation or a previous history of destructive behavior;
3. patients with treatment-resistant depression;
4. diagnostic discrimination of depression from other medical and neurological (e.g., dementia) entities; and
5. patients whose medical condition is threatened because of depressive symptoms or antidepressant interventions.

However, many elderly depressives can be managed successfully by their primary providers. As previously noted, primary care physicians are likely to be the only practitioners whom depressed geriatric patients will accept to provide their psychiatric care.[6]

Heterocyclic (tricyclic and tetracyclic) antidepressants can effectively treat geriatric depression (Table 5). Most of these agents have been in use since the late 1950s, and they appear to have similar efficacy. However, the ability of elderly patients, many of whom are already somatically preoccupied, to tolerate these

TABLE 5. Antidepressant Drug Treatment[31,27]

Drug	Starting Dose	Incremental Change	Approximate Maximum Dose
Nortriptyline (Aventyl, Pamelor)	10 mg/day	10 mg/2–3 days	100 mg/day (check blood level: 50–150 ng/ml)
Desipramine (Norpramin, Pertofrane)	10–25 mg/day	10 mg/2–3 days	150–200 mg/day
Doxepin (Sinequan, Adapin)	10 mg/day	10 mg/2–3 days	150–200 mg/day
Maprotoline (Ludiomil)	25 mg/day	25 mg/2–3 days	150–200 mg/day
Trazadone (Desyrel)	25 mg/day	25 mg/2–3 days	400 mg/day
Phenelzine (MAOI) (Nardil)	15 mg/day	15 mg/5–6 days	60–75 mg/day

agents varies widely. The tricyclics are the most widely prescribed antidepressants. They are notorious for side effects, including cardiotoxicity (arrhythmias, prolonged PR and QT intervals), anticholinergic effects and orthostatic hypotension. Of the large group of agents available, the secondary amine active metabolites of parent drugs amitriptyline (nortriptyline) and imipramine (desipramine) are best tolerated by the elderly. These drugs should be started in extremely low doses and slowly titrated against side effects to a therapeutic level.[31] Assays of blood levels of nortriptyline and desipramine are readily available at commercial laboratories and are useful in titration. Conventional wisdom is that appropriate therapeutic geriatric dosages are about half of usual adult doses (i.e., 25–100 mg per day of nortriptyline and 25–150 mg per day of desipramine). Additionally, doxepin is moderate in anticholinergic effects. However, this tricyclic is associated with significant sedation and orthostatic hypotension and, like the others, should be used with substantial caution. The tetracyclic antidepressant maprotoline was touted initially as having more rapid onset than the tricyclics. Like its predecessors, this drug requires a full two- to six-week trial (geriatric dose range 50–150 mg). However, its low side effect profile makes it attractive for the treatment of geriatric depression.[31]

Chemically unique pharmaceuticals have been marketed more recently. Trazadone has relatively few anticholinergic effects and causes arrhythmias only rarely. Its extreme sedative and hypotensive effects demand slow titration (to doses of 50–400 mg per day).

Monamine oxidase inhibitors (MAOIs) are effective antidepressants, well tolerated by older depressives who are capable of complying with the required tyramine-limited diet. These drugs are generally less anticholinergic than the heterocyclics but cause both supine and orthostatic hypotension.[36] Inasmuch as they are ordinarily employed as "second line" drugs for treatment-resistant patients, institution of MAOIs is best left to the psychiatric consultant. Similarly, electroconvulsive treatment (ECT) for depression can be safe and effective. However, this modality has no place in primary care settings.

All somatic treatments for depression should be supplemented by changes in support network, structured daily activities, and perceived level of function.[31,32] Involvement in senior adult programs, volunteer programs, and active family roles can "speed" the work of antidepressants. Treatment participation by key caregivers or family members can be enormously helpful.

COGNITIVE IMPAIRMENT

Dementia. The prevalence of intellectual impairment among the elderly necessitates appropriate assessment of complaints of memory loss, confusion, and deteriorating functional ability. The purpose of a comprehensive evaluation is to determine whether dementia is present, whether it can be reversed or, if not, how deterioration can be slowed as much as possible.[38] The recommendation for this rigorous workup by a National Institute on Aging task force is based upon numerous reports that between 10 and 30% of cognitively impaired patients suffer from treatable entities.[39] Equally convincing is a large, well-controlled study that indicated that in over 30% of a series of geriatric patients properly evaluated, more than one illness was contributing to the dementia state. Treatment of concomitant medical, neurological, and psychiatric disorders provided at least temporary improvement in 27.5% and sustained gains in 14% of the study group. While improvement was not defined as reversibility, amelioration in quality of life was appreciated by patients and their families (for a complete discussion, see Larson et al., 1985).[10]

The recommended dementia evaluation includes a complete medical and psychiatric history, a review of all medications, a physical examination, a complete neurologic examination, and a mental status exam, including rating with an instrument like the *Mini-Mental-Status*. Laboratory screening includes a complete blood count, electrolytes and liver function tests, VDRL (or RPR), assessment of serum B_{12} and folate levels, CT scan of the head without IV contrast, and a chest x-ray. Admittedly, this is a costly workup. However, the cost savings associated with improvement in intellectual ability and prolongation of relative autonomy is estimated to be considerable.[39]

In Larson's study, the most common "treatable" illnesses associated with or causing dementia were drug toxicity, hypothyroidism and other metabolic diseases, and depression. In all, more than 250 medical illnesses were recognized in 60% of the 200 patients studied. Treatment for many of these entities improved outcome.[10]

The vulnerability of older adults to even the rarest toxic effects of medications must be recognized (see Chapter 5). The sparsest possible pharmaceutical regime—one lacking direct CNS toxins—is recommended for all older patients, and particularly for those with cognitive impairment. All medications should be considered suspect, and agents whose necessity is in doubt should be eliminated whenever possible.

Other medical illnesses that may cause or complicate dementia—including thyroid disease, neurosyphilis, vitamin B_{12} or folate deficiencies, azotemia, hypercalcemia, iron deficiency anemia, substance use disorders (including alcohol), thiamine deficiency, subdural hematoma, CNS tumor, normal pressure hydrocephalus, and depression—should be treated in standard fashion, but with as much cooperation from caregivers as possible.[10]

Most dementias are irreversible. Between 60 and 70% of elderly patients with global cognitive disability suffer senile dementia of the Alzheimer's type.

Another 5% to 15% probably have multi-infarct dementia or questionably reversible normal pressure hydrocephalus.[38] Early recognition of these dementias is important in preventing unnecessary rapid deterioration and in helping families and caregivers to make short-term and long-term plans.

By definition, the clinical diagnosis of a primary degenerative dementia of the Alzheimer's type is one of exclusion. The workup already discussed should identify tangible lesions responsible for cognitive decline. Because of the uncertain nature of the diagnosis and the unpredictibility of the course of the disease, clinicians must be cautious about labeling possibly affected individuals. The mean life expectancy of patients with SDAT from the time of symptom onset is between three and five years.[18] Similarly, patients with MID may sustain long periods of consistent levels of disability before suffering classic "stepwise" deterioration.[40]

Patients with dementia are extremely susceptible to alterations in cognition and function when they become medically ill.[10] Infections, metabolic disturbances, and changes in medication regimens can cause rapid changes in mental status. Any rapid change in function in a patient with a slowly progressive dementia should raise suspicion of the presence of a secondary medical process. Aggressive management of medical illnesses is likely to lead to elimination of "excess disability." Similarly, discontinuation of potentially toxic medications (e.g., anticholinergics, antidepressants [anticholinergic effects may cause confusion and/or delirium], sedative hypnotics, some antihypertensives and antiarrhythmics, digitalis, antiparkinsonians, analgesics, antineoplastics and H_2 antagonists, to name a few) can effect a return to the patient's baseline level of disability.[41]

The primary care physician is likely to be a most important source of information and support for patients and their families. The physician can be supported in this task by well-informed nonphysician providers. Demented individuals often deny their symptoms and are unable to integrate the ramifications of the diagnosis.[18] However, family members and other caregivers can benefit enormously from education about the illness, its possible course, associated symptoms, and available community resources. Appropriate family support can prolong care in noninstitutional settings, protect hard-earned financial resources, and promote prevention and early detection of medical or psychiatric illnesses in the patient. Family members should be encouraged to attend support groups. Family meetings held by the primary physician or other closely involved providers can educate "en masse" all potential caregivers and provide direction for optimal care. Respite for caregivers should be encouraged. Community and private senior adult programs and/or day-care settings (depending upon the level of patient impairment) can supplement available family care. Where resources are available, companions and other home health aides may also be employed. Long-term care provided by family caregivers is not without substantial indirect and direct costs. Depending upon the level of support necessary, home health and respite care may approach institutionalization in actual dollar costs. Additionally, family members may miss days of work, be forced to early retirement, and sustain substantial stress. Renovations of the home environment and the purchase of medical equipment can be quite expensive. As a dementia progresses, these must be weighed against the costs of institutionalization.

Psychiatric symptoms often complicate cognitive decline. In the earliest phases of dementia, moderate anxiety and depression are not uncommon.[42] As the illness progresses, paranoia, hallucinosis, agitation, and insomnia may become prominent. These latter symptoms may be the most difficult for families to manage and may precipitate hospitalization or institutionalization.[42] Any psychiatric symptoms in these patients must be managed holistically. Medical and toxic contributions must be ruled out prior to intervention. Remaining "excess" psychiatric symptoms may respond to pharmacologic intervention. The treatment of concomitant depression in patients with dementia can be very complicated and should be provided by a psychiatrist.

Patients with dementia and agitation or psychosis often have no access to psychiatric care and may respond rapidly to cautious intervention by a primary care practitioner. Very-low-dose neuroleptic medications can be employed successfully in outpatient settings. Haloperidol (Haldol), starting with doses of 0.5 mg per day, is minimally sedative and is low in anticholinergic potency.[43] This drug is usually well tolerated but is associated with a high incidence of extrapyramidal side effects (EPS). Lower potency medications, like thioridazine (Mellaril) (starting at 5–10 mg/day), provide more sedation and less EPS but are more anticholinergic than haloperidol.[41] Any of the neuroleptics should be started at minimal available dosages and increased very cautiously. Notably, they are all associated with reversible and irreversible movement disorders (i.e., EPS and tardive dyskinesias, respectively).[44] Benzodiazepine drugs and other sedative hypnotics should be employed only transiently, as they may promote more confusion and even agitation.[39]

Delirium. Delirium is a "transient organic brain syndrome characterized by acute onset, global impairment of cognitive functions (i.e., perceiving, thinking, remembering) and widespread derangement of cerebral metabolism."[45] This disorder is of extreme importance to the primary care provider. Reports estimate that between 15 and 40% of hospitalized elderly medical patients suffer a delirium of some severity and that delirium is associated with significant morbidity and mortality.[45] It is essential to recognize this mental status change as acute and labile in nature so that proper treatment interventions may be made rapidly. It is particularly important to distinguish delirium from the more chronic dementias. While these entities may coexist, acute changes must be addressed in all patients to ensure return to baseline function.

While delirium and dementia both cause disorientation and memory impairment, other symptoms are not necessarily shared. Delirious patients may also suffer a clouding of consciousness; decreased ability to shift, focus and sustain attention; perceptual disturbances, including illusions and hallucinations; disturbances of the sleep/wake cycle; and changes in psychomotor activity. These symptoms develop within hours or days and can fluctuate over the course of a day.[45] Table 6 provides a straightforward comparison of dementia and delirium.

Detailed descriptions of the etiology of delirium and appropriate treatment strategies are available in Lipowski[41] and Beresin.[43,45] Needless to say, correction of the organic etiology, aggressive medical support, including nutritional and electrolyte maintenance, discontinuation of all possible medications, and constant supervision are necessary. All CNS toxins should be avoided. However, if agitation becomes severe, low dose haloperidol (0.5 mg po or IM q12h) is the treatment of choice.[41,43,45] Ward management of the delirious patient can be simple and effective. The patient's room should be quiet and well lit. A calendar, clock, and chart of the day's schedule should be clearly posted. Patients with eyeglasses and hearing aids should wear them at all times. Familiar possessions

TABLE 6. Delirium vs. Dementia*

Features	Delirium	Dementia
Onset	Acute	Usually insidious
Duration	Brief	Chronic, unless reversible
Consciousness	Fluctuation	Static
Orientation	Abnormal; mistake familiar for unfamiliar	May be normal in mild cases
Memory	Recent defective (registration, retention and recall)	Recent and later remote defective
Attention	Always impaired	May be intact
Perception	Frequently disturbed; contents vivid	Misperceptions may be absent; contents less florid
Thinking	Disorganized; contents rich	Impaired; contents empty and stereotyped
Judgment	Poor	Poor
Insight	May be present in lucid intervals	May be absent
Sleep	Always disturbed	Variable
EEG	Invariably abnormal (slow: fast in withdrawal)	Normal or mild slowing

* From Beresin EV: Delirium in the Elderly: Assessment and Management. Clinical Perspectives on Aging No. 3. Philadelphia, Wyeth Laboratories, 1985, with permission.

from home can help orient the patient and family members should be asked to stay by the bedside as long as possible. Consistency in staff caretakers should be maintained. The patient should be as free to move as possible and should be able to communicate freely with staff members.[45]

PRACTICE RECOMMENDATIONS

1. Incorporate questions about living situations, work, relationships, recent losses, function, interest, activity, appetite and sleep in the medical history and review of systems. This will require little time and provide helpful data.

2. When extensive workups for somatic complaints (especially GI and pain syndromes) are negative, be suspicious about depression, even in the absence of depressed mood.

3. Set up a system so that self-administered rating scales for depression can be distributed and completed in the patient waiting area and scored by administrative personnel before the beginning of an office visit (see Appendix A).

4. Bear in mind that cognitive screening can be performed by any health care personnel. Required training is minimal, and structured instruments like the Mini-Mental-State (see Appendix A) can be integrated with routine triage and recording of vital signs. If nursing personnel are readily available, a standard functional assessment can be added (see Chapter 11).

5. Include forms to record the MMS in the chart. Formal mental status examination requires only a small amount of physician time and various elements can be obtained during routine history taking and the physical examination.

6. Establish a relationship with a single psychiatric consultant who is skilled in dealing with medically frail populations and the elderly, in particular. In this way, informal consultation can supplement formal evaluations and ongoing mutual education can improve clinical practice.

7. Use all available social work support to establish a resource data base. Closely allied social workers from local hospitals, social and private agencies, and those employed by group medical practices can be enormously helpful in the management of older medical patients. They may be key figures in providing support and counselling for family caregivers.

8. Have each patient's medication regimen listed on the front of the chart. This will allow rapid scanning and scrutiny if changes in mental function occur. Ask the patient and family about over-the-counter medications and drugs prescribed by other physicians.

REFERENCES

1. Whitney FW: Alzheimer's disease: Toward understanding and management. Nurse Practitioner 1985; 10(9):25–36.
2. Myers JK, Weissman MM, Tischler GL, et al: Six-month prevalence of psychiatric disorders in three communities. Arch Gen Psychiatry 1984; 41:959–967.
3. Brody EM, Kleban MH: Physical and mental health symptoms in older people: Who do they tell? J Am Geriatr Soc 1981; 29:442–449.
4. Haas WH, Crandell LA, Bain DJ: Characteristics of family practitioners with large geriatric practices. J Am Geriatr Soc 1980; 28:289–293.
5. Nixon SA: The family physician's role in the care of the elderly. J Am Geriatr Soc 1982; 30:417–420.
6. Waxman WM, Carner EA: Physicians' recognition, diagnosis and treatment of mental disorders in elderly medical patients. The Gerontologist 1984; 24:593–597.
7. Waxman HM, Carner EA, Klein M: Underutilization of mental health professionals by community elderly. The Gerontologist 1984; 24:23–30.
8. Conrad K: Compliance with drug therapy. In Conrad K, Bressler R (eds): Drug Therapy in the Elderly. St. Louis, C.V. Mosby Co., 1982.
9. Waxman HM, Carner EA, Blum A: Depressive symptoms and health service utilization among community elderly. J Am Geriatr Soc 1983; 31:145–149.
10. Larson EB, Reifler BV, Sumi SM, et al: Diagnostic evaluation of 200 elderly outpatients with suspected dementia. J Gerontol 1985; 40:536–543.
11. Gallagher DE, Thompson LW: Effectiveness of psychotherapy for both endogenous and non-endogenous depression in older outpatients. J Gerontol 1983; 38:707–712.
12. Weiner RD: The role of electroconvulsive therapy in the treatment of depression in the elderly. J Am Geriatr Soc 1982; 30:710–712.
13. Koch-Weser J: Psychotropic drug use in the elderly (Part 2). N Engl J Med 1983; 308:194–199.
14. Stoudemire A, Thompson TL: Recognizing and treating dementia. Geriatrics 1981; 36:112–120.
15. Butler RN: Psychiatry and the elderly: An overview. Am J Psychiatry 1975; 32:899–900.
16. Goldman H, Feder J, Scanlon W: Chronic mental patients in nursing homes: Re-examining data from the National Nursing Home Study. Hosp Commun Psychiatry 1986; 37:269–272.
17. Secretary's Task Force on Alzheimer's Disease, U.S. Dept. of Health and Human Services, DHHS Publication No. (ADM) 84-1323. Washington, D.C., 1984.
18. Schneck MK, Reisberg B, Ferris SH: An overview of current concepts of Alzheimer's disease. Am J Psychiatry 1982; 139:165–173.
19. Gurland B, Dean L, Cross B: The epidemiology of depression and dementia in the elderly: The use of multiple indicators of these conditions. In Cole JD, Barrett JE (eds): Psychopathology in the Aged. New York, Raven Press, 1980.
20. Murrell SA, Himmelfarb S, Wright K: Prevalence of depression and its correlates in older adults. Am J Epidemiol 1983; 117:173.
21. Frederick CJ: Current trends in suicidal behavior in the United States. Am J Psychother 1978; 32:172–200.
22. Arie T: Prevention of mental disorders of old age. J Am Geriatr Soc 1984; 32:460–465.
23. Murphy E: Social origins of depression in old age. Br J Psychiatry 1982; 141:135.

24. Brown GW, Harris TD: Social Origins of Depression. London, Tavistock Press, 1978.
25. Beck AT, Ward CH, Mendelson M, et al: An inventory for measuring depression. Arch Gen Psychiatry 1961; 4:561.
26. Nielson AC, Williams TA: Depression in ambulatory medical patients. Arch Gen Psychiatry 1980; 37:999–1004.
27. Gallagher D, Nies G, Thompson LW: Reliability of the Beck Depression Inventory with older adults. J Consult Clin Psychol 1982; 50:152–153.
28. Zung WW: A self-rating depression scale. Arch Gen Psychiatry 1965; 12:63–70.
29. Folstein MF, Folstein SE, McHugh PR: Mini-Mental State: A practical method for grading the cognitive state of patients for the clinician. J Psychiatr Res 1975; 12:189–198.
30. Kahn RL, Goldfarb AL, Pollack M, Peck A: Brief objective measures for the determination of mental status in the aged. Am J Psychiatry 1960; 117:326–328.
31. Busse EW, Simpson D: Depression and antidepressants and the elderly. J Clin Psychiatry 1983; 44:5 (Sec.2):35–39.
32. Fogel BS, Fretwell M: Reclassification of depression in the medically ill elderly. J Am Geriatr Soc 1985; 33:446–448.
33. McAllister TW, Price TR: Severe depressive pseudodementia with and without dementia. Am J Psychiatry 1982; 139:626–628.
34. Kramer BA: Depressive pseudodementia. Psychiatry 1982; 23:538.
35. Snyder S: Application of neurology to psychiatry. In Kaplan HI, Sadock BJ (eds): Comprehensive Textbook of Psychiatry, 4th ed. Williams and Wilkins, Baltimore, 1985.
36. Goldman LS, Alexander RS, Luchins DL: Monoamine oxidase inhibitors and tricyclic antidepressants: Comparison of their cardiovascular effects. J Clin Psychiatry 1986; 47:225–229.
37. Winograd CH, Jarvik LF: Physician management of the demented patient. J Am Geriatr Soc 1986; 34:295–308.
38. Larson EB, Reifler BV, Featherstone HJ, English DJ: Dementia in elderly outpatients: A prospective study. Ann Intern Med 1984; 100:417–423.
39. National Institute on Aging Task Force: Senility reconsidered: Treatment possibility for mental impairment in the elderly. JAMA 1980; 244:259–263.
40. Hachinski V: Cerebral blood flow: Differentiation of Alzheimer's disease from multi-infarct dementia. In Katzman R, Terry RD, Bick KL (eds): Alzheimer's Disease: Senile Dementia and Related Disorders. New York, Raven Press, 1978.
41. Lipowski ZJ: Transient cognitive disorders in the elderly. Am J Psychiatry 1983; 140:1426–1436.
42. Winograd CH, Jarvik L: Physician management of the demented patient. J Am Geriatr Soc 1986; 34:295–308.
43. Beresin EV: Delirium. In Sederer LI (ed): Inpatient Psychiatry: Diagnosis and Treatment. Baltimore, Williams and Wilkins, 1983.
44. Ayd FJ: Haloperidol: Twenty years' clinical experience. J Clin Psychiatry 1978; 39:807–814.
45. Beresin EV: Delirium in the elderly: Assessment and management. Clinical Perspectives on Aging No. 3. Philadelphia, Wyeth Laboratories, 1985.

13
PREVENTING ELDER ABUSE
AND NEGLECT

Elizabeth Capezuti, RN,C, MSN

The identification of the abused patient, regardless of age, is one of the most difficult tasks in clinical practice. Most older adults live at home because of support by family caregivers; it is mostly a myth that the American family has abandoned its aged members. When an older person is in need of assistance to continue living independently, he or she is quite likely to turn first to the family for help. Few older people receive assistance from formal social service or health organizations. It is the informal support system, i.e., the family, that provides a wide variety of assistance ranging from transportation and shopping to complete 24-hour-per-day care of all basic needs. Despite the strain of some of these tasks, most families accept these responsibilities. Unfortunately, some caregivers do abuse and neglect the elderly. Since the only contact outside of the home for some of these older persons may be visits to the family physician, it is essential that physicians be able to detect abuse accurately and intervene appropriately for the elder abuse victim.

Recently, the Council on Scientific Affairs of the American Medical Association issued a resolution for the development of diagnostic and treatment guidelines concerning elder abuse and neglect by a multidisciplinary task force (Table 1). Additionally, the AMA has distributed to state medical associations model state legislation for mandatory physician reporting of elder abuse.[1] These actions indicate recognition by the medical profession of the problem's significance and the role of the physician in prevention, identification an management of abuse and neglect.

DEFINITIONS AND CATEGORIES

Categories of abuse include material, physical, sexual, and psychological/ emotional categories. **Material or financial abuse** is the misappropriation of funds or other resources.[2] This can include failure to disburse available funds for needed services or equipment because the caregiver refuses to deplete the elder's assets. **Physical abuse** is the "infliction of physical pain or injury as well as physical coercion such as confinement against one's will."[3] Physical abuse includes being slapped, hit, cut, burned or physically restrained. In discussions of elder abuse, it is physical abuse that usually comes to mind because of its obvious manifestations. In contrast, **sexual abuse,** particularly if the victim is elderly, is a form of abuse most people, including physicians, are reluctant to acknowledge. This avoidance, unfortunately, results in decreased recognition of its occurrence. Sexual abuse is defined as "any form of sexual intimacy between two persons

TABLE 1.   Resolution 112 (adopted June, 1986)
by The American Medical Association*

Recommends the AMA:

1. To initiate the establishment of a multidisciplinary task force to develop preventive, diagnostic and management strategies specific to elder abuse and neglect.

2. To organize a national program addressing elder abuse and neglect through state medical societies.

* Source: Council on Scientific Affairs: Elder abuse and neglect. JAMA 1987; 257(7):966-971.

either without consent or by force or the threat of force."[4] It is also the inability to give adequate consent, as may be seen with chronic dementia or the older mentally retarded person. **Psychological/emotional abuse** is the infliction of mental anguish, which includes yelling, insulting, threatening or silence. Psychological abuse is difficult to assess and therefore difficult to manage appropriately. The manifestations are more subtle, unlike the bruise or burn associated with physical abuse. It is also easier to intervene with a caregiver who feels guilt because of a physical injury inflicted on an older person. The results of psychological/emotional abuse, i.e., humiliation, intimidation, isolation and infantilization,[4,5,6] may not be as obviously damaging as a fractured rib. Psychological abuse often plays a significant role with other types of abuse, as well. Regardless of type, abuse implies an active intervention by the abuser.

Neglect, on the other hand, can be either a passive or active failure by a caregiver to provide adequate care. **Passive neglect** occurs when caregivers lack knowledge about proper care, for example, the caregiver who is unaware of the need for ambulation or change in position to prevent decubiti, contractures or pneumonia. In contrast, **active neglect** occurs when the caregiver understands how to properly care for the older person, or is aware of resources, and yet does not "intervene to resolve a significant need."[7] Neglect indirectly produces physical manifestations, as compared to physical abuse that directly results in objective changes. One might assume that neglect is not as serious a problem as abuse, but if undetected or untreated neglect may have life-threatening consequences.[8] Inadequate nutrition, misuse of medications or oversedation with tranquilizers, inappropriate treatment of decubiti, urinary tract infections, and fecal impaction are all examples of caregiving failures that lead to a chronic decline in the older person's ability to combat serious illness. Pneumonia or sepsis secondary to infected decubiti may become more resistant to treatment. Neglect may initially appear less serious compared to abuse, yet over time it may in fact have more deleterious effects.

SIGNIFICANCE OF THE PROBLEM

It is believed that about 4% of elderly Americans or about 1.1 million older persons are victims of abuse each year.[9] Accurate statistics are not available because a national survey has never been conducted, and, in truth, actual figures would no doubt be impossible to obtain. Figures are derived from a few studies with small samples. The majority of these involved interviewing professionals or reviewing records instead of direct interviews with the abused or the abusers, thus further weakening their usefulness.[9]

Nonetheless, the elder-abuse literature, coupled with the substantial data on child and spouse abuse, indicates that primary care physicians and emergency rooms are important gatekeepers in the recognition and follow-up of victims of domestic violence.[11,12] The elderly visit physicians' offices more frequently than younger persons due to the greater likelihood of chronic illness. These continued contacts with the older person over time places the physician in an ideal position to detect signs of abuse and neglect as well as identify potential victims. Although emergency room staff may witness the more obvious signs of abuse, it is through a long-term physician-patient relationship that the clinician has an advantage in observing subtle changes in health status and can therefore play a significant role in preventing serious illness or injury.

PREVENTION

Nationally, violence has been recognized as a major cause of early or premature death. Projects such as the violence epidemiology program at the Center for Disease Control and the Surgeon General's inclusion of violence as a priority in the national prevention strategy of the U.S. Public Health Service challenge both researchers and clinicians to confront the issue of abuse. Instead of viewing violence as solely a law enforcement problem, the current view is that abuse is a public health problem.[13]

Increasing the awareness and knowledge of physicians and other health professionals is the initial step in addressing abuse as a public health problem.[14] Such education contributes to primary prevention of abuse and neglect through identification of high-risk older persons and families. Secondary and tertiary prevention, especially through early recognition of abuse or neglect, can prevent further harm to the victim and serious illness. Preventive and screening strategies decrease the likelihood of multiple emergency room visits, hospitalization, and death. The chronically abused or neglected older person may, over time, decline to such a poor state of health that standard medical intervention will not resolve an acute illness. The costs of community resources such as respite care, in-home services, and counseling may be considerably less than acute-care hospitalization or long-term nursing home placement. Promotion of the integrity of family relationships is the underlying concern of these efforts. The physician needs to be keenly aware of middle aged family caregivers and the potential for abuse and neglect in order to facilitate independence and health for all aging family members.

EVALUATION OF ABUSE AND NEGLECT

Direct observation of abuse is unlikely, making careful assessment of physical and behavioral indicators of abuse or neglect imperative. The detection of actual or potential abuse is difficult because the symptomatology is rarely clear-cut or easily available. Most elderly persons would prefer to hide acts of abuse against them by family members or other caregivers on whom they depend for their daily care. For elderly persons, identification by their physicians of abuse by children or other family members is extremely embarrassing. In fact, older persons may blame themselves for the abuse. In addition, some older persons are unable to communicate the problem due to dementia or expressive aphasia. To complicate the picture further, it is not always easy to distinguish some signs of abuse from normal age changes. For example, ecchymosis may be related to capillary fragility, or a fractured bone to osteoporosis.[15] Nevertheless, current research efforts have uncovered significant indicators for the evaluation of abuse and neglect. The unique approach of geriatric practitioners of focusing on functional assessments and viewing the older person within the context of the family or possibly caregiver relationship facilitates both the screening for and prevention of abuse and neglect.

FUNCTIONAL AND CAREGIVER ASSESSMENT

Although the elderly are more likely to have at least one chronic illness and many will have two or more health problems, it is the effect of those illnesses on daily living that is most important when evaluating an older person. Questions regarding the ability to perform activities of daily living (see Chapter 11) give the physician information about the level of dependency of an older person on the caregiver. Functional assessment may reveal problems that can be corrected through treatment or rehabilitation services; for example, weakness in a wheelchair-bound older person may be relieved with a change in medication or through ambulation training. Problems with eating or dressing secondary to stroke may be decreased with assistive devices. Functional assessment provides information about both the current level of functioning as well as potential areas for improvement in independent activity.

Asking the older person to describe a typical day may shed some light on how much an individual is stimulated versus neglected. For example, is the person physically restrained in a chair or left to stare out a window all day when the caregiver goes to work? Description of one's day also reveals important information affecting health such as frequency of meals, toileting and exercise. The caregiver's role, and his or her possible need for assistance, also becomes more apparent with careful, yet probing, questions.

Whenever suspicion of abuse or neglect exists, the older person and caregiver need to be interviewed separately to allow each person an opportunity to describe perceptions of the situation. Ascertaining role expectations, that is, what both expect their parts in the relationship to be, is essential if problems such as caregiver burnout are to be recognized. Caregivers who never seek assistance from other family members or "outside" community resources, and never take time for personal needs, can eventually come to the end of their rope. This selfless style of caregiving can lead to frustration with a potential for abuse.

Understanding how each family member views the illness and subsequent functional abilities is also helpful in uncovering actual or potential problems. For example, an elderly person who perceives himself as a "cardiac cripple" may place unfounded demands on caregivers. The caregiver may feel used or manipulated and respond with anger. The physician can intervene through patient and family education. Explaining the realistic limitations of the older person's illness can prevent some of the miscommunication that contributes to abuse. Thus, the assessment of functional status, description of a typical day, and the perceptions and attitudes of the older person and the caregiver are all essential components of the interviewing process when abuse or neglect is suspected.

RISK ASSESSMENT

Abuse or neglect is rarely presented as the "chief complaint." It is much more likely that the older person will attempt to hide abuse or neglect by family members or other caregivers on whom they depend for assistance.[16] Despite the sparcity of research, studies have revealed some consistent findings regarding risk factors for abuse and neglect. These factors may help identify those suffering from abuse and neglect as well as identify the characteristics of those families with the potential to abuse.

The High Risk Older Person. Most investigations have found that the abused are more likely to be women and the "old-old," i.e., 75 years of age or older.[17,18,19] Due to gender differences in life expectancy, men are less likely to live as long as women or to live alone. Elderly men are likely to have younger, healthier wives who care for them. On the other hand, these same women will eventually be widowed. Elderly women more often are poorer and have a higher potential for dependency on adult children or other family members for assistance. With increasing age comes the increased likelihood of physical or mental impairments that impede the ability to function independently. The dependent, older woman is more at risk for neglect, especially if her needs exceed the caregiver's resources.[20,21] The abused older person frequently lives with the abuser.

The High-Risk Abuser. First of all, caregivers suffering from physical or mental problems are less likely to care adequately for an older person and are more likely to be neglectful or abusive. At particular high risk are those suffering from psychopathology, drug addiction or alcoholism.[22] In addition, emotional immaturity, coupled with unresolved dependency issues, may have implications for abuse.

Second, elder abuse may be one of many types of family violence within the home. Verbal and physical abuse in reaction to stress may be acceptable behavior in the family system. Therefore a history of child or spouse abuse needs to be considered in assessing the abilities of families to care for their elders. A history of other abusive or violent behavior such as homicide or suicide also provides significant data.

A third consideration regarding the caregiver's manifestation of anger toward the older person through abuse is dependency. Recent evidence suggest abusers are more likely to be dependent on their elderly victims in cases of abuse (vs. neglect).[23,24,25] Frequently, the abuser may depend on the victim for financial support. The abuser can be an adult who has never been able to separate from his or her parent. He or she feels powerless in the relationship and displays his or her anger in a variety of abuses: physical, psychological/emotional, sexual or financial. This type of dependency-related abuse has also been seen in marriages in which the husband is severely disabled because of dementia or stroke. The wife who is the primary caregiver is abused by the husband, who feels frustrated and powerless by his decreasing physical and/or mental abilities.[26] However, situations in which the abuser is dependent on the victim have not been linked to cases of neglect.

The manifestations of neglect such as dehydration, malnutrition, frequent UTIs, multiple decubiti, etc. may go unrecognized as indicators of inadequate care. In these cases the neglected older adult usually depends on the caregiver for assistance, yet the caregiver cannot meet the elder's needs for a variety of reasons. Frequently, the caregiver receives little respect or understanding from other family members. A number of studies have documented the social, emotional, physical and financial stresses of caregiving.[27,28,29] Data derived from the 1982 National Long-Term Care Survey[30] reveal a committed caregiving population with multiple responsibilities. Caregivers are more likely to be women, either wives or daughters.

The average age is 57, although one fourth are over 65. Almost three fourths live with the care recipient. One third have family incomes in the poor or near-poor category. Many female caregivers have stopped working or reduced their working hours in order to assist a relative at home. With respect to other commitments, one fourth of caregiving children have children under the age of 18 in the same household. Brody[31] has described these women as "in the middle," i.e., middle-aged women with responsibility for caring for children and parents. Caregiver stress or "burnout" is considered a significant risk factor in neglect.

Demands of caregiving may result in increasing isolation for the caregiver, who may have fewer outlets for enjoyment and receive little or no recognition for their difficult work. Frequently, families are not aware of the extensive time and energy required to care for an ill family member at home. Particularly with demented elders, problems like wandering, insomnia, incontinence, agitation and paranoia are disturbing for the caregiver and other members of the household. Formal support systems such as visiting nurse services and adult day care are not used by the majority of caregivers, probably due to high out-of-pocket expenses as well as lack of knowledge about such services.

Risk factors are indicators of potential or actual abuse or neglect. When one's suspicion is raised, more substantial assessment of abuse and neglect needs to take place.

SIGNS AND SYMPTOMS

Identifying those at risk for abuse and neglect is critical before a thorough evaluation of this problem can be addressed. The interview should then proceed from the least threatening questions, i.e., functional assessment and caregiver supports, to a more directed inquiry. Obviously, a long-term physician-patient/family relationship makes this task easier.

History.[32] When seeing an elderly patient for the first time, carefully review any past medical records. A history of "doctor shopping or hopping" may be as indicative of a family's attempt to hide a pattern of repetitive injuries as are multiple emergency room visits to different hospitals. Such behavior is characteristic of a family in an abusive cycle. Such families do not establish a relationship with one physician, thereby preventing the opportunity for the physician to uncover the abusive situation.

Whenever delays have occurred between onset of trauma or illness and presentation to the physician, suspicions about abuse or neglect should increase. A caregiver may initially think the problem will resolve without medical care. When the caregiver realizes the problem is not resolving, i.e., the older person cannot ambulate or has lost the function of an arm, help is sought. It is also suspicious when someone other than the primary caregiver brings the person to the physician's office or the emergency room. This "other" person knows little of the older person's health status, medications, daily functioning, and so forth. The inability to answer questions may be a way to block the physician's probing of the etiology of an injury or of inadequate care. Any history that is incompatible with the extent of injury or illness needs further exploration. For example, symmetrical bruises on the upper arms are highly unlikely with a fall from bed. Also, a decubitus exposing the bone does not develop over a few days. This incomplete or questionable history should always alert the physician to a situation requiring close scrutiny and follow-up (Table 2).

TABLE 2.   "Red Flags": Signs and Symptoms Specific to Elder Abuse*

Any history incompatible with the injury or illness.

Older person is overly anxious only in presence of caregiver.

Symmetrically located bruises or injuries.

Imprint injuries.

Rope burns on ankles or wrists.

Unusually located burns or bruises

* Sources: Tomita S: Detection and treatment of elderly abuse and neglect: A protocol for health care professionals. Physical and Occupational Therapy in Geriatrics 1982; 2(2):37–51.

Johnson D: Abuse of the elderly. Nurse Practitioner 1981; 6(1):29–34.

Mental Status.[33]   An older person who presents as fearful or overly anxious during the history or the examination may be afraid to "say the wrong thing." Again, interviewing and/or examining the person separately from the caregiver may provide a safe environment for expression of one's real fears. Separating the older person and the caregiver is also indicated when the caregiver answers all the questions for the parent and/or belittles his or her ability to remember or to present an adequate health history.

The depressed or withdrawn caregiver may indicate a lack of interest in the care of the older person. Exploration of issues during the interview should proceed with caution, since probing may spark anger or discontinuation of future visits to the physician. The physician needs to establish trust with the abuser before he or she will admit the abuse or will accept help. This is also true with the abused older adult. Depression or passive behavior on the part of the elder may be an indicator of resignation to the abusive situation. Therefore, the admittance of abuse or neglect may take several interviews.

The older person presenting with disorientation, confusion or extreme lethargy may be the victim of chemical restraints (tranquilizers or hypnotics), or of malnutrition or dehydration. Displays of paranoia and anxiety in the presence of the caregiver, as in true dementia, need careful assessment. Such behaviors may be related to fear of the abusive caregiver. At this point, the physician needs to make inquiries of other family members or friends who are able to provide further information regarding the older person-caregiver relationship.

Physical Examination.[34,35]   Occasionally elderly persons may refuse to disrobe completely due to embarrassment or difficulty in removing clothes, e.g., tight-fitting girdles or corsets. Such behavior may also indicate an attempt to hide injuries located centrally on the body. Sometimes, abusers will only inflict bruises in areas covered by clothing. Similarly, the elderly woman who refuses a pelvic and/or rectal exam may be hiding injuries related to sexual abuse. Hematomas located on the inner thighs strongly suggest forced intercourse. Decreased vaginal and rectal sphincter tone are also highly suspicious signs. With recurrent vaginal and urinary tract infections, sexually transmitted disease secondary to abuse should be considered.

Bilateral, symmetrical injuries such as hematomas on upper arms and axillae or rib fractures are important clues of forceably holding, grabbing or shaking a person. Fractures, dislocations and sprains need to be explored within the context of other signs and symptoms suspicious of abuse. Imprint injuries (bruises that retain the shape of the object) are strong physical indicators of

TABLE 3. Potential Signs of Neglect*

Decubiti

Dehydration

Malnutrition

Urine burn excoriations

Frequent urinary tract infections

Contractures

Oversedation

Over or under use of medications

Inappropriate clothing

Untreated medical problems

* Sources: O'Malley TA: Identifying and preventing family mediated abuse and neglect of elderly persons. Ann Intern Med 1983; 98(6):998–1005.

O'Malley TA: Categories of family mediated abuse and neglect of elderly persons. J AM Geriatr Soc 19 ; 32(5):362–369.

abuse. Examples include a belt buckle and an iron. A person physically restrained will have rope burns or marks of the ankles or wrists. A bruise across the cheeks or the mouth may be the result of forced feedings or being gagged to silence. Several hematomas and/or injuries in different stages of resolution may reflect abuse over a long period of time.

Burns in an unusual location, such as cigarette burn on the back, is highly significant. Spotty absence of hair as opposed to the usual hair loss pattern of central alopecia of aging men can be due to vigorous hair pulling.

The signs of neglect are often more subtle (Table 3). It is easier to attribute signs of inadequate care to increasing age. Although it is true that falls may be due to a variety of neurological and cardiac causes and may have serious consequences secondary to osteoporosis, the frequency and/or poor explanation for causes can point to abuse. Dehydration and malnutrition and less clear-cut problems, often explained as the older person's lack of appetite. Poor personal hygiene can be presented as lack of interest or refusal to be cleaned by others. Frequent urinary tract infection and/or fecal impaction may be attributed to the effects of age, because under or overuse of medications or not seeking medical attention for illness or injury can be easily labelled as "noncompliance."

Poor muscle tone and stiff joints need evaluation before atrophy or contractures occur. Such signs may be secondary to physical restraint or confinement to a chair or a bed for long periods of time. Intervening when decubiti are in the early stage may prevent further neglect as well as significant life-threatening illness such as sepsis. Although neglect and abuse are difficult to assess, each needs to be included as a "rule out" in a large variety of presentations for physical and psychological problems.

DIAGNOSIS

With such an exhaustive review of behavioral and physical indicators of abuse and neglect, excessive or premature suspicion regarding abuse and neglect may occur. Inclusion of suspicious historical or physical findings in the differential diagnosis, however, may in fact prove useful in the observation of the older person and caregiver over time. As with other health problems, no one sign or symptom can be used to diagnose definitively.[36] Therefore, a cluster of signs and symptoms over time is more helpful in evaluating abuse and neglect. Primary prevention includes increasing the awareness of health care providers;[37] listing as a problem "suspicious for neglect or abuse" contributes to such awareness. Every bruise is not abuse, yet integrating abuse into the list of possible causes increases the likelihood of recognition, and therefore treatment of abuse and neglect.

DOCUMENTATION

Essential for diagnosis, as well as potential intervention by legal and/or social service agencies, is accurate and comprehensive documentation. Suspicious symptoms elicited from interviews in the office, emergency or hospital room and from telephone interviews should be in the chart. Any time the older person or caregiver admits to abuse or neglect, a direct quote should be recorded.

Physical findings need to be described specifically. For example, instead of documenting "hematoma of upper left arm," an accurate description of the size, color and shape of the bruise should be noted. Adding to the description, sketches of the injury provide graphic illustration; a full-body sketch is necessary in cases of multiple injuries.

The best depictions of injuries are photographs. A close-up of the injury next to a coin demonstrates size. Similar to the drawing, a full-body picture should also be taken to demonstrate both the exact location and its placement among other injuries, if applicable. A full-length photograph also confirms identity of the victim in case the photograph's veracity is challenged. Both sketches and photographs should always be signed and dated.

Additionally, interventions, consultations and referrals should be recorded. Careful documentation will prove helpful if the physician is later asked to offer testimony at legal proceedings.[38]

MANAGEMENT OF ABUSE AND NEGLECT

MANDATORY/VOLUNTARY REPORTING LAWS

Prior to intervention, a diagnosis of actual or suspicious abuse or neglect must be established. Frequently, the physician may be hesitant to make a diagnosis fearing a suit for defamation of character by the accused caregiver.[39] Despite this fear of retribution, 37 states have laws that mandate such reporting, many without requiring the older person's consent.[40,41] With few exceptions, the abuse only need be suspected, not fully substantiated. The assurance of immunity is part of most abuse reporting statutes. In fact, in some states, failure to report may result in fines, licensing penalties or jail.[42] Even in states without such laws the judicial system is likely to protect the physician reporting suspicious abuse and neglect. The ethical principle of beneficence, i.e., removing or preventing harm, is considered essential to sound clinical decision-making in professional medical practice.[43,44]

It is controversial whether mandatory reporting actually limits the ability of the physician to intervene successfully prior to an investigation. Many mandatory reporting laws of the states are meant to provide health and social services to assist the older person to maintain independence and prevent abuse.[45] Unfortunately, the funding in many states is inadequate to allow for effective interventions. The physician or agencies known to the physician in the community may be able to alleviate the situation without the additional stress of an investigation on the family. The reporting of abuse or neglect may sever the trust between the physician and patient and family and therefore hinder the process of treatment of the problem. On the other hand, many individuals and families would not admit a problem or accept intervention without the threat of government agency action. Those in crisis have also benefited greatly from such agencies. Despite the content of mandatory reporting law (or lack of it) in one's state, the decision of how to proceed in a case of abuse and neglect is as individualized as the persons and resources involved.

INTERVENTION STRATEGIES

Elder abuse and neglect is not clear-cut in either diagnosis or treatment. No one clinician can intervene as effectively as a group of health and social service practitioners familiar with this problem. However, the role of detection of actual or potential cases by the primary physician is essential before clinicians specialized in abuse and neglect can intervene successfully. Community resources can also give assistance with detection of abuse and neglect when the office-based data collection is inconclusive. For example, a home visit from a visiting nurse service can uncover the extent of a poor living situation suspected by the physician.

The physician needs to determine emergency situations requiring immediate attention. Lastly, and most importantly, the primary care physician sets the tone for acceptance of treatment of the abused and the abuser. Emphasizing the positive aspects of intervention (i.e., a better quality of life for all involved), the physician demonstrates his or her concern.[46] Counseling the victim and the abuser regarding the need for change facilitates the process of ending the abusive situation.

EMERGENCY SITUATIONS

When the abuse or neglect results in illness or injury requiring hospitalization, medical intervention takes precedence. The danger of recurrence upon return to the home is high and, therefore, individuals representing resources within the hospital need to be contacted immediately. This early contact promotes a successful plan upon discharge. Some acute care settings (for example, the Beth Israel Hospital in Boston[47]) have elder abuse assessment teams. Geriatric physicians, multidisciplinary inpatient consultation teams,[48,49] and/or geriatric clinical nurse specialists are important resources as well. Even if such specialists are not available, hospital social workers and discharge planners are usually available for follow-up of abuse cases.

For those outpatient situations in which the abused or neglected older person is believed to be in imminent danger, the local adult protective services unit of the area agency on aging needs to be contacted. Adult protective service units are mandated to investigate and intervene in crisis situations; the amount of nonvoluntary intervention is dependent on individual state laws. Additionally, many police departments and district attorney's offices have special domestic violence units to handle cases of abuse or neglect.

For abusers requiring immediate mental health services, crisis intervention units are available as part of emergency room departments in many hospitals. The easiest way for a primary physician to refer cases appropriately in both emergent and nonemergent situations is to identify a few local community sources that can provide information and referral.

RESOURCES TO PREVENT OR ALLEVIATE
ABUSE AND NEGLECT

Referral Agencies. Geriatric and geropsychiatric programs and clinics are staffed with an interdisciplinary team of professionals familiar with difficult problems of aging, such as abuse and neglect. The geriatric nurse practitioner or social worker can assist in suggesting referral sources as well as long-term follow-up. The nurse or social worker can work with the family to facilitate change in a variety of ways: counseling, direct services and referrals.

If such specialized geriatric health services are not available, every community is served by a local area agency on aging. These agencies are federally mandated to act as coordinators of aging services. If direct social service consultation is unavailable, hospital social workers can be contacted. Additionally, nonprofit social service agencies and visiting nurse associations will also provide coordination and referral services. The aforementioned groups serve as linkages for physicians in identifying appropriate referrals for their patients and families.

Counseling. Abused older persons benefit from both individual and group counseling. Counseling can help the abused person to feel better and more able to make decisions based on his or her best interests. It can also be educative, providing information about legal rights as well as services and techniques of self-care to reduce dependency on the caregiver. Individual counseling can be obtained from traditional mental health services or from geriatric and geropsychiatric programs, social service agencies, rape counseling groups, women's organizations dealing with abuse, and advocacy groups for older persons. Group counseling may also be available by organizations such as the Elder Abuse Victim's Support Group in New York City.[50] Legal counseling is usually provided by private lawyers, the district attorney's office, or special legal service programs through the local bar association.

Potential or actual abusers can also receive individual counseling from the same resources as older persons. Caregivers who are stressed with the burdens of caregiving may also benefit in a group with other caregivers in similar situations. Organizations such as Children of Aging Parents and the Alzheimer Disease and Related Disorders Association organize hundreds of caregiver support groups across the country. Actual or potential abusers whose problems stem from dependency on the older person instead of the stresses of caregiving would probably profit more from individual therapy. Therapy with a psychiatrist or therapist can facilitate insight into the nature of the relationship and assist the adult child to live independently. For some, more direct therapeutic techniques emphasizing self-control may be necessary to prevent further violence. Regardless of type, counseling can be the initial step in self-recognition of a conflict in the family and can lead to alleviation of the abuse or neglect.

Prevention of abuse and neglect begins with the physician counseling families regarding realistic caregiving responsibilities. Frequently older persons and their families look to the physician for "approval" to receive "outside" assistance. Many American families perceive their role as providing for all the needs of the older adult. "Prescribing" or suggesting to families to seek support services may change the families viewpoint and thus lead to a reduction of caregiver strain. Primary prevention, i.e., identifying high-risk families and recommending changes before abuse occurs, is the most important role in office practice.

Support Services.   Referral to agencies that provide in-home or community services for the aged can decrease caregiver strain as well as increase the older person's quality of life. Visiting Nurse Services (VNS) can provide a variety of professional services in the home, treating illness or preventing deterioration through rehabilitative efforts. VNS and social service agencies provide home health aides, personal care attendants, companions, friendly visitors, housekeeping, and meal preparation or delivery. These services provide temporary respite for the caregiver as well as facilitate the older person's ability to remain at home. Senior centers provide stimulating activities, trips and meals. For those with a physical or mental impairment, adult day care centers are excellent resources. Many families find it easier to care for an older person in the evening and the weekends instead of round the clock. Adult day care provides a protective environment with structured activities, physical exercise, and opportunities for socialization. Other providers of respite include nursing homes that accept residents for short temporary stays. Services that assist the older person directly and, therefore, the caregiver indirectly can prevent or alleviate abuse and neglect.

Alternative Living Arrangements.   Frequently the family physician's opinion is sought when adults are considering the move of a parent into their home or to a nursing home or other long-term care setting. It is assumed the move will relieve any problems the older person is experiencing, since assistance will be more easily available. The implications of a change in living arrangements, such as issues of personal space and perceptions regarding needs as well as changes in responsibilities, are all important considerations. The physician needs to provide anticipatory guidance or referral to health professionals experienced in counseling older persons and their families. The prevention of problems related to a poorly made decision is one way to prevent abuse or neglect.

Through discussion with the family it may be discovered that other living arrangements, such as a boarding home, a retirement or life care community, or nursing home placement, may be the most appropriate choice. The older person's right to make an informed decision is essential throughout the process. Obviously, the bulk of services described is not specific to abuse or neglect. However, these community resources for the older person and his or her family are the essential components needed to intervene successfully.

CONCLUSION

Abuse and neglect of older persons is an unfortunate occurrence in our society. Physicians are in a critical position to confront this problem in their practice.

At the primary prevention level, the resources described assist older persons to live as independently as possible and supplement familial support to older persons. Once an at-risk family is identified, more active intervention through referral is needed.

The other very important role of the primary care provider is to identify actually abused or neglected older victims. With increased awareness of signs and symptoms, it is assumed that early detection of abuse and neglect will take place.

Finally, no one provider or profession is solely responsible for assessment or intervention. Multidisciplinary consultation should be employed to stop or prevent abuse or neglect. Ethically, and in some instances, legally, it is one's professional responsibility to assess and confront problems of this nature. Patient advocacy is the cornerstone of professional practice.

PRACTICE RECOMMENDATIONS

1. Include abuse as a "rule out" in all older persons presenting with injury.
2. Consider neglect when there is evidence of poor care.
3. Interview older persons separately from caregivers when one suspects abuse or neglect.
4. Collect a functional assessment to determine degree of dependency of older person.
5. Determine when adults are dependent on an older person, especially for financial support.
6. Screen for familial violent behavior, e.g., homicide, suicide, child and spouse abuse.
7. Check for psychopathology, drug addiction and alcoholism.
8. Ask nonthreatening questions (e.g., description of typical day) before direct questions regarding abuse or neglect.
9. Ask probing questions when answers regarding injury are vague.
10. Examine all parts of the older patient's body (he or she may be hiding bruises).
11. Look for highly suspicious signs such as imprint injuries and symmetrical or unusual locations of bruises or burns.
12. Document all signs and symptoms specifically.
13. Sketch injuries or take a photograph.
14. Report cases to an appropriate agency, usually adult protective services.
15. Select local agencies and health facilities for emergency referrals.
16. Refer to geriatric programs or community social service groups for assistance in case management.
17. Explain to older persons and their families the usefulness of counseling.
18. Utilize formal support services to decrease caregiver burn-out.
19. Facilitate the older person to make decisions in his or her best interests.

REFERENCES

1. Council on Scientific Affairs: Elder abuse and neglect. JAMA 1987; 257(7):966–971.
2. Wolf R, Godkin M, Pillemer K: Maltreatment of the elderly: A comparative analysis. Pride Institute Journal of Long Term Home Health Care 1986; 5(4):10–17.
3. Ibid., 11.
4. Council on Scientific Affairs: Elder abuse and neglect. JAMA 1987; 257(7):966–971.
5. Tomita S: Detection and treatment of elderly abuse and neglect: A protocol for health care professionals. Physical and Occupational Therapy in Geriatrics 1982; 2(2):45.
6. Hickey T, Douglass R: Mistreatment of the elderly in the domestic setting: An exploratory study. Am J Public Health 1981; 71(5):500–507.
7. O'Malley T, Everitt D, O'Malley H, Campion E: Identifying and preventing family-mediated abuse and neglect of elderly persons. Ann Intern Med 1983; 98:998–1005.
8. Fulmer T, Ashley J: Neglect: What part of abuse. Pride Institute Journal of Long Term Home Health Care 1986; 5(4):18–24.
9. House Select Committee on Aging, Subcommittee for Health and Long-Term Care: Elder Abuse: A National Disgrace (Executive Summary), May 10, 1985.
10. Pillemer K: Elder Abuse and Neglect: Recommendations From the Research Conference On Elder Abuse and Neglect. University of New Hampshire, June 1986.

11. Pillemer K: Domestic violence against the elderly. Background document for the Surgeon General's workshop on violence and public health. Leesburg, Virginia, October 1985.
12. Taler G, Ansello E: Elder abuse. Am Fam Phys 1985; 32(2):107–114.
13. Foege W: Violence and Public Health. Report from the Surgeon General's Workshop on Violence and Public Health. Leesburg, Virginia, October 1985.
14. Council on Scientific Affairs: Elder abuse and neglect. JAMA 1987; 257(7):966–971.
15. Sengstock M, Hwalek M: A critical analysis of measures for the identification of physical abuse and neglect of the elderly. Home Health Care Services Quarterly 1986; 6(4):27–39.
16. Council on Scientific Affairs: Elder abuse and neglect. JAMA 1987; 257(7):966–971.
17. Block M, Sinnett J (eds): The Battered Elder Syndrome. University of Maryland Center on Aging. College Park, Maryland, 1979.
18. O'Malley H, Segars H, Perez R, et al: Elder abuse in Massachusetts: A survey of professionals and paraprofessionals. Legal Research and Services for the Elderly. Boston, Massachusetts, 1979.
19. Lau E, Kosberg J: Abuse of the elderly by informal care providers. Aging Sept/Oct 1979; 10–15.
20. O'Malley T: Abuse and neglect of the elderly: The wrong issue? Pride Institute Journal of Long Term Home Health Care 1986; 5(4):25–28.
21. Council on Scientific Affairs. Elder abuse and neglect. JAMA 1987; 257(7):966–971.
22. Hickey T, Douglass R: Mistreatment of the elderly in the domestic setting: An exploratory study. Am J Public Health 1981; 71(5):500–507.
23. Pillemer K: Risk factors in elder abuse: Results from a case-control study. In Pillemer K, Wolf R (eds): Elder Abuse: Conflict in the Family. Dover, Massachusetts, Auburn House, 1986, pp 239–263.
24. Wolf R, Godkin M, Pillemer K: Maltreatment of the elderly: A comparative analysis. Pride Institute Journal of Long Term Home Health Care 1986; 5(4):10–18.
25. Kimsey L, Tarbox A, Bragg D: Abuse of the elderly—The hidden agenda: I. The caretakers and the categories of abuse. J Am Geriatr Soc 1981; 29(10):465–472.
26. Pillemer K: The dangers of dependency: New findings on domestic violence in the elderly. Social Problems 1985; 33(2):146–158.
27. Brody E: Women in the middle and family help to old people. The Gerontologist 1981; 21(5):471–480.
28. Brody S, Poulshock W, Masciochi C: The family caring unit: A major consideration in the long term support system. The Gerontologist 1978; 18(6):556–561.
29. Philip L, Rempusheski: Caring for the frail elderly at home: Toward a theoretical exploration of the dynamics of poor quality family caregiving. Advances in Nursing 1986; 8(4):62–84.
30. Stone R, Cafferata G, Sange J: Caregivers of the Frail Elderly: A National Profile. National Center for Health Service Research and Health Care Technology Assessment, Rockville, Maryland, 1982.
31. Brody E: Women in the middle and family help to old people. The Gerontologist 1981; 21(5):471–480.
32. Tomita S: Detection and treatment of elderly abuse and neglect: A protocol for health care professionals. Physical and Occupational Therapy in Geriatrics 1982; 2(2):37–51.
33. Rathbone-McCuan E, Goodstein R: Elder abuse: Clinical considerations. Psychiatric Ann 1985; 15(5):331–339.
34. Tomita S: Detection and treatment of elderly abuse and neglect: A protocol for health care professionals. Physical and Occupational Therapy in Geriatrics 1982; 2(2):45.
35. Fulmer T, Ashley J: Neglect: What part of abuse. Pride Journal of Long Term Home Health Care 1986; 5(4):18–24.
36. Pies T: Elder abuse: Clinical detection and intervention. Geriatric Medicine Today 1987; 6(1):24–31.
37. Council on Scientific Affairs: Elder abuse and neglect. JAMA 1987; 257(7):966–971.
38. Pies T: Elder abuse: Clinical detection and intervention. Geriatric Medicine Today 1987; 6(1):24–31.
39. Ibid.
40. Thobaben M, Anderson L: Reporting elder abuse: It's the law. Am J Nurs 1985; 85(4):371–374.
41. Gilbert DA: The ethics of mandatory elder abuse reporting statutes. Advances in Nursing Science 1986; 8(2):51–62.
42. Thobaben M, Anderson L: Reporting elder abuse: It's the law. Am J Nurs 1985; 85(4):371–374.
43. Gilbert DA: The ethics of mandatory elder abuse reporting statutes. Advances in Nursing Science 1986; 8(2):51–62.
44. Council on Scientific Affairs: Elder abuse and neglect. JAMA 1987; 257(7):966–971.
45. Regan JJ: Intervention through adult protective services programs. The Gerontologist 1978; 18(3):250–254.

46. Pies T: Elder abuse: Clinical detection and intervention. Geriatric Medicine Today 1987; 6(1):24–31.
47. The Beth Israel Hospital Elder Assessment Team: An elder abuse assessment team in an acute hospital setting. The Gerontologist 1986; 26(2):115–118.
48. Epstein AM, et al: The emergence of geriatric assessment units: The "new technology of geriatrics." Ann Intern Med 1987; 106(2):299–303.
49. Williams ME: Outpatient geriatric evaluation. Clin Geriatr Med 1987; 3(1):175–183.
50. Breckman R: Starting an Elder Abuse Victims' Support Group: A Guide for Facilitators. New York, Victim Services Agency, 1986.

14

URINARY INCONTINENCE

Laurence H. Beck, MD

Urinary incontinence in the elderly is an important problem that has only recently begun to be well understood, described, and managed. It is appropriate to include incontinence in a text on prevention not so much because the condition itself can be prevented but because proper diagnosis and management may prevent serious functional decline and maintain independence in elderly individuals. Management of urinary incontinence, therefore, represents an important example of *tertiary* prevention.

The prevalence of urinary incontinence in the elderly has been difficult to measure, in large part due to reluctance of patients to volunteer that they have urinary incontinence but also to physicians' and other health care providers' failure to ask specifically about the condition. A useful definition of clinically significant urinary incontinence is "a condition in which involuntary loss of urine is a social or hygienic problem and is objectively demonstrable."[1] Using such a definition, the prevalence of urinary incontinence has been estimated to be from 5 to 15% of elderly living in the community.[2] The prevalence is much higher, around 50%, in institutionalized elderly individuals.[3]

The costs of urinary incontinence can be measured in monetary and, equally importantly, in *social* terms. A number of detailed and more informal studies of the dollar cost of urinary incontinence have indicated that the total cost of the condition is staggering. One careful analysis estimates the total direct and indirect economic cost at $8 billion, with about 75% of this attributed to elderly individuals living in the community.[4] In this study, the average annual cost to the incontinent person living in the community, for supplies and laundry alone, was $912 per year. These costs, of course, are usually *not* reimbursable through third-party carriers. Needless to say, substantial reduction in the prevalence of urinary incontinence could result in reallocation of large dollar amounts toward other health or social problems for the individual as well as society.

As impressive as is the economic impact of urinary incontinence, it is the social impact on the individual and his or her family that warrants a vigorous management and preventive approach. Urinary incontinence is considered by most individuals as an indignity and an embarrassment. Many elderly individuals with urinary incontinence deny their incontinence in an attempt to maintain self-respect. However, as control of micturition worsens, the fear of an accident, the concern about odors, and the diminution in self-esteem often lead to a vicious cycle of social isolation. The elderly individual becomes afraid to go out of the house and is embarrassed to have friends or family in to visit. The consequences can be psychological, in the form of anger, depression, or apathy. These psychological changes and self-imposed isolation often lead to more global functional decline, so that the elderly individual becomes less and less independent in activities of daily living. Urinary incontinence is often described as the "straw that broke the camel's back" in terms of the decision by family to seek nursing home placement of an elderly individual.[5] For families who are able to cope with elderly relatives with multiple functional impairments, therefore, effective management of urinary incontinence can be viewed as an important preventive strategy, by delaying or eliminating the need for nursing home placement.

PHYSIOLOGY

Although the precise physiology of micturition is complex and still incompletely understood, the system can be divided roughly into three components: the central nervous system (CNS), which provides both voluntary and involuntary mechanisms to store urine and, when appropriate, to urinate; the bladder itself, which is a large muscle (detrusor) under complex neurologic and pharmacologic control; and the bladder outlet, which is a coordinated series of functional sphincters and conduits which must act synergistically in order for the micturition cycle to work normally (Fig. 1).

The main portion of the bladder muscle (detrusor) is predominantly cholinergic, i.e., acetylcholine-like drugs (bethanecol; Urecholine) cause contraction and atropine-like drugs (oxybutinin; Ditropan) inhibit contraction. The bladder neck and internal sphincter are predominantly alpha-adrenergic, i.e., sympathetic agonists (phenylpropanolamine; Ornade) cause contraction (closure). In addition, the internal and external sphincter muscles in the female are somewhat estrogen-dependent, so that estrogen lack can contribute to decreased sphincteric competence.[6]

Wein has stressed the two discrete phases of micturition: the urine storage function and the bladder-emptying function.[7] Normally, as the bladder fills with urine, local (spinal cord) and distant (brain) reflexes allow concomitant bladder relaxation (to accommodate the increasing volume of urine) and closure of the sphincters (to prevent leakage). As the bladder volume reaches a certain threshold, sensory neurons signal the central nervous system, producing an awareness of bladder fullness. Parallel reflex arcs are poised to initiate contractions of the bladder; normally, however, these contractions are overcome by inhibitory neurons from the central nervous system, which remain dominant until the appropriate time and place for micturition have presented themselves. Additional reflex mechanisms cause instantaneous increased sphincteric resistance whenever intraabdominal (and thereby intravesical) pressure is increased by a cough, straining, lifting, etc.; this mechanism prevents the involuntary loss of urine under such circumstances (stress incontinence).

Interruption of or interference with the normal functioning of any of these three components (central nervous system, bladder, or bladder outlet) can cause or contribute to urinary incontinence. The major types of urinary incontinence, discussed in a following section, can be easily understood by keeping these principles in mind.

Although a number of classifications of urinary incontinence have been proposed, the most useful system for the practitioner separates the condition into four types: urge incontinence, stress incontinence, overflow incontinence, and functional incontinence.

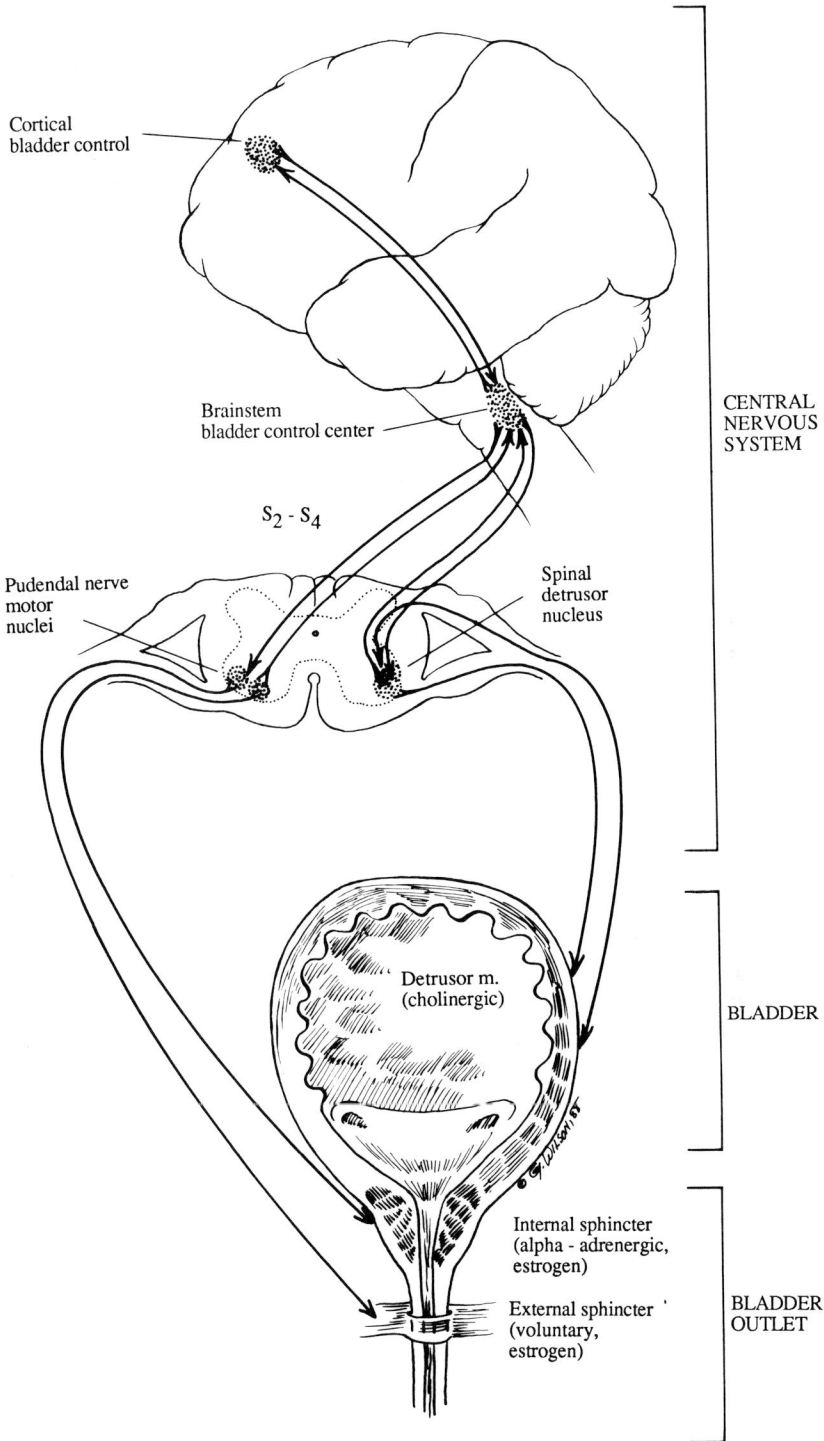

Cortical
bladder control

Brainstem
bladder control center

$S_2 - S_4$

Pudendal nerve
motor
nuclei

Spinal
detrusor
nucleus

CENTRAL
NERVOUS
SYSTEM

Detrusor m.
(cholinergic)

BLADDER

Internal sphincter
(alpha - adrenergic,
estrogen)

External sphincter
(voluntary,
estrogen)

BLADDER
OUTLET

FIGURE 1. Simplified diagram of neurologic bladder control.

Urge Incontinence. Also known as detrusor instability, urge incontinence has been noted to be the most common type of urinary incontinence in elderly individuals of both sexes, accounting for 40 to 70% of cases. Urge incontinence occurs when uninhibited bladder contractions happen with great enough force to overcome urethral resistance. The usual history, in aware patients, is the feeling of an urge to void, followed shortly thereafter by a large involuntary micturition. Since the interval between sensation and voiding is often too brief for the individual to reach the toilet or commode, wetting occurs. Urge incontinence can result from increased excitability of the bladder, as may occur with inflammatory bladder conditions (bacterial cystitis, bladder stone, neoplasm) or, more commonly, by decreased cortical (CNS) inhibition. The latter mechanism is responsible for urge incontinence in many elderly patients with stroke, dementia, Parkinson's disease, or central nervous system tumors.

Stress Incontinence. Stress incontinence results from urethral sphincter weakness, with small-volume urine leakage occurring whenever there is a sudden increase in intraabdominal pressure, such as with lifting, laughing, coughing, etc. This form of incontinence is much more common in women than in men and, in elderly women, may be associated with large-volume leakage.[8] The competence of the sphincteric mechanism depends, in part, upon the angle formed between the bladder and urethra. This angle becomes less acute with normal aging and following some pelvic surgery, and this change alone may account for some cases of stress incontinence. In addition, decreased internal sphincter strength is an important cause of stress incontinence and can occur with normal aging (particularly when associated with estrogen lack), with lumbosacral spondylosis, or from peripheral (pudendal) neuropathy. Finally, the external sphincter, which is striated muscle, can become weak due to age, surgery, or perhaps multiparity, resulting in a diminished pelvic floor competence and leading to stress incontinence.

Overflow Incontinence. This condition occurs primarily due to motor weakness of the bladder muscle or from bladder outlet obstruction. Detrusor weakness may result from diabetic neuropathy or lower motor neuron disease, and sometimes from anticholinergic medications. Similarly, loss of sensation of bladder fullness (sensory atonic bladder) may occur in diabetes mellitus and lead to overflow. The most prevalent cause of partial bladder outlet obstruction is prostatic hypertrophy, leading to gradual bladder distention. In all these situations, there are few or no detrusor contractions despite high bladder volume. Frequently, there is no urge to void. Physical examination usually reveals a large distended bladder. Urine "leaks" out of the overfilled bladder in small amounts with changes in abdominal pressure or posture.

As indicated, diabetic patients with peripheral or autonomic neuropathy are at particularly high risk for this type of incontinence, since they may develop a combination of motor *and* sensory defects leading to impaired bladder emptying. Diabetic patients of this sort and elderly men with benign prostatic hypertrophy (BPH) may develop acute decompensation of the bladder-emptying mechanism, resulting in overflow incontinence, at the time of medical illness. This is thought to be due to general loss of muscle tone associated with illness, as well as to enforced supine posture preventing upright voiding. In addition, anticholinergic side effects of many drugs used in the elderly (particularly neuroleptic drugs such as phenothiazines and antidepressants) may tip the pharmacologic balance in the bladder toward urinary retention, resulting in overflow incontinence.

Functional Incontinence. Functional incontinence occurs when a continent individual is unable to get to the toilet in time to prevent an accident. This is usually caused by musculoskeletal disability (such as arthritis, stroke, etc.), or severe psychologic impairment (depression with indifference, hostility or severe anxiety). Occasionally, cerebrovascular disease or dementing illness leads to an apraxia preventing locomotion or the ability to initiate the physical act of micturition. In institutionalized patients, iatrogenic functional incontinence sometimes occurs from prolonged restraint usage or from passive neglect of bedbound patients. In addition, the prescription of rapidly-acting potent diuretics may create incontinence in a normally continent individual, as may the use of sedatives and hypnotics.

DIAGNOSIS

Since many elderly patients do not seek care for incontinence either because of shame or the mistaken but common assumption that incontinence is "part of getting old," the physician must specifically ask about urinary incontinence ("Do you ever have accidents? Do you have trouble getting to the bathroom in time? Do you sometimes wet yourself when you cough?", etc.). Further questioning about the volume of urine lost, the sensation of an urge or lack thereof, and the circumstances in which accidents occur, are usually adequate to classify the patient into stress, urge, or functional incontinence categories (see flow diagram, Fig. 2). The physical examination should include a careful palpitation of the lower abdomen (to detect the large bladder of overflow incontinence), as well as a pelvic examination in the woman. The latter should be carried out to note evidence of uterine or bladder prolapse, atrophic vaginitis, or other local anatomic abnormalities. In addition, this is an efficient way of obtaining a post-void residual volume (PVR), which should normally be less than 50 mL. Evidence of urinary tract infection (UTI) should prompt a course of specific antibacterial therapy before further evaluation or treatment, since UTI is an important cause of *transient* urge incontinence.

Patients with large residual volumes should routinely be referred to a urologist for more extensive investigation. Most men with a high PVR have outlet obstruction from BPH. Some men and women with a high PVR may have the recently described entity "detrusor hyperactivity with inadequate contractile force."[9] This condition, which Resnick feels may be an advanced stage of urge incontinence, does not respond well to the usual anticholinergic medications used in urge incontinence (see below). Specific therapy for these patients, as well as those with bladder outlet obstruction, requires urologic evaluation with cystoscopy, cystometrogram, and often urine flow studies. Therefore they should be regularly referred from the generalist to the urologist for management. However, most other patients can be classified by history and physical examination alone and can be managed empirically, based on physiologic principles. It should be noted that intravenous urogram (IVU) is *not* a routine part of the evaluation of urinary incontinence.

Prior to initiation of any management strategy, it is useful to have an objective record of the incontinence pattern, so that trials can be evaluated for effectiveness. A standardized incontinence record has been found to be of value;

FIGURE 2.   Flow diagram for urinary incontinence.

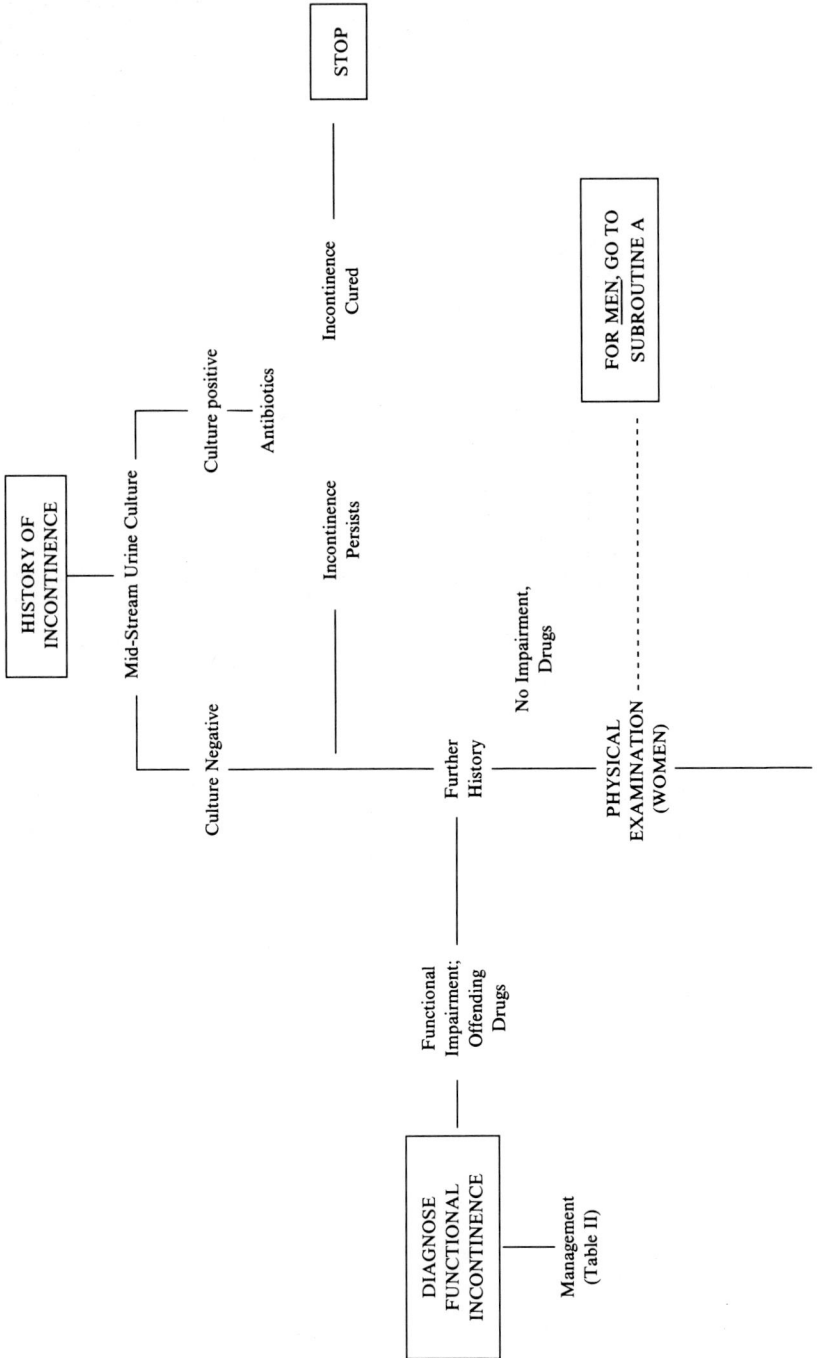

HISTORY OF
INCONTINENCE

Mid-Stream Urine Culture

Culture Negative

Culture positive

Antibiotics

Incontinence
Persists

Incontinence
Cured

STOP

Further
History

No Impairment,
Drugs

PHYSICAL
EXAMINATION
(WOMEN)

FOR MEN, GO TO
SUBROUTINE A

Functional
Impairment;
Offending
Drugs

DIAGNOSE
FUNCTIONAL
INCONTINENCE

Management
(Table II)

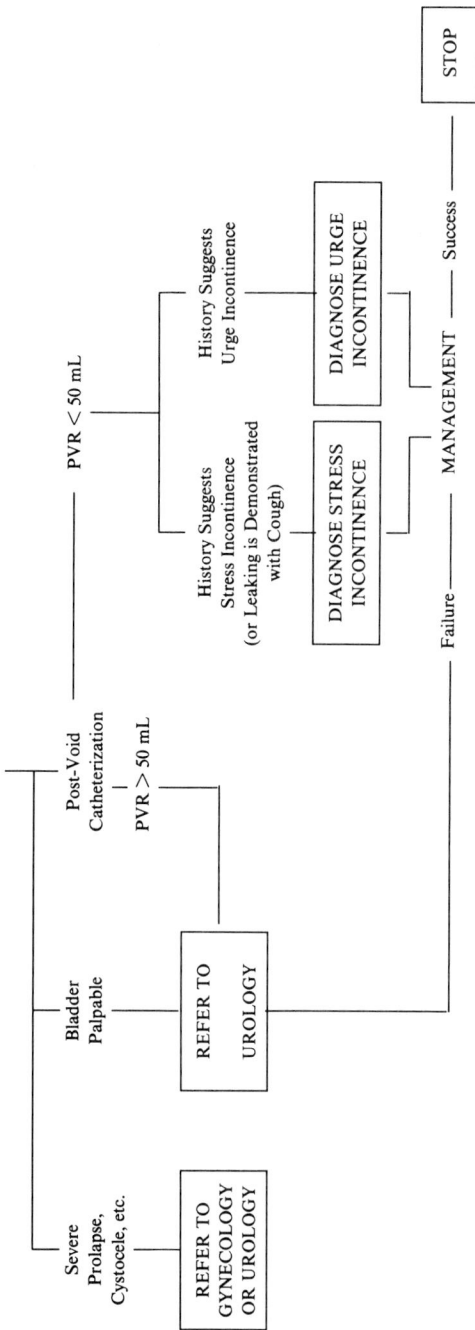

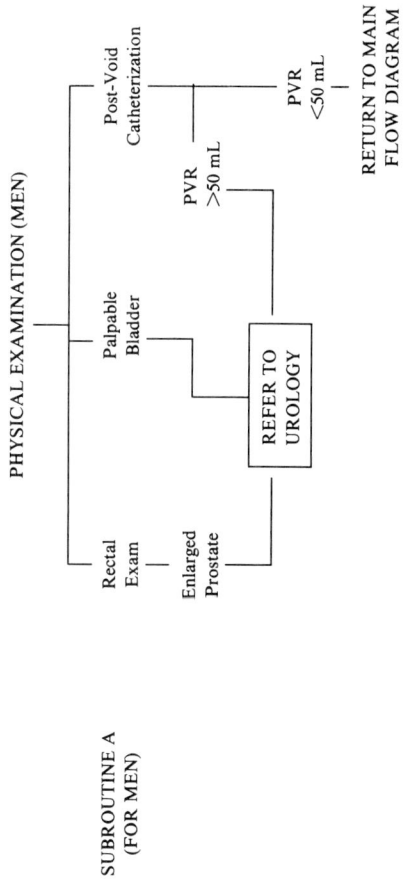

TABLE 1. Kegel's Exercise

For people who have difficulty controlling urination when coughing, sneezing, laughing, etc., the following exercise is recommended:

> You may sit, stand, or lie down to do this exercise. Without tensing muscles of your buttocks (seat), abdomen, or legs, tighten all your muscles in the pelvic floor as if you were preventing the passage of gas or urine. Hold tight for 10 seconds and then relax for 10 seconds.
>
> Repeat this exercise 20 times three times a day or a total of 60 times a day.
>
> Increase gradually until you can do 100 a day

patients are asked to fill it out for one week *prior to* the onset of any management regimen in order to document the frequency and volume of accidents, as well as the circumstances surrounding each episode. These data forms can be used as additional evidence for the physician in assigning patients to one of the physiologic categories of incontinence.

Following the initiation of management, the patient is asked to continue using the incontinence record for several weeks in order to measure response. Not only is such a record valuable for the physician in determining whether to stay with or change a particular therapy, but the record often is a strong motivating factor for the patient to continue the management regimens, some of which, such as Kegel's exercise (Table 1), require continued work on the part of the patient. An example of a simple incontinence record is shown as Figure 3.

MANAGEMENT OF URINARY INCONTINENCE (Table 2)

Functional Incontinence. Management of patients with functional incontinence should include measures that will remove impediments to successful micturition. These can sometimes be as simple as providing a nighttime urinal or bedside commode, or rearranging furniture so that the toilet is closer or more accessible to the patient. Medications that may decrease orientation or level of alertness (benzodiazepines, hypnotics, other centrally-acting agents such as alpha-methyldopa) should be eliminated or replaced, if possible, as should conditions (hyperglycemia) or drugs (diuretics) leading to increased urine flow.

Some patients become so completely functionally impaired or immobile that one has to choose between the risks of continued incontinence (wet bed clothes, macerated skin, pressure ulcers) versus the infectious risk of long-term urinary bladder catheterization. Unless the patient can be changed almost immediately after every accident, an indwelling catheter is probably preferable in these extreme cases where incontinence cannot be eliminated or managed in another way.

Overflow Incontinence. As indicated above, all patients with overflow incontinence should be referred to the urologist for evaluation, since many of these patients, particularly men, have surgically correctable causes of the overflow. In patients in whom the cause of the overflow is clearly neurologic (e.g., spinal injury, sensory atonic bladder, or detrusor weakness due to diabetic autonomic neuropathy), a trial of a direct cholinergic stimulant such as bethanechol chloride (Urecholine) may be attempted. Unfortunately, high doses, 50 to 100 mg per day, may be required and are often associated with intolerable side effects.[10]

Name ______________________ Week starting ________/________/________
Month Day Year

Instructions:

- Mark **D** for **Dry** each time urination occurs without leakage.
- Mark **W** for **Wet** each time leakage occurs.

  (If you cannot tell when the leakage occurred, Mark **W** at the time closest to when you find the wetness).
- Record circumstances accompanying each **Wet** recording in lower half of box (e.g., heavy lifting; during sleep; couldn't reach toilet).

Example:

W / coughing

	7 am	8 am	9 am	10am	11am	12n.	1 pm	2 pm	3 pm	4 pm	5 pm	6 pm	7 pm	8 pm	9 pm	10pm	11pm	12am	1 am	2 am	3 am	4 am	5 am	6 am
Mon																								
Tue																								
Wed																								
Thu																								
Fri																								
Sat																								
Sun																								
	Morning					**Afternoon**						**Evening**					**Night**							

FIGURE 3. Bladder Record. Adapted from Ouslander JG: Diagnostic evaluation of geriatric urinary incontinence. Clin Geriatr Med 1986; 2:715–730.

TABLE 2. Management of Urinary Incontinence

Type of Incontinence	Causes	Management Regimens
Functional	CNS disease (paresis, apraxia)	Remove or replace offending drugs
	Apathy (depression)	Improve patient mobility
	Musculoskeletal disease with immobility	Provide appropriate receptacles (urinals, commodes)
	Medications	
	Restraints	
	Neglect	
Overflow	Bladder outlet obstruction (BPH, urethral stricture)	Refer to urologist
		Trial of cholinergic drug
	Autonomic neuropathy (especially in diabetes)	Urinary catheterization: intermittent or continuous
Urge	CNS disease (stroke, dementia, tumor, Parkinson's)	Bladder antispasmodics (oxybutinin, flavoxate, dicyclomine, propantheline)
	Spinal cord injury	Imipramine
	Cystitis	Kegel's exercise
	Bladder stone, tumor	Bladder retraining
Stress	Estrogen lack	Adrenergic agents (pseudoephedrine, phenylpropanolamine)
	Pelvic surgery	Imipramine
	Multiparity	Estrogen
	Aging	Kegel's exercise
	Spondylosis	Surgery (in minority)

Although patients with uncorrectable bladder disease and overflow incontinence may eventually need long-term urinary catheterization, those patients with upper extremity dexterity (or a responsible caregiver) can be successfully managed with intermittent straight catheterization. The self-catheterization is carried out using a clean (not sterile) technique 2–4 times per day, and can be taught to patients through many urologists' offices. Intermittent catheterization has a lower rate of urinary tract infection than does chronic indwelling catheterization.

Stress Incontinence. The management options for stress incontinence are somewhat broader than for other types and depend, in part, on patient motivation and preferences. In the older female, with evidence of estrogen deficiency on vaginal exam, the use of topical estrogen cream or an oral estrogen preparation (e.g., Premarin 0.625 mg per day) should be tried initially. In the younger woman, a trial of an alpha-adrenergic agent is warranted. Successful treatment of stress incontinence has been reported with pseudoephedrine (Sudafed) 30–60 mg QID, with ephedrine 25–50 mg QID,[12] and with phenylpropanolamine (as the combination Ornade capsule) twice a day.[13] All three drugs share the same potential side effects: blood pressure elevation, insomnia, anxiety and, rarely, cardiac arrhythmias. Similar success has been reported with imipramine 25 mg BID to QID,[14] due to its alpha-adrenergic effect on the urethral sphincter. The bladder relaxant properties of imipramine offer an added beneficial effect in those patients with a component of urge incontinence (see below). The potential side effects of imipramine are principally related to its anticholinergic properties (dry mouth, blurry vision, sedation), although these side effects are usually not prominent at such low doses.

A widely used approach for both stress and urge incontinence is Kegel's exercise (Table 1). This method can be recommended particularly to younger women and well-motivated individuals of either sex. The purpose of the exercise is to strengthen the pelvic floor muscles, which contribute to competence of the urethral sphincter. The exercise involves voluntary tensing of the perineal muscles for 20–30 repetitions two to three times a day. The location of the proper muscles can be taught by asking the patient to attempt to stop urination mid-stream, or by asking a woman patient to squeeze a finger inserted into the vagina during pelvic exam. In many communities, nurse-managed incontinence clinics are available for teaching these techniques; in some clinics, the exercises are coupled with biofeedback devices, and reported results are often dramatically successful.[15] Kegel's exercise can be combined with estrogen cream for added benefit in older women.

Although various surgical approaches ("bladder suspension" procedures) have been used extensively in younger women, there has been less experience and less success in elderly patients. Since nonsurgical regimens are usually successful in reducing incontinence, surgery should be utilized only in patients with a severe anatomic abnormality such as marked uterine or bladder prolapse with associated stress incontinence.

Urge Incontinence. Urge incontinence can often be controlled pharmacologically with antispasmodic drugs that inhibit contraction of the bladder smooth muscle. The drugs commonly used are propantheline (Pro-Banthine) 15–30 mg q 6h, oxybutinin (Ditropan) 5 mg 3–4 times daily, dicyclomine (Bentyl) 20 mg TID, and flavoxate (Urispas) 100–200 mg TID. Propantheline has the most pronounced anticholinergic side effects of the group and therefore is least preferred in elderly patients. The other three are about equal in terms of efficacy in urge incontinence and in their anticholinergic side effects. Elderly patients should be started on a low dose, e.g., 5 mg oxybutinin once a day, and then the dose slowly increased, depending upon urinary response and side effects.

Imipramine has a strong antispasmodic effect on the bladder, as noted above, and should be considered a second-line drug in urge incontinence. It is particularly useful when there is also an element of stress incontinence. Its important side effects are principally related to its anticholinergic activity.

A number of newer drugs are currently being tested and developed for activity in urge incontinence. Perhaps the most promising are the calcium channel blockers, such as nifedipine, which has been shown to be effective in small numbers of patients.[16]

Kegel's exercise can be recommended as adjunctive therapy for well-motivated patients with urge incontinence and may contribute to urinary control.

Behavioral therapy, such as bladder retraining, has also been reported to be successful in as many as 50% of patients with urge incontinence.[17] The principle behind such training is the development of a very regular toileting schedule, with gradual increase in the interval between voidings. The patient must learn to control the urge to void voluntarily. These approaches can be taught in the office and are also commonly employed in nurse-managed incontinence clinics in the community.

The approach outlined in the preceding pages should be successful in reducing or eliminating urinary incontinence in the majority of patients. Most patients will have such dramatic improvement, over time, that they will easily be able to report their improvement. In others with less striking results, the Bladder Record (Figure 3) will be used as a measure of partial success or failure of a given regimen. A given trial should last a full 6 to 8 weeks before concluding that it has not been successful. For patients who fail one attempt, it is often reasonable to try an alternative regimen (Table 2) before referring the patient to the urologist for more specific investigation.

PRACTICE RECOMMENDATIONS

1. Ask every patient about presence of incontinence: Do you always make it to the toilet? Do you sometimes have accidents? Do you have such an urge to void that you can't get to the bathroom?

2. Ask for the details of accidents: Is it only with cough or straining? Does it occur in certain situations? Is it always present? How long has it been present?

3. Get a urinalysis (and culture, if indicated). If UTI is present, treat and re-evaluate before further investigation/management of incontinence.

4. Do a pelvic examination in women and obtain catheterized post-void residual (PVR) urine volume in men and women.

5. If PVR is greater than 50–100 mL, refer to urologist.

6. If PVR is less than 50 mL, classify patient, according to history and physical examination, into urge, stress, or functional incontinence.

7. Provide patient with a Bladder Record for one week prior to initiation of any treatment.

8. Use management approach for each type as shown in Table 2.

9. Allow 6–8 weeks of medical therapy or exercises before assigning as success or failure.

10. If one regimen fails, try another or refer to urologist for more intensive bladder evaluation.

REFERENCES

1. Mohide EA: The prevalence and scope of urinary incontinence. Clin Geriatr Med 1986; 2:639–655.
2. Yarnell JWG, St. Leger AS: The prevalence, severity, and factors associated with urinary incontinence in a random sample of the elderly. Age Aging 1979; 8:81–85.
3. Ouslander JG, Kane RL, Abrass IB: Urinary incontinence in elderly nursing home patients. JAMA 1982; 248:1194–1198.
4. Hu T: The economic impact of incontinence. Clin Geriatr Med 1986; 2:673–687.
5. Weissert W, Scanlon W: Determinants of institutionalization of the aged. Working paper no. 1466-21, Washington, D.C. The Urban Institute, November 1982.
6. Reed T: The effects of estrogens and gestagens on the urethral pressure profile in urinary continent and stress incontinent women. Acta Obstet Gynecol Scand 1980; 59:265–270.
7. Wein AJ: Physiologic of micturition. Clin Geriatr Med 1986; 2:689–699.

8. Wells TJ, Brink CA, Diokno AC: Urinary incontinence in elderly women: clinical findings. J Am Geriatr Soc 1987; 35:933–939.
9. Resnick NM, Yalla SV: Detrusor hyperactivity with impaired contractile function. JAMA 1987; 257:3076–3081.
10. Williams ME, Pannill FC: Urinary incontinence in the elderly. Ann Intern Med 1982; 93:895–907.
11. Wein AJ, VanArsdalen KN: Nonsurgical management of neuropathic voiding dysfunction. Semin Urol 1985; 3.
12. Diokno A, Taub M: Ephedrine in treatment of urinary incontinence. Urology 1975; 5:624.
13. Montague DK, Steward BH: Urethral pressure profiles before and after Ornade administration in patients with stress urinary incontinence. J Urol 1976; 122:198–199.
14. Edwards LE: The investigation and management of incontinence of urine in women. Ann R Coll Surg Engl 1973; 84:505–507.
15. Burgio KL, Robinson JC, Engel BT: The role of biofeedback in Kegel exercise training for stress urinary incontinence. Am J Obstet Gynecol 1986; 154:58–64.
16. Rudd T, Andersson KE, Ulmsted U: Effects of nifedipine in women with unstable bladders. Urol Int 1979; 34:421–429.
17. Jarvis G, Millar DR: Controlled trial of bladder drill for detrusor instability. Br Med J 1980; 281:1322–1323.
18. Ouslander JG: Diagnostic evaluation of geriatric urinary incontinence. Clin Geriatr Med 1986; 2:715–730.

15
THE ECONOMICS OF
PREVENTION IN THE ELDERLY

John M. Eisenberg, MD, MBA

On his 82nd birthday, Theodor Seuss Geisel, better known as Dr. Seuss, published *You're Only Old Once,* a tongue-in-cheek story of an elderly man's screening examination at the Golden Years Clinic. After walking along Stethoscope Row, passing the Wuff-Whiffer test, and scoring well on the Pill Drill, the elderly man greets with pleasure the reassurance of a clean bill of health, as he is told, "You're in pretty good shape for the shape you are in!"[1]

Earlier, when the examination started, the elderly man had been asked to read an eyechart in which the letters spelled out, "Have you any idea how much money these tests are costing you?" Although Dr. Seuss did not include a cost-benefit analysis of the screening examination as an appendix to *You're Only Old Once,* the grin on the protagonist's face at the book's end suggests that the exams were worth the cost.

As Americans like Dr. Seuss become more willing to question the value of medical care in the face of its increasing cost, critical attention is focused on ways to avoid preventable diseases and their attendant expense. This chapter discusses different approaches that have been used to assess the economic implications of preventive care for the elderly. Full mastery of the technical and analytic methods of health economics is not mandatory for the practice of clinical medicine. However, policy decisions based on these analyses have a great impact on medical practice. In addition, the clinical decision-maker will often find these techniques useful in weighing the value of different clinical options. The discussion in this chapter of how these analyses are performed and how they are applied to clinical issues will help clinicians to evaluate published studies and to understand the ways in which certain of these economic approaches may be biased against the elderly. The message is that prevention might save money on occasion, but reducing future expenditures is not the main reason for spending now on prevention. The main economic attraction of preventive services is that they accomplish their goal and the goal of all medical care—improved health—at a cost that is often a bargain compared with the improvement in health obtained from the cost of other medical services.

PAYING FOR DISEASE OR PREVENTION?

The U.S. Public Health Service reports that four major causes of death, each at least partially preventable, account for about half of this country's total cost of illness each year.[2] These are diseases of the circulatory system (particularly coronary artery disease and stroke); neoplasms; the combination of accidents, poisonings, and violence; and diseases of the respiratory system.

197

Despite the high cost of preventable diseases, less than 4 percent of current health expenditures are spent on disease prevention.[3,4] Third-party payers have been particularly reluctant to pay for preventive services. The federal government is no exception. Ironically, despite recommendations from the National Institutes of Health to screen for diseases such as breast cancer and from the Centers for Disease Control to immunize the elderly against influenza, another branch of the Department of Health and Human Services does not pay for these services. The Health Care Financing Administration—which operates Medicare, the federal health plan for the elderly—is instructed by the statute establishing Medicare's covered services not to pay for most prevention. The law specifically bans payment for periodic examinations: for eye, hearing and dental examinations; and for immunizations except for pneumococcal vaccine.

Therefore, Medicare pays for illness rather than prevention. In fact, Somers has pointed out elsewhere that under the existing benefit structure, 39 percent of elderly Medicare enrollees received no reimbursement at all in 1982; 54 percent received less than $100 and accounted for 0.4 percent of all reimbursements. At the other extreme, 14 percent of Medicare enrollees accounted for 70 percent of the total reimbursements.[5] This policy and the resulting allocation of funds, suggests Somers, reveal the financial disincentives to the elderly who might benefit from preventive services; these preventive services are less well covered by Medicare, and most Medicare outlays are for curative services. With the advent of improved Medicare coverage for catastrophic illness, this curative rather than preventive orientation of Medicare will be reinforced.

Somers has also pointed out the curious double standard applied to Medicare's decisions about whether to cover preventive services. Although Medicare prohibits consideration of cost in evaluating whether to cover new diagnostic or therapeutic procedures, cost considerations are routinely used to forestall the coverage of preventive services.[5] The message from Washington seems to be, prevent disease in the elderly but don't ask us to pay for it.

Somers blames the poor Medicare coverage of preventive services for the elderly on the view that the elderly are "too old or too disabled for effective prevention."[5] However, while it may be true that Medicare's coverage decisions were founded on the biases of ageism, it is also true that solid evidence supporting the effectiveness, cost effectiveness, and cost benefit of prevention for the elderly has been lacking. Even the literature that is available on prevention's cost-effectiveness has been found deficient, with few notable exceptions.[3,6] If the evidence for prevention is tenuous in general, the challenge is even greater with regard to prevention for the elderly.[7,8] In his review of geriatric screening, Freer argued that "the effectiveness of geriatric screening is perhaps the least well-established of all types of screening."

Although there is cause for skepticism about the value of preventive medicine for the elderly, evidence is emerging that a targeted program of risk reduction to prevent disease, as well as screening to detect disease early, can be effective in reducing morbidity and mortality.[9]

COST-EFFECTIVENESS ANALYSIS: COMPARING PREVENTION ALTERNATIVES

The principal goal of preventive medicine is to improve and maintain the health of its recipients. However the improvement is measured, an evaluation of prevention must compare the resources spent and the outcomes obtained for different ways of preventing disease. This is the essence of cost-effectiveness analysis—a comparison of alternatives.

In order to compare alternatives, the units of measurement for the costs and the outcomes of each alternative must be the same. The cost of an intervention is usually expressed in units of currency: how many dollars does it cost? However, the input of other resources could be used as well, for example, the number of minutes of provider time that are consumed giving care. Since most preventive measures require a variety of resources—professionals, support staff, equipment—the units of these resources must be translated into a common unit of value. Most of these services are purchased, so the logical unit of value is currency, and cost is generally measured in dollars in the U.S.

Although outcomes may be expressed in different terms than costs, the outcomes of each alternative must all be measured alike. It may be difficult to find a common unit of measurement to compare what two different preventive interventions provide, for example, in both years of life saved and suffering avoided. One approach that is currently popular is to express the outcome as years of life adjusted for their quality. These quality-adjusted life years (QALYs) provide a common unit of measurement whereby an intervention that saves 10 years of life can be compared with one that improves the quality of life for 20 years. By placing a value on the quality of life in different conditions, researchers can calculate the equivalent number of healthy years of life. For example, one might use a survey to determine that 10 years of life with moderate angina pectoris is equivalent to 5 years of life without angina. The methods of making these conversions are being improved, and this approach of valuing outcomes of medical care in units of healthy years of life is becoming increasingly popular.[10]

The cost-effectiveness evaluation of the North Karelia Hypertension Program is a good example of the use of quality-adjusted life years.[11] The investigators modified an approach developed by Weinstein and Stason to add the costs in the numerator and to add the quality-adjusted life years in the denominator (Table 1). This enabled them to calculate the cost per quality-adjusted life year for the prevention program.

The results of the cost-effectiveness analyses of the North Karelia project suggest a cost per quality-adjusted life year between $3,612 and $5,830. The authors conclude that the intensified hypertension control in North Karelia had costs per unit of effectiveness that were more favorable than those of other heart disease interventions.[11]

Other analysts have used quality-adjusted life years in cost-effectiveness analyses. For example, about 10 years ago Weinstein and Stason estimated the cost per year of healthy life gained from reducing diastolic blood pressure from 110 to 90 mmHg in 60-year-old men to be $16,330; for women, $5,030.[12] Another example applied to prevention of disease in older individuals was the cost-effectiveness of pneumococcal vaccine for adults 65 or older, which was calculated to be $1,000 per year of healthy life.[13] This figure compared favorably to the cost per year of healthy life added by pneumococcal vaccine for a 2–4 year-old child of $77,000.

Because one of the goals of special interest in prevention of disease in the elderly is the prolongation of active life, Katz and colleagues have suggested a new measure of outcome. They have proposed that "active life expectancy" be used to evaluate the impact of preventive services, recognizing that simply prolonging life may not be as valuable a contribution to the health of the elderly as assuming that those years are functional.[14] This measure of active life

TABLE 1.   Cost Effectiveness Equation Used by
the North Karelia Hypertension Program*

$$\frac{C}{E} = \frac{CRx + CSE + CRxLE - Cmorb - CLL}{YLE + Ymorb - YSE}$$

Numerator (costs):

> CRx = incremental cost of case finding and treatment
> CSE = costs of side effects of treatment
> CRxLE = cost of treating any illness in added years of life
> Cmorb = treatment costs saved by avoiding cardiovascular morbid events
> CLL = decline in livelihood losses offset by increase in costs to maintain
> increased number of retired persons due to decreased mortality

Denominator (outcomes valued in quality adjusted life years):

> YLE = increase in life expectancy
> Ymorb = value of improved quality of life due to decreased morbidity
> YSE = reduction in quality of life resulting from side effects of antihypertensive
> treatment

* From Nissinen A, et al: Cost-effectiveness of the North Karelia Hypertension Program, 1972–1977. Med Care 1986; 24:767–780.

expectancy, like quality-adjusted life-years, considers not only the years of life but the person's health status during those years.

The gain in life expectancy from prevention may be especially cherished by the elderly. Hazzard has shown how the elimination of certain diseases adds almost as many years to the life of a 65-year-old as to the life of a newborn. For example, elimination of heart disease would add an average of 4.9 years to the life of a 65-year-old, compared with 5.9 years for a newborn. The elimination of malignant neoplasms would add an average of 1.2 years to the life of a 65-year-old, 2.3 years to the life of a newborn.[15] For the average 65-year-old, these additional years of life offered by preventive care may be more valuable than the years would be to a young adult, since they represent a larger proportionate improvement in years of life remaining.

Since only a limited amount of money is available to pay for medical care, cost-effectiveness analysis offers clinical decision-makers an opportunity to compare the costs of alternative approaches in the same units and their outcomes in the same units. By choosing interventions with the best cost-effectiveness, policy-makers and physicians can obtain more health with the resources available. For example, one study of the cost-effectiveness of glaucoma screening found that the most cost-effective strategy differs for different age groups. While tonometry provides the lowest cost per year of vision saved for persons aged 40 to 44, ophthalmoscopy and field of vision measurements are the most cost-effective ways to screen for glaucoma in the elderly.[16]

COST-BENEFIT ANALYSIS:
DOES PREVENTION SAVE MONEY?

Instead of asking how much health is obtained by spending money on medical care as in cost-effectiveness analysis, a different approach is to ask how much money is saved by spending some. This approach, which is called cost-benefit analysis, requires that the cost and the outcome be measured in the same units so that a net cost or net benefit can be calculated. Generally, cost and benefit are described in monetary terms, so the economic consequences of an intervention's contribution to health (i.e., the benefit) must be calculated from the clinical consequences. While no single intervention can be described as cost effective without being compared to another, cost-benefit analysis enables a single intervention to be evaluated by itself. Is its benefit greater than its cost?

When cost-benefit analysis has been applied to preventive medicine, the results have been mixed. Economist Louise Russell warns against claiming that prevention will save money. She argues that "prevention usually adds to medical expenditures, contrary to the popular view that it reduces them."[17] Even if prevention does not save money, Russell points out that it can still be a worthwhile investment in better health and this, not the dollar savings, is the criterion on which its success should be judged. Her arguments suggest that it would be nice for a preventive program or clinical intervention to save money (for the patient, the health care system, or society as a whole), but inability to meet the cost-benefit criterion should not squelch the idea. If cost-effectiveness analysis suggests that the intervention is a less expensive way to achieve a favorable health outcome (e.g., years of healthy life gained), then the preventive measure should be adopted.

While Russell's book, *Is Prevention Better Than Cure?*, reminds us that the most important contribution of economic analysis of medical care is to guide clinicians in obtaining the greatest contribution to health from the available resources, others who have studied the economic impact of prevention have been more optimistic about the possibility of savings from prevention. Still, results of cost-benefit of prevention for the elderly generally suggest that it may provide improved health but may not save money. For example, Oster and Epstein have found that the expenses saved by reduction of serum cholesterol range from $1 to $321, but are smallest for the elderly.[18]

In another cost-benefit analysis, Oster and colleagues assessed the economic benefits that result when two-pack-a-day smokers quit smoking. They demonstrated that for all consequences of smoking (including lung cancer, chronic obstructive pulmonary disease, and coronary heart disease), the economic benefits from smoking cessation decrease with age. They calculated the savings in medical care costs (called direct costs) as well as the avoided loss of productivity due to acute illness, disability, and premature death (called indirect costs). For example, the direct economic benefits of quitting due to reduction in the risk of chronic obstructive lung disease in heavy smokers ranged from $808 in men aged 75 to 79 to $1,537 in women aged 60 to 64.[19]

Similarly, routine childhood immunization is not only more cost effective than many other health care services, but it is also cost saving, or cost beneficial.[6] Among adults, influenza vaccine offers savings because of its prevention of lost productivity (indirect costs), but neither influenza nor pneumococcal vaccine can claim to save direct medical care expenses.[6,13] Influenza immunization results in savings to society only if both direct and indirect costs are included.[6]

The measurement of indirect costs as the value of lost productivity in the cost-benefit or cost-effectiveness equation causes difficulty in assessing prevention for the elderly. The argument is an old one, the same as that put forth by Richard Petty, the 17th century English physician, who proposed that more should be spent for medical care since the saved earnings of those whose health would be improved exceeds the costs.[20] When indirect costs are included in most economic analyses of medical care, the savings from prevention appear to be much larger than when only direct costs are included. Similarly, in cost-effectiveness analyses, when saved indirect costs are subtracted from the net medical care expenses (direct costs), the net total cost is reduced. This results in a lower cost per unit of outcome for the preventive measure. However, the elderly are less often employed, so the method of analysis that uses lost earnings as a cost of illness will suggest smaller savings for the elderly. This method of analysis therefore would bias clinicians and policy-makers away from providing preventive and curative services to the elderly.[21]

An example of the bias that is introduced by using lost earnings is evident in Oster and Epstein's analysis of cholesterol reduction. For example, they calculate that a 25 percent reduction in cholesterol from an initial level of 340 mg/dL will provide $12,849 in indirect benefits for a 35 to 39-year-old man, but only $3 for a 70- to 74-year-old man. Although the savings in medical expenses are lower for the elderly than for younger age groups, the difference is much greater in indirect benefits.[18]

Oster and colleagues used similar methods in their analysis of the savings to be gained from smoking cessation, and similar differences in savings were seen for the elderly. While the direct saving that stems from avoiding the risk of chronic obstructive pulmonary disease for heavy smokers was about the same for men aged 35 to 39 ($1,030) and those aged 75 to 79 ($808), the indirect savings were vastly different—$24,831 for men aged 35 to 39 but only $573 for those aged 75 to 79.[19] Therefore, prevention for the elderly seems much less economically advantageous when indirect costs (calculated as lost productivity or wages) are included than when only direct costs are considered.

Another technique that is used in economic analyses of medical care diminishes the calculated benefit of preventing diseases that will be suffered by the elderly. Since dollars that are to be gained in the future are not worth the same as dollars gained today, the procedure of discounting is employed. By using a discount rate, which adjusts for the changing worth of the dollar with time (e.g., 5 percent), this technique can calculate the value today of a future benefit or cost. In cost-benefit analysis discounting helps quantify the natural preference for immediate returns. Our preference to have something today instead of in the future can be measured by a rate called the social rate of time preference, and this applies to health outcomes as well as to monetary gains. Since we value today's gains more than tomorrow's, and since we cherish today's money more than tomorrow's, it follows that social preferences might make us reluctant to spend today's money for tomorrow's beneficial outcomes. Hence, we may be reluctant to spend on medical care for the young to prevent illness that will occur in the elderly. Even behavioral changes, which require nonmonetary sacrifice today for tomorrow's gains, may not be adopted despite impressive cost-benefit calculations. Similarly, health education, which cannot even claim substantial documented savings,[22] might not be adopted because of the delay between the cost of intervention and the savings from improved health.

WHO IS PAYING THE BILL AND WHO IS BENEFITING?

One important controversy in analyzing cost-benefit or cost-effectiveness data revolves around the point of view of the analyst. What is good for the goose is not necessarily good for the gander, and one person's cost may be another's savings.

Economics suggest that the social perspective is usually the preferred one, because it allows costs and benefits to be counted only if they are not offset by someone else's benefit or cost. However, it is difficult—and some would argue unethical— for a clinician to make a decision from the societal perspective if that decision is clearly in conflict with the best decision from the patient's viewpoint.

Four principal points of view are considered in economic analysis of medical care: those of the individual (the patient, consumer, or client), the provider (e.g., the physician, hospital, or nursing home), the payer (e.g., Medicare or Blue Cross/Blue Shield) and society as a whole. For example, imagine that Medicare is deciding whether to pay for a preventive measure that has a favorable net benefit only when avoided indirect costs are considered, but that does not save Medicare money in medical costs. An alternative decision for Medicare might be to pay for another preventive service that has large direct medical savings but little indirect savings. Which will Medicare choose? From the perspective of its own self-interest, Medicare would pay for the second service and enjoy the larger savings in covered medical expenses. However, the policy-makers at Medicare should realize their responsibility to beneficiaries who would benefit from the indirect savings, as would society as a whole.

Imagine the dilemma for another policy-maker, the clinician working in a health maintenance organization (HMO), who must decide whether to offer a preventive service to a patient. Again, the different points of view may come into conflict, since the HMO will gain only the direct savings but the patient will benefit from the indirect savings (as well as nonmedical direct savings such as avoided expenses for transportation). The clinician, with a commitment to both the HMO and the patient, must weigh the two perspectives if they would lead to different conclusions about the net benefit of the preventive service.

In several economic analyses that provide data about prevention, the perspective that is taken determines the conclusion. For example, pneumococcal immunization for high-risk persons (including those over 50 years of age) was found to have a benefit-to-cost ratio of 2.32 when both direct costs and indirect costs were included.[23] In contrast, when only direct costs were included, the benefit-to-cost ratio was 0.338.

Similarly, hypertension treatment only pays back about 25 percent of its direct cost in reduced costs of caring for persons with stroke and coronary heart disease.[24] However, when absenteeism is reduced with a work-site hypertension program, it may be possible to reduce expenses to the employer, for whom reduced health care costs and averted lost productivity are meaningful benefits.[25]

The question of whether reductions in indirect costs provided by prevention programs have enough economic benefit to save societal resources is probably not relevant for most of the elderly. If a person is not working, then the method of valuing indirect costs by lost wages (the "human capital approach") suggests that there can be no savings in lost productivity. For the elderly, most prevention programs are probably not cost saving even if they do improve the quality of life or longevity.

In addition to being reluctant to subsidize the patient, the employer, or society as a whole, third-party payers may have reasons other than the discounting of future gains to be reluctant to pay now to avoid a disease that may not occur for decades. By then, the patient may live elsewhere, or may have gone from Blue Cross or HMO coverage to Medicare, or from Medicare to other coverage.[6] For example, Medicare pays a large portion of the elderly's hospital and outpatient bills but very little of the nursing home bills. Why should a self-interested Medicare program spend large amounts of money now to prevent disease or disability that would require admission to a nursing home years from now when another payer, such as Medicaid, is likely to be the one to benefit from the saved long-term care costs?

Another economic dimension of prevention programs in the elderly is that they may induce additional costs. One way in which prevention might induce unnecessary costs is by generating large numbers of false-positive results.

False-positive results were a problem in one screening program at the Kaiser-Permanente Plan. Over 40 percent of persons screened had a follow-up encounter, and 10 percent had additional tests. New diagnoses were made in far less than 1% of patients.[26] While the screening may be worthwhile for the individual with disease, the costs and risk of tests that are induced by the false-positive result can be considerable.

In the cost-effectiveness analysis of glaucoma performed by Gottlieb and colleagues, a referral cutoff of 21 mmHg on tonometry was preferred to a cutoff of 24 mmHg.[16] For those aged 75 to 79, for example, the average cost per year of vision saved with a cutoff of 21 mmHg would be $2,170; with a cutoff of 24 mmHg, the cost per year of vision saved would be $2,280. However, the investigators suggest that the number of referrals that might result from mass screening with a cutoff of 21 mmHg to evaluate whether the screening revealed truly abnormal ocular pressures would probably overwhelm the nation's ophthalmologists, who would either turn them away or ignore other important work.[16] No matter what the screening program, the risk of false-positive results could make the program unrealistically expensive or unmanageable.

THE COST OF PREVENTION'S SUCCESS— THE PRICE OF LONGER LIFE

A successful prevention program has two potential costs to society that we have not yet addressed: the cost of diseases that the aged live to develop, and the added cost of old-age pensions.

Not all health economists agree, but often cost-benefit and cost-effectiveness analyses include, as a cost of successful prevention or treatment that extends longevity, the expenses incurred in the future because the person lives long enough to undergo further routine medical care or to acquire more diseases that require treatment. Russell suggests that a simple rule be used: if the question is, what will the program mean for medical expenditures now and in the future, then these induced costs of successful care and increased longevity should be included. On the other hand, if the purpose of the analysis is to determine whether the program is a good investment, only the costs of the preventive program should be counted and the induced costs should be ignored.[17] In neither case would the effects of prolonged life on expenses for food, clothing, housing, and other nonmedical consumption be included.

An example of the cost of longer life was provided by Wright's study of smoking cessation. Wright found that when future medical care expenses of persons who quit smoking are calculated, the increased medical expenses that result from greater longevity fall to the Medicare budget, since the additional years are often those after the age of 65.[27] Because of these additional years under Medicare and the attendant expenses, the present value of Medicare's added future expenditures for a 45-year-old light smoker who quits is between $204 and $2,745.

Some suggest that future medical costs need not be considered since they are not relevant to the question of the intervention's effects on the cost of caring for the illness of concern. In any case, the future costs, if counted, should be discounted to the present, which will decrease their impact on the calculus of the analysis.

A second issue, that of old-age pensions, is also of direct importance to the elderly. Gori and Richter used the Wharton econometric model to predict the effect of successful prevention programs with resultant prolonged life expectancy.[28] Their conclusions are most sobering. Initially, they suggest, the gross national product and government revenues would grow as a result of increased productivity and survival among the work force. However, an increase in survival would soon have a profound demographic effect, with an increase in the size of the retired population. The elderly would be eligible for pension funds and social security payments, and there would be increased taxes or debt to cover the retirement expenditures. In contrast, Warner and Murt suggest that the retirement age may be postponed (witness recent Social Security legislation) and that productive years of labor may be prolonged along with survival.[29]

Depending on how these factors of induced medical care expenses and pension benefits due to improved longevity are handled in economic analyses of prevention, substantial differences in results, their interpretations, and their policy implications may occur.

PROSPECTS

Among the many obstacles to preventive care of the elderly, one that looms large is the present-day economic barrier. The American Cancer Society described in 1980 the national cost of following its set of recommendations.[30]

For a 65-year-old woman to follow the recommendations of the American Cancer Society and the Centers for Disease Control (influenza immunization, mammography, Papanicolaou test every third year, physician examination, sigmoidoscopy) alone would cost $158.90 yearly according to Medicare's prevailing fees for Philadelphia internists. When the INSURE Project on Lifecycle Preventive Health Services paid for preventive services in its trial, the cost for adults 75 and older was $131.80.[31] Because Medicare's deductible is $75 and most Medicare-eligible persons receive less than $100 per year of medical care paid by Medicare,[5] these costs fall largely to the individual elderly person.

However, with the INSURE project, patients expressed a willingness to pay extra for preventive care insurance if it were available.[31] Similarly, in HMOs and in situations where care is free, there is greater utilization of preventive services.[29] Even if the programs do not save money for Medicare, selected preventive services may be a more effective way to use the constrained Medicare dollar.

If all 31 million women over age 50 were screened, for example, the cost in 1980 dollars would be about 1.5 billion each year. To examine all Americans over 40 annually with sigmoidoscopy would cost about $2.75 billion. To perform sputum cytology and chest radiographs every 4 months to detect lung cancer (as has been done in a major ongoing trial of lung cancer screening) would have a direct cost of approximately $3 billion per year. For a population of 100,000 average-risk women, the present value of the cost (discounted to 1980 dollars) for every-3-year cervical cancer screening with Papanicolaou tests would be about $10 million. The present value of an every-6-month screening program would be about $55 million.

Prevention can be a costly business, and taking a bookkeeper's approach to medical care may suggest that prevention is not a profitable investment. But the bookkeeper's perspective, counting only dollars, is a narrow one. Even if prevention only occasionally saves money, it is often the most productive way to spend limited resources in medical care. Even if the cost-benefit calculus falls short of profitability, cost-effectiveness analysis often reveals the wisdom of the commitment to prevention. As new measures of functional status and health outcomes in the elderly are developed, the economic evaluation of preventive services will become more clinically meaningful. In preserving the longevity and activity of the elderly, a targeted approach to prevention is good medical practice.

REFERENCES

1. Geisel TS: Dr. Seuss: You're Only Old Once. A Book for Obsolete Children. New York, Random House, 1986.
2. U.S. Public Health Service: The economic burden that prevention could reduce. In Health US, 1980. Washington, DC, Department of Health and Human Services, 1980; 285–290. PHS#81-1232.
3. Rogers PJ, Eaton EK, Bruhn JG: Is health promotion cost effective? 1981; 10:324–339.
4. Sheffler RM, Paringer L: A review of the economic evidence on prevention. Medical Care 1980; 18:473–484.
5. Somers A: Why not try preventing illness as a way of controlling Medicare costs? N Engl J Med 1984; 311:853–856.
6. Banta HD, Luce BR: Assessing the cost-effectiveness of prevention. J Community Health 1983; 9:145–165.
7. Stults BM: Preventive health care for the elderly. West J Med 1984; 141:832–845.
8. Freer CB: Geriatric screening: A reappraisal of preventive strategies in the care of the elderly.
9. Collen MF, Feldman R, Siegelaub AB, Crawford D: Dollar cost per positive test for automated multiphasic screening. N Engl J Med 1970; 283:459–463.
10. Weinstein MC: Cost-effective priorities for cancer prevention. Science 1983; 221:17–23.
11. Nissinen A, Tuomilehto J, Kottke TE, Puska P: Cost-effectiveness of the North Karelia Hypertension Program, 1972–1977. Med Care 1986; 24:767–780.
12. Weinstein MC, Stason WB: Hypertension: A Policy Perspective. Cambridge, MA, Harvard University Press, 1976.
13. Willems JS, Sanders CR, Riddough MA, Bell JC: Cost-effectiveness of vaccination against pneumococcal pneumonia. N Engl J Med 1980; 303:553–559.
14. Katz S, Branch LG, Branson MH, et al: Active life expectancy. N Engl J Med 1983; 309:1218–1224.
15. Hazzard WR: Preventive gerontology. Strategies for healthy aging. Postgrad Med 1983; 74:279–287.
16. Gottlieb LK, Schwartz B, Pauker SG: Glaucoma screening. A cost-effectiveness analysis. Surv Ophthalmol 1983; 28:206–226.
17. Russell LB: Is Prevention Better Than Cure? Washington, DC, The Brookings Institution, 1986, p 134.
18. Oster G, Epstein AM: Primary prevention and coronary heart disease: The economic benefits of lowering serum cholesterol. Am J Public Health 1986; 76:647–656.
19. Oster G, Colditz GA, Kelly NL: The Economic Costs of Smoking and Benefits of Quitting. Lexington, MA, Lexington Books, 1984.
20. Fein R: On measuring economic benefits of health programs. In Veatch R, Branson R (eds): Ethics and Health Policy. Cambridge, MA, Ballinger, 1986.
21. Avorn J: Benefit and cost analysis in geriatric care; turning age discrimination into health policy. N Engl J Med 1984; 310:1294–1301.
22. Engleman SR, Forbes JF: Economic aspects of health education. Soc Sci Med 1986; 22:443–458.
23. Patrick KM, Woolley FR: A cost-benefit analysis of immunization for pneumococcal pneumonia. JAMA 1981; 245:473–477.
24. Weinstein MC, Stason WB: Cost-effectiveness of interventions to prevent or treat coronary heart disease. Annu Rev Public Health 1985; 6:41–63.
25. Shephard RJ: Employee health and fitness: The state of the art. Prev Med 1983; 12:644–653.
26. Friedman GD, Goldberg M, Ahuja JN, et al: Biochemical screenings tests: Effect of panel size on medical care. Arch Intern Med 1972; 129:91–97.

27. Wright VB: Will quitting smoking help Medicare solve its financial problems? Inquiry 1986; 23:76–82.
28. Gori GB, Richter BJ: Macroeconomics of disease prevention in the United States. Science 1978; 200:1124–1130.
29. Warner KE, Murt HA: Economic incentives for health. Annu Rev Public Health 1984; 5:107–133.
30. American Cancer Society. ACS Report on the cancer-related health check-up. CA 1980; 30:194–240.
31. Logsdon DN, Rosen MA, Demak MM: The INSURE Project of lifecycle preventive health services: Cost containment issues. Inquiry 1983; 20:121–126.

16
THE HOME TEAM

Risa Lavizzo-Mourey, MD, MBA

Geriatrics is often described as a team endeavor. The multiple problems of frail elderly, which require the expertise of many disciplines, are best addressed through the efforts of an interdisciplinary team. The benefits of such a team approach have been widely described in inpatient, long-term care, and academic ambulatory settings. However, the vast majority of geriatric patients do not receive their medical care in these settings. They are cared for, in most cases, by internists and family practitioners working in solo or group practices. Thus, primary care physicians may spend as much as 60% of their time attending to the problems of the elderly. Often it is these committed physicians and their patients who would most benefit from the interdisciplinary team approach. Yet, such an approach may seem least accessible to these physicians. Therefore, this chapter will develop the notion of a traveling interdisciplinary team and will discuss strategies to facilitate a team approach using home health agencies.

The core members of a team caring for geriatric patients include a physician, a nurse practitioner and a social worker.[1,2] This group provides the initial assessment of a frail elderly person's medical, functional, and social needs, and subsequently develops a plan that may enlist the services of other professionals such as physical therapists, occupational therapists, psychiatrists and speech therapists. The team approach is based on the recognition that, among frail elderly, problems are frequently multifactorial with the different factors being interrelated. Thus, in a Geriatric Evaluation Unit or Clinic, patients are typically seen by each member of the team, and plans reflecting and combining the group's expertise are carried out. Ideally, the provider taking the lead varies, depending on the patient's needs. Sometimes the physician plays the central role, and other times it is the social worker. Such a multidisciplinary approach has been pioneered in rehabilitation units, long-term care settings, and, increasingly, in acute care settings.

The outcomes associated with geriatric teams and their assessments have been studied in all of the above settings and generally seem to provide more accurate and complete diagnoses, better assessment of function, a decrease in the rate of nursing home placement, a decrease in the number of medications prescribed with a concomitant increase in compliance, and improved cognition.[2-9] Although it has not been formally studied, anyone who has tried to provide care to very needy elderly in both a team setting and as an individual would agree that the individual provider's effectiveness is increased when a team approach is used. Trying to address medical problems when there are contributory social and psychological problems, all of which must be faced with limited family and financial resources, is extremely frustrating for patient and physician alike. The team approach allows segmentation of the patient's problems and delegation to individual members with the team. Thus everyone's frustration is probably decreased.

So, how can a primary care physician reap the benefits of a team approach for his or her patients without adding several salaries to the payroll? First, part of a team is better than no team. Physicians who see a large number of elderly, particularly those working within group practices, should consider the benefits of adding a nurse practitioner, particularly one trained in geriatrics, to their practice. In several states the nurse practitioner can bill for services rendered, and, in the remainder, the physician can bill for services provided by the nurse practitioner under the physician's supervision. Thus, functional status assessments, medication reviews and counselling, and often-neglected preventive measures can be provided by someone who may be better trained to provide these services than the physician. Some experts in the field feel that nurse practitioners are the ideal professionals to provide case management. As the case manager, the nurse practitioner assesses the multi-dimensional needs of the patient, develops a dynamic plan, and coordinates the resources necessary to implement that plan. The nurse practitioner's role can be augmented with periodic social service consultations.

As attractive as this geriatric duo may be, it is still not feasible for many physicians. However, the concept of a traveling team, where all of the personnel with the exception of the physician are employees of one or more home health agencies, is attractive and feasible for the majority of community-based physicians. In 1983 Medicare began reimbursing a more diverse mix of skilled in-home services. Since that time, the number of home health agencies has increased dramatically, as has the proportion that can provide interdisciplinary care. Home care, which used to be synonymous with visiting nurse services, now routinely provides skilled nursing care, custodial nursing care, physical therapy, occupational therapy, speech therapy, social services, venipuncture, and parenteral and enteral nutrition, as well as other intravenous therapies.

To illustrate the point, consider an 87-year-old patient with osteoporosis and arthritis who sees her physician for a compression fracture of T10 and, as a result, has the home care team activated. Initially, she requires bed rest and pain control. The nurse and nurse's aide supervise her medications, monitor the side effects of the analgesics and keep her bathed, fed and comfortable. During this time, the physical therapist evaluates her and her environment, is able to recommend several simple modifications to reduce the risk of falling, and begins therapeutic exercises. The patient progresses slowly and, probably as a result, begins to show signs of depression. She is started on a tricyclic antidepressant, without complication, by the physician, largely because drug levels can be routinely drawn and orthostatic blood pressures checked by the nurse. After about 2½ months she is walking again and back to her baseline functioning. This potentially devastating episode does not necessitate hospitalization or nursing home placement. However, without the effective use of a home care team, both probably would be necessary.

Under current Medicare guidelines, homebound Medicare recipients requiring skilled care may well be eligible for home care benefits. Hospital discharge planners are aware of these benefits and, consequently, are the main source of referrals for home health agencies. Yet, any physician *could* be a part of this traveling team. Effective participation in such an interdisciplinary team does not require money or much time. It does require identification of appropriate patients, interactive clinical participation, and the commitment to keeping the team functioning.

STRATEGY FOR TEAM PARTICIPATION

1. *The Right Patients*

Since the only glue holding a traveling team together is a shared commitment toward the patient, it is important to strengthen this bond by referring appropriate patients to interdisciplinary care. Patients who require multiple skilled services, who have experienced recent functional decline, who have a reasonable probability of attaining treatment goals, and who can be described as homebound are ideal candidates.

It is important also to mention the family's role. If the patient is fortunate enough to have family members who can participate in the case, it should be made clear that they are considered members of the team. Efforts should be made to keep them informed and to complement the family-provided care rather than interfere with or duplicate it. This often involves something as simple as scheduling home visits of patients with working family members, such that the amount of time the elderly person is left alone is minimized. For patients and families who have the means to pay for home services out of pocket, only the clinical issues are relevant. However, the majority of elderly rely on Medicare for financial access to home care.

In order to qualify for Medicare reimbursement, the case must be made that the patient is homebound *and* requires skilled services. It is not enough to describe the elder as homebound; documentation must be provided to indicate that leaving the home is difficult due to the patient's inability to negotiate stairs or to walk more than 15 feet without exhaustion, shortness of breath, or angina. Requiring assistance with ambulation and special transportation are also acceptable indicators of homebound status. Specific types of skilled services will be discussed later in the chapter but, in general, skilled services are those that are provided by specially trained professionals, such as a registered nurse, physical therapist, or speech therapist. However, being homebound and requiring skilled services does not mean the physician must make home visits.

Setting appropriate goals can be done best by considering deficits in activities of daily living and instrumental activities of daily living. For example, patients with Alzheimer's disease often develop incontinence. Early on, the etiology may be multifactorial—there may be a functional component due to the patient's inability to get to the toilet quickly, there may be an element of detrusor instability due to the central nervous system changes associated with Alzheimer's disease, and there may be an iatrogenic component due to the patient's specific medications. After an initial office evaluation to rule out reversible causes of urinary incontinence, involvement with the home care team would be very appropriate. The goal would be a bladder training program that the patient and his family would carry out and would keep him dry throughout most of the day. The home team would then evaluate the environment for contributors to functional incontinence, initiate an incontinence chart, and teach the patient's family an appropriate toileting schedule.

Similarly, a patient having difficulty with medication compliance due to a dementia-related swallowing apraxia could also benefit from the expertise of a home care team. The nurse also could do a complete functional assessment, because the patient with dementia is very likely to have other significant functional deficits. The speech therapist may be able to teach a family member ways to overcome this apraxia, such as inducing the swallowing reflex by mixing the medicines with a cold substance such as sherbet. Gains such as these may be viewed as small accomplishments, but they do improve the patient's and the family members' quality of life, are satisfying for the team and, therefore, are worthwhile. It is doubtful that even the most dedicated physician could make these improvements in a patient's life without the help of other professionals.

2. *To the Physician: Be Available Clinically*

The physician's only interaction with the home care team may be over the telephone and should not be viewed negatively; rather, it should be viewed as a characteristic of these kinds of teams. Obviously, the effectiveness of the team will improve if there is good communication. Therefore:

• Take care in filling out referral forms. A recent study indicated that as many as 50% contain inaccurate information.[10]

• Make yourself available to members of the home care team, especially during the assessment period. Studies indicate that the most cost effective consultations are ones where the consulting physician and the consultant address the same issues and problems because *they have talked.*[11] Often when a member of the home care team calls, he or she is doing so from the patient's home and with specific questions. So, whenever possible, try to take these calls when they come. The alternative is to schedule these calls just as a team working within an institution would schedule team meetings. Early in the morning, 7:30–9:00, before the home visits are made is a particularly good time to schedule calls.

• Integrate the assessments of the home care team into your overall plan. Often these assessments are the physician's only access to an accurate appraisal of the home environment and, therefore, are essential in developing strategies for injury prevention and environmental change. Similarly, these assessments may allow realistic goals to be set regarding patient and family education.

In incorporating the home care team's assessments into your plan, be sure to consult with them and agree on priorities. Often, a frail elderly patient and his or her family are just as overwhelmed by the multitude of problems as the physicians are. If priorities are not set and adhered to, the patient's frustration will potentially be exacerbated.

• Communicate with the team. This is especially important for group practices where several physicians may be interacting with the home care team. Just photocopying an office note may be enough to update the home care team on your latest plan and, more importantly, the rationale for that plan.

• Limit the number of home care agencies you interact with to one or two and get to know the personnel at those agencies. It may be possible to request that the same nurse take care of several of your patients. Many home health agencies begin the morning with "sign-in rounds." Try to stop by during one of these times and introduce yourself. Next, familiarize yourself with the particular strengths and weaknesses of your home health agency. Home health agencies may have geriatric nurse practitioners or geriatric social workers or speech therapists with particular interests and areas of expertise that might be especially beneficial to certain patients. Similarly, nurse clinical specialists with psychiatric training can work in home health agencies under the supervision of a psychiatrist.

3. *Keep the Team Working Smoothly*

Home health agencies work on a very small profit margin. Therefore, the physician's attention to administrative details can literally keep an agency afloat, and will certainly make that agency much more willing to accommodate your special needs and those of your patients. Points to remember:

● Sign orders and care plans right away. In most cases, the agencies cannot bill without these signatures. The wording of your referral and assessments can have important billing implications for the agency. Certain words like "stable" and "status quo" are often interpreted by intermediaries to mean that the patient no longer has rehabilitation potential or an acute process and therefore is ineligible for services. If in doubt, ask the agency for guidance. The wrong words can sometimes lead to Medicare denying payment for services already provided. Needless to say, a high denial rate can be devastating for an agency, and they may request your support in appealing the denial. Orders for venipunctures and injections must have a supporting diagnosis. For example, Medicare will not reimburse a venipuncture for fasting blood sugar if there is no accompanying diagnosis of diabetes or hypoglycemia. In general, write orders for evaluation *and* therapy, because an order for evaluation only will require a subsequent therapy order if any treatments are to be given.

● Keep in mind these commonly ordered services that are not reimbursed:
1. Pre-pouring medications
2. Pre-filling insulin syringes
3. Prevention of injury or illness **unless** reasonable probability that a change may occur (for example, a patient with a recent hip fracture is just beginning to walk again)
4. Skin care, bathing, foot care, and social services or supportive therapy
5. Occupational therapy for employment purposes or without other skilled services being necessary
6. Physical therapy for maintenance range of motion
7. Family counseling by the social worker

One of our colleagues, in describing the flexibility of the well-functioning geriatric team, drew analogies between a relay team and a basketball team. On a relay team, each person's job is well-defined. Each person runs a good race and then passes the baton without missing a step. A basketball team, on the other hand, is made up of five people with well-defined functions that sometimes overlap and always interact. If a traditional geriatric team is analogous to a regular-season basketball team, then the traveling home team is analogous to an all-star basketball team. Both the all-star team and the traveling home team come together for a purpose, quickly decide on their roles, work together toward achieving their goal, and then disband. Better geriatric care can surely be provided if more physicians become linked to traveling home teams.

PRACTICE RECOMMENDATIONS

1. Patients most likely to benefit from a home team's involvement include (a) patients with multiple deficits, (b) patients with recent functional decline who have potential for improvement, and (c) patients who are homebound.

2. Involve the family as team members.

3. Set realistic goals for the patient.

4. The physician should be available clinically and participate actively in the team.

5. The physician should incorporate the home team's assessment in his or her plan and communicate his or her assessment and plan to the team.

6. Work with the team to set and follow mutually agreed priorities.

7. The physician should become familiar with the clinical assets of the home care agencies to which you regularly refer.

8. Learn the relevant Medicare regulations and try to use terminology that will not be misinterpreted by the Medicare intermediaries.

REFERENCES

1. Williams ME: Outpatient geriatric evaluation. Clin Geriatr Med 1987; 3:175–183.
2. Barker WH, Williams TF, Zimmer JG, et al: Geriatric consultation teams in acute hospitals: Impact on back-up of elderly patients. J Am Geriatr Soc 1985; 33:422–428.
3. Lefton E, Bonstelle S, Frengley JD: Success with an inpatient geriatric unit: A controlled study. J Am Geriatr Soc 1983; 31:149–155.
4. Popplewell PY, Henschke PJ: What is the value of a geriatric assessment unit in a teaching hospital? A comparative study. Aust Health Rev 1983; 6:23–25.
5. Rubenstein LZ, Josephson KR, Wieland GD, et al: Effectiveness of a geriatric evaluation unit: A randomized clinical trial. N Engl J Med 1984; 311:1664–1670.
6. Rubenstein LZ, Josephson KR, Wieland GD, et al: Geriatric assessment on a subacute hospital ward. Clin Geriatr Med 1987; 3:131–143.
7. Teasdale TA, Schuman L, Snow E, et al: A comparison of outcomes of geriatric cohorts receiving care in a geriatric assessment unit and on general medicine floors. J Am Geriatr Soc 1983; 31:529–534.
8. Berkman B, Campion EW, Swagerty E, et al: Geriatric consultation team: Alternative approach to social work discharge planning. J Gerontol Soc Work 1983; 5:77–88.
9. Allen CM, Becher PM, McVey LJ, et al: A randomized controlled clinical trial of a geriatric consultation team: Compliance with recommendations. JAMA 1986; 255:2617–2621.
10. Lavizzo-Mourey R, Laskowsky RJ, Harris MD, Parente CA: Improving drug regimens for the homebound. Am J Nurs May 1987; 593–596.
11. Lee T, Pappius E, Goldman L: Impact of inter-physician communication on the effectiveness of medical consultation. Am J Med 1983; 74:106–112.

APPENDIX A

ASSESSMENT AND SCREENING INSTRUMENTS

The following pages present several established instruments that can be used by the clinician to facilitate screening of elderly patients for a variety of problems. Many of the questionnaires are self-administered (i.e., the patient can complete the questionnaire on his or her own while in the waiting room before an appointment). However, it should be remembered that patients with visual, reading or other language difficulties may need assistance in completing the questionnaires. Other instruments, such as those related to functional status and balance, provide guides for conducting such evaluations in the standard history and physical examination.

A brief description of administration instructions, as well as instrument characteristics, scoring and interpretation, is presented with each instrument. Further information about how best to integrate information gained from the instruments is presented in various chapters in this book. In addition, selected references in the literature are indicated where further information about each instrument is available.

The following instruments are presented and discussed:

Scored instruments	Related information:
Michigan Alcoholism Screening Test	Chapter 8
Nutritional Risk Index	Chapter 8
Zung's Self-Rating Depression Scale	Chapter 12
Beck Depression Inventory	Chapter 12
Short Portable Mental Status Questionnaire	Chapter 12
Mini-Mental State Examination	Chapter 12
Non-scored instruments	**Related information:**
Balance and Gait Test	Chapter 10
Functional Status Scales	Chapter 11

For more information including other potentially useful instruments, we recommend Israel L, Kozarevic D, Satorius N: Source Book of Geriatric Assessment. Basel, Karger, 1984.

MAST

(MICHIGAN ALCOHOLISM SCREENING TEST)

General Instructions.   This is a self-administered questionnaire that can be completed by the patient in 15 minutes or less. The patient is asked to indicate a "yes" (Y) or "no" (N) answer for each of the questions.*

Instrument Characteristics.   This 24-item instrument has recently been validated in the elderly and is most useful as a screening test. There are two shorter versions that have not been validated in the elderly.

Scoring.   The direction and scoring weights are shown next to each question on the next page. A score of 3–4 indicates "possible alcoholism" and a score of 5 or more indicates "definite alcoholism." No significant differences between men and women have been identified.

For more information:

Selzer ML: The Michigan Alcoholism Screening Test (MAST): The quest for a new diagnostic instrument. Am J Psychiatry 1971; 127:1653–1658.

Willenbring: Alcoholism screening in the elderly. J Am Geriatr Soc 1987; 35:869.

---

* See Chapter 8 for further discussion.

MICHIGAN ALCOHOLISM SCREENING TEST (MAST)

	Scoring Weights
1. Do you feel you are a normal drinker?	N-2
2. Have you ever awakened the morning after some drinking the night before and found that you could not remember a part of the evening before?	Y-2
3. Does your wife/husband/companion ever worry or complain about your drinking?	Y-1
4. Can you stop drinking without a struggle after one or two drinks?	N-2
5. Do you ever feel bad about your drinking?	Y-1
6. Do friends or relatives think you are a normal drinker?	N-2
7. Are you always able to stop drinking when you want to?	N-2
8. Have you ever attended a meeting of Alcoholics Anonymous (AA)?	Y-5
9. Have you gotten into fights when drinking?	Y-1
10. Has drinking ever created problems between you and your wife/husband?	Y-2
11. Has your wife/husband (or other family member) ever gone to anyone for help about your drinking?	Y-2
12. Have you ever lost friends or girlfriends because of your drinking?	Y-2
13. Have you ever gotten into trouble at work because of drinking?	Y-2
14. Have you ever lost a job because of drinking?	Y-2
15. Have you ever neglected your obligations, your family or your work for two or more days in a row because you were drinking?	Y-2
16. Do you ever drink before noon?	Y-1
17. Have you ever been told you have liver trouble? Cirrhosis?	Y-2
18. Have you ever had delirium tremens (DTs), severe shaking, heard voices or seen things that weren't there after heavy drinking?	Y-2
19. Have you ever gone to anyone for help about your drinking?	Y-5
20. Have you ever been a hospital because of drinking?	Y-5
21. Have you ever been a patient in a psychiatric hospital or on a psychiatric ward of a general hospital where drinking was a part of the problem?	Y-2
22. Have you ever been seen at a psychiatric or mental health clinic or gone to a doctor, social worker or clergyman for help with an emotional problem in which drinking has played a part?	Y-2

NUTRITIONAL RISK INDEX

General Instructions.   This is a self-administered questionnaire containing 16 items taking 2 to 3 minutes to complete. The patient is asked to indicate a "yes" or "no" answer for each of the questions.*

Instrument Characteristics.   This test was designed to identify patients at high risk for malnutrition associated conditions or impairments. The reliability and validity against other instruments have been assessed. However, they have not been validated against serum albumin, anthropomorphic measurements and other clinical signs of malnutrition. This test is best used as a screening test.

Scoring.   Each "yes" answer is given 1 point. Patients with a score 8 or greater are at high risk whereas patients scoring 7 or below are not considered at risk for developing nutritionally related conditions.

For more information:

Wolinsky F, Rodney M, Coc M, et al: Further assessment of the reliability and validity of a nutritional index: Analysis of a three way panel study of elderly adults. Health Serv Res 1986; 20:6977–990.

---

* See Chapter 8 for further discussion.

NUTRITIONAL RISK INDEX

1.	Do you have an illness or condition that interferes with your eating?	YES	NO
2.	Do you have an illness that has cut down on your appetite?	YES	NO
3.	Do you have trouble biting or chewing any kind of food?	YES	NO
4.	Are there any kinds of foods that you don't eat because they disagree with you?	YES	NO
5.	Do you wear dentures?	YES	NO
6.	Have you had any spells of pain or discomfort for 3 days or more in your abdomen or stomach in the past month?	YES	NO
7.	Did you have any trouble swallowing at least 3 days in the last month?	YES	NO
8.	Did you have any vomiting at least 3 days in the last month?	YES	NO
9.	Do you have any trouble with your bowels that makes you constipated or gives you diarrhea?	YES	NO
10.	Have you gained or lost any weight in the last 30 days? (Note: net gain/loss must have exceeded 10 pounds.)	YES	NO
11.	In the past month, have you taken any medicines prescribed by a doctor?	YES	NO
12.	Have you ever been told by a doctor that you were "anemic" (had iron poor blood)?	YES	NO
13.	Do you smoke cigarettes regularly now?	YES	NO
14.	Have you ever had an operation on your abdomen?	YES	NO
15.	In the past month, have you taken any other medicines that were not prescribed by a doctor?	YES	NO
16.	Are you now on any kind of a special diet?	YES	NO

Reproduced from Wolinsky F, Rodney M, Coc M, et al: Further assessment of the reliability and validity of a nutritional index: Analysis of a three way panel study of elderly adults. Health Serv Res 1986; 20:6977-990, with permission

ZUNG'S SELF-RATING DEPRESSION SCALE

General Instructions. This is a self-administered questionnaire in which the patient is asked to answer 20 questions using the previous week as the time reference. There are four possible answers to each question: (a) none or little of the time, (b) some of the time, (c) good part of the time, (d) most or all of the time.*

Instrument Characteristics. The questionnaire requires approximately 3 minutes to complete and is written in simple language. The test has been used with hospitalized as well as ambulatory subjects. It has been validated against other instruments and is most useful as a screening tool.

Scoring. Each item is scored 1, 2, 3, 4, yielding a maximum raw score of 80 points. The scoring of each question is shown on the next page. The raw score is converted to an index by dividing the raw score by 80 and converting to a percentage (e.g., raw score/80 × 100). The higher the index the greater the probability of depression. An index score greater than 50 indicates depression.

For more information:

1. Hedlund JL, Vieweg BW: The Zung Self-Rating Depression Scale: a comprehensive review. Journal of Operational Psychiatry 1979; 10:51–64.

2. Zung WWK: A Self-Rating Depression Scale. Arch Gen Psychiatry 1965; 12:63–70.

---

* See Chapter 12 for further discussion.

SELF-RATING DEPRESSION SCALE

W.W.K. ZUNG

Name _____ Age _____ Sex _____ Date _____	None OR a Little of the Time	Some of the Time	Good Part of the Time	Most OR All of the Time	
1. I feel down-hearted, blue and sad	1	2	3	4	
2. Morning is when I feel the best	4	3	2	1	
3. I have crying spells or feel like it	1	2	3	4	
4. I have trouble sleeping through the night	1	2	3	4	
5. I eat as much as I used to	4	3	2	1	
6. I enjoy looking at, talking to and being with attractive women/men	4	3	2	1	
7. I notice that I am losing weight	1	2	3	4	
8. I have trouble with constipation	1	2	3	4	
9. My heart beats faster than usual	1	2	3	4	
10. I get tired for no reason	1	2	3	4	
11. My mind is as clear as it used to be	4	3	2	1	
12. I find it easy to do the things I used to	4	3	2	1	
13. I am restless and can't keep still	1	2	3	4	
14. I feel hopeful about the future	4	3	2	1	
15. I am more irritable than usual	1	2	3	4	
16. I find it easy to make decisions	4	3	2	1	
17. I feel that I am useful and needed	4	3	2	1	
18. My life is pretty full	4	3	2	1	
19. I feel that others would be better off if I were dead	1	2	3	4	
20. I still enjoy the things I used to do	4	3	2	1	
				Sds raw score	
				Sds index	

BECK DEPRESSION INVENTORY

General Instructions. This is a self-administered questionnaire, with 21 questions. Each question has four possible responses. The patient should circle the one which best describes how he/she has been feeling during the previous week.*

Instrument Characteristics. This instrument was designed to measure the severity of depressions. It takes <5 minutes to complete. It discriminates between groups with differing severity of depression and is sensitive to changes in the severity of depression.

Scoring. The scoring of each item is indicated on the questionnaire. There is a maximum score of 63. Patients scoring above 22 are probably depressed and should be further evaluated.

For more information:

Beck AT, Beanesdenfer A: Assessment of depression: The Depression Inventory. In Pichot P (ed): Psychological Measurements in Psychopharmacology. V.7, Basel, Switzerland, Karger 1974, pp 151–169.

---

* See Chapter 12 for further discussion.

BECK DEPRESSION INVENTORY (B.D.I.)

A.T. BECK

On this questionnaire are groups of statements. Please read each group of statements carefully. Then pick out the one statement in each group which best describes the way you have been feeling during the PAST WEEK, INCLUDING TODAY. Circle the number beside the statement you have chosen. Be sure to read all the statements in each group before making your choice. If several in the group seem to apply equally well, circle each one.

1. 0 I do not feel sad.
   1 I feel sad.
   2 I am sad all the time and I can't snap out of it.
   3 I am so sad or unhappy that I can't stand it.

2. 0 I am not particularly discouraged about the future.
   1 I feel discouraged about the future.
   2 I feel I have nothing to look forward to.
   3 I feel the future is hopeless and that things cannot improve.

3. 0 I do not feel like a failure.
   1 I feel I have failed more than the average person.
   2 As I look back on my life, all I can see is a lot of failures.
   3 I feel I am a complete failure as a person.

4. 0 I get as much satisfaction out of things as I used to.
   1 I don't enjoy things the way I used to.
   2 I don't get real satisfaction out of anything anymore.
   3 I am dissatisfied or bored with everything.

5. 0 I don't feel particularly guilty.
   1 I feel guilty a good part of the time.
   2 I feel quite guilty most of the time.
   3 I feel guilty all of the time.

12. 0 I have not lost interest in other people.
    1 I am less interested in other people than I used to be.
    2 I have lost most of my interest in other people.
    3 I have lost all of my interest in other people.

13. 0 I make decisions about as well as I ever could.
    1 I put off making decisions more than I used to.
    2 I have greater difficulty in making decisions than before.
    3 I can't make decisions at all anymore

14. 0 I don't feel I look any worse than I used to.
    1 I am worried that I am looking old or unattractive.
    2 I feel that there are permanent changes in my appearance that make me look unattractive.
    3 I believe that I look ugly.

15. 0 I can work about as well as before.
    1 It takes an extra effort to get started at doing something.
    2 I have to push myself very hard to do anything.
    3 I can't do any work at all.

16. 0 I can sleep as well as usual
    1 I don't sleep as well as I used to.
    2 I wake up 1–2 hours earlier than usual and find it hard to get back to sleep.
    3 I wake up several hours earlier than I used to and cannot get back to sleep.

17. 0 I don't get more tired than usual.
    1 I get tired more easily than I used to.
    2 I get tired from doing almost anything.
    3 I am too tired to do anything.

18. 0 My appetite is no worse than usual.
    1 My appetite is not as good as it used to be.
    2 My appetite is much worse now.
    3 I have no appetite at all anymore.

19. 0 I haven't lost much weight, if any, lately.
    1 I have lost more than 5 pounds.
    2 I have lost more than 10 pounds.
    3 I have lost more than 15 pounds.

    I am purposely trying to lose weight by eating less.

    _____ Yes;   _____ No.

20. 0 I am no more worried about my health than usual.
    1 I am worried about physical problems such as aches and pains; or upset stomach; or constipation.
    2 I am very worried about physical problems and it's hard to think of much else.
    3 I am so worried about my physical problems that I cannot think about anything else.

21. 0 I have not noticed any recent change in my interest in sex.
    1 I am less interested in sex than I used to be.
    2 I am much less interested in sex now.
    3 I have lost interest in sex completely.

6. 0 I don't feel I am being punished.
   1 I feel I may be punished.
   2 I expect to be punished.
   3 I feel I am being punished.

7. 0 I don't feel disappointed in myself.
   1 I am disappointed in myself.
   2 I am disgusted with myself.
   3 I hate myself.

8. 0 I don't feel I am any worse than anybody else.
   1 I am critical of myself for my weaknesses or mistakes.
   2 I blame myself all the time for my faults.
   3 I blame myself for everything bad that happens.

9. 0 I don't have any thoughts of killing myself.
   1 I have thoughts of killing myself, but I would not carry them out.
   2 I would like to kill myself.
   3 I would kill myself if I had the chance.

10. 0 I don't cry any more than usual.
    1 I cry more now than I used to.
    2 I cry all the time now.
    3 I used to be able to cry, but now I can't cry even though I want to.

11. 0 I am no more irritated now than I ever am.
    1 I get annoyed or irritated more easily than I used to.
    2 I feel irritated all the time now.
    3 I don't get irritated at all by the things that used to irritate me.

SHORT PORTABLE
MENTAL STATUS QUESTIONNAIRE

General instructions. The patient is asked each of 10 questions by an interviewer. There is no time limit. If the answer is only partially correct, it is considered an error.*

Instrument Characteristics. This instrument was designed to detect the presence and intensity of cognitive disorders in the elderly. It takes approximately 2 minutes to administer and it has been validated against the other established and respected instruments. (It is best used as a screening test for cognitive loss.)

Scoring. Each error is given one point. The total score is interpreted as follows:

0 – 2 errors = intact.
3 – 4 errors = mild intellectual impairment.
5 – 7 errors = moderate intellectual impairment.
8 –10 errors = severe intellectual impairment.
Allow one more error if subject has only grade school education.
Allow one fewer error if subject has had education beyond high school.
Allow one more error for blacks, regardless of education criteria.

For more information:

Pfeiffer E: A short portable mental status questionnaire for the assessment of organic brain deficit in elderly patients. J Am Geriatr Soc 1975; 23:433–441.

---

* See Chapter 12 for further discussion.

SHORT PORTABLE MENTAL STATUS QUESTIONNAIRE (S.P.M.S.Q.)

E. PFEIFFER

Instructions: Ask questions 1–10 in this list and record all answers. Ask question 4a only if patient does not have a telephone. Record total number of errors based on ten questions.

Allow one more if subject has had only a grade school education.
Allow one less error if subject has had education beyond high school.
Allow one more error for black subjects, using identical education criteria.

+	-	
		1. What is the date today? _____ Month Day Year
		2. What day of the week is it? _____
		3. What is the name of this place? _____
		4. What is your telephone number? _____
		4a. What is your street address? _____ *(Ask only if patient does not have a telephone)*
		5. How old are you? _____
		6. When were you born? _____
		7. Who is the President of the U.S. now? _____
		8. Who was President just before him? _____
		9. What was your mother's maiden name? _____
		10. Subtract 2 from 20 and keep subtracting 3 from each new number, all the way down.

TOTAL NUMBER OF ERRORS

0– 2 Errors	*Intact Intellectual Functioning*
3– 4 Errors	*Mild Intellectual Impairment*
5– 7 Errors	*Moderate Intellectual Impairment*
8–10 Errors	*Severe Intellectual Impairment*

To be completed by interviewer

Patient's Name _____   Date: _____

Sex: 1. Male   Race: 1. White
     2. Female   2. Black
                            3. Other

Years of education: _____   1. Grade School
                               2. High School
                               3. Beyond High School

Interviewer's Name: _____

Source: Pfeiffer E, J Am Geriatr Soc 1975; 23, 10:433–441.

MINI-MENTAL STATE EXAMINATION

General Instructions. The patient should be seated in a quiet, well lighted room. Instruct the patient to listen carefully and then answer each question as accurately as possible. This test may not be accurate in patients with severe hearing or visual deficits. Specific instructions are included adjacent to each question.*

Instrument Characteristics. This instrument measures cognitive impairment relating to orientation, registration recall, attention concentration, calculations, language and motor skills. It is useful in quantifying cognitive skills and screening for cognitive loss. It has been extensively validated and the 24 hour test-retest reliability has been documented.

Scoring. One point is given for each correct answer yielding a maximum score of 30. Generally, a score below 24 indicates cognitive impairment. However, this may not be the best cutoff for very highly educated or very poorly educated individuals.

For more information:

Folstein MF, Folstein SE, McHugh PR: Mini-Mental State: a practical method for grading the cognitive states for the clinician. J Psychiatric Res 1975; 12:188–198.

---

* See Chapter 12 for further discussion.

MINI-MENTAL STATE EXAMINATION

I. Orientation (Maximum score 10)
   Ask "What is today's date?" Then ask specifically for parts omitted; e.g., "Can you also tell me what season it is?"

Date (e.g., January 21)	1 ——
Year	2 ——
Month..................	3 ——
Day (e.g., Monday)	4 ——
Season	5 ——

   Ask "Can you tell me the name of this hospital?"
   "What floor are we on?"
   "What town (or city) are we in?"
   "What county are we in?"
   "What state are we in?"

Hospital	6 ——
Floor	7 ——
Town/City	8 ——
County	9 ——
State	10 ——

II. Registration (Maximum score 3)
   Ask the subject if you may test his/her memory. Then say "ball," "flag," "tree" clearly and slowly, about one second for each. After you have said all 3 words, ask subject to repeat them. This first repetition determines the score (0–3) but keep saying them (up to 6 trials) until the subject can repeat all 3 words. If (s)he does not eventually learn all three, recall cannot be meaningfully tested.

"ball"	11 ——
"flag"	12 ——
"tree"	13 ——
Record number of trials:	_____

III. Attention and calculation (Maximum score 5)
   Ask the subject to begin at 100 and count backward by 7. Stop after 5 subtractions (93, 86, 79, 72, 65). Score one point for each correct number.

"93"	14 ——
"86"	15 ——
"79"	16 ——
"72"	17 ——
"65"	18 ——
	OR

   If the subject cannot or will not perform this task, ask him/her to spell the word "world" backwards (D, L, R, O, W). The score is one point for each correctly placed letter, e.g., DLRORW = 5, DLORW = 3. Record how the subject spelled world backwards:

   D L R O W

Number of correctly- placed letters	19 ——

IV. Recall (Maximum score 3)
Ask the subject to recall the three words you previously asked him/her to remember (learned in Registration)

"ball" .... 20 ——
"flag" .... 21 ——
"tree" .... 22 ——

V. Language (Maximum score 9)
Naming: Show the subject a wrist watch and ask "What is this?" Repeat for pencil. Score one point for each item named correctly.

Watch .... 23 ——
Pencil .... 24 ——

Repetition: Ask the subject to repeat, "No ifs, ands, or buts." Score one point for correct repetition.

Repetition .... 25 ——

3-Stage Command: Give the subject a piece of blank paper and say, "Take the paper in your right hand; fold it in half and put it on the floor." Score one point for each action performed correctly

Takes in right hand ...... 26 ——
Folds in half .... 27 ——
Puts on floor .... 28 ——

Reading: On a blank piece of paper, print the sentence "Close your eyes." in letters large enough for the subject to see clearly. Ask subject to read it and do what it says. Score correct only if (s)he actually closes his/her eyes

Closes eyes .... 29 ——

Writing: Give the subject a blank piece of paper and ask him/her to write a sentence. It is to be written spontaneously. It must contain a subject and verb and make sense. Correct grammar and punctuation are not necessary

Writes sentence .... 30 ——

Copying: On a clean piece of paper, draw intersecting pentagons, each side about 1 inch, and ask subject to copy it exactly as it is. All 10 angles must be present and two must intersect to score 1 point. Tremor and rotation are ignored.
E.g.,

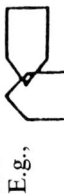

Draws pentagons .... 31 ——

Total score ——

Score: Add number of correct responses. In section III include items 14–18 or item 19, not both. (Maximum total score 30)

Rate subject's level of consciousness: ——— (a) coma, (b) stupor, (c) drowsy, (d) alert

Reprinted with permission from Folstein MF, et al: Mini-mental state: A practical method of grading the cognitive state of the patient for the physician. J Psychiatr Res 1975; 12:189.

BALANCE AND GAIT TEST

INSTRUCTIONS TO EXAMINERS

General Instructions.   Explain to subjects that you are going to ask them to perform several maneuvers that reflect activities they perform during their daily activities. Let them know you will explain each thing you want them to do or let them know what you are going to do. Inform each subject that he or she can decline to perform any maneuver, but also reassure them that you will be there and be watching them carefully and that you will not ask them to perform any unsafe maneuvers. The following list of instructions refer to individual balance maneuvers or gait observations.*

These maneuvers are best used as a structured evaluation of gait and balance.

For more information:

Tinetti ME: Performance-oriented assessment of mobility problems in elderly patients. J Am Geriatr Soc 1986; 34:119–126.

Tinetti ME, Ginter SF: Identifying mobility dysfunctions in elderly patients: standard neuromuscular examination or direct assessment? JAMA 1988; 259:1190–1193.

---

* See Chapter 10 for further discussion.

BALANCE AND GAIT

Subject is seated in hard armless chair.

Maneuver	Instructions
1. Sitting balance • leans or slides in chair. • steady, safe.	
2. Arise • unable without help. • able, but uses arms to help. • able without use of arms.	Attempt to get up with arms folded. Subject should fold arms and then get up from the chair. Note the number of attempts.
3. Attempts to arise • unable without help. • able, but require more than one attempt. • able to arise with one attempt.	
4. Immediate standing balance (first 5 seconds) • unsteady (staggers, moves feet, marked trunk sway). • steady, but uses walker or cane, or grabs other object for support. • steady without walker or cane or other support.	With arms folded the patient should rise and stand.

Maneuver	Instructions
10. Able to stand on one leg for 5 seconds • symptoms or staggering with lateral movement or extension. • marked decreased R.O.M. but without symptoms or staggering. • at least moderate R.O.M. and steady.	Subject instructed to turn head from side to side as far as possible and look up as far as possible.
11. Back extension (let patient alone) • refuses to try or no extension or uses walker while doing it. • tries but little extension. • good extension.	Patients are instructed to extend backward as far as possible.
12. Reaching up (have subject reach to a high shelf) • unable or unstable, needs to hold on to steady self. • able to reach up and is stable.	Have patient actually take something down from a high shelf.
13. Bending over (place pen on floor and ask subject to pick it up) • unable or is unsteady. • able and is steady.	Self-explanatory.

5. Standing balance

Give patient a chance to gain balance while standing and then instruct him or her to put his or her feet as close as possible.

- unsteady.
- steady, but wide stance (medial heels more than 4" apart), or uses cane, walker or other support.
- narrow stance without support.

6. Nudge (subject at maximum position with feet as close together as possible; examiner pushes lightly on subject's sternum with palm of hand 3 times).

Instruct patient to stand with feet as close as possible. Then lightly push for about 2 seconds over the sternum. Do not use sudden jerky motions.

- begins to fall.
- begins to fall, staggers, grabs, but catches self.
- steady.

7. Neck (document exact symptoms)

Subject instructed to turn head from side to side as far as possible and look up as far as possible.

- symptoms or staggering with lateral movement or extension.
- marked decreased R.O.M. but without symptoms or staggering.
- at least moderate R.O.M. and steady.

8. Eyes closed

- unsteady.
- steady.

9. Turn 360°

Self-explanatory.

- discontinuous steps.
- continuous.
- unsteady (grabs, staggers).
- steady.

14. Sit down

Self-explanatory.

- unsafe (misjudged distance; falls into chair).
- uses chair.
- uses arms or not a smooth motion.
- safe, smooth motion.

15. Turning

- staggers, unsteady.
- discontinuous, but no staggering or uses walker or cane.
- steady, continuous.

16. Able to pick up walking speed (tell subject to walk as fast as he or she can—a pace at which he or she feels safe)

- None.
- Some.
- Marked.

17. Is walking aid used appropriately.

- No.
- Yes.
- Not applicable.

18. Trunk

- Asymmetrical.
- Symmetrical.

FUNCTIONAL STATUS

PHYSICAL AND SOCIAL SKILLS

General Instructions. These four sets of questions are best used as guidelines to structure an interview on social and physical functioning. Each area of function is assessed with a series of questions aimed at defining exactly what the patient can do within a given activity area. The first series of questions is appropriate for self-sufficient elderly, the second, third, and fourth progress to levels appropriate for more dependent elderly. The last two are both measures of activities of daily living (ADL). The physical maintenance scale was discussed in Chapter 11, and the index of ADL represents an alternative. While these questions can be scored, scoring is probably not necessary in clinical settings. The questions, however, do provide a useful format and framework for recording data in the clinical record.*

For more information:

Lawton MP, Brody EM: Assessment of older people. Self maintaining and instrumental activities of daily living. Gerontologist 1969; 9:177–186.

Lawton MP: The functional assessment of elderly people. J Am Geriatr Soc 1971; 19:465–481.

Katz S, Downs TD, Cash HR, Grotz RC: Progress in development of the index of ADL. Gerontologist Spring 1970; Part 1:20–30.

---

* See Chapter 11 for further discussion.

PHYSICAL SELF-MAINTENANCE SCALE (ADL)*

A. Toilet

  1. Cares for self at toilet completely; no incontinence.
  2. Needs to be reminded, or needs help in cleaning self, or has rare (weekly at most) accidents.
  3. Soiling or wetting while asleep, more than once a week.
  4. No control of bowels or bladder.

B. Feeding

  1. Eats without assistance.
  2. Eats with minor assistance at meal times, with help in preparing food or with help in cleaning up after meals.
  3. Feeds self with moderate assistance and is untidy.
  4. Requires extensive assistance for all meals.
  5. Does not feed self at all and resists efforts of others to feed him.

C. Dressing

  1. Dresses, undresses and selects clothes from own wardrobe.
  2. Dresses and undresses self, with minor assistance.
  3. Needs moderate assistance in dressing or selection of clothes.
  4. Needs major assistance in dressing but cooperates with efforts of others to help.
  5. Completely unable to dress self and resists effort of others to help.

D. Grooming (neatness, hair, nails, hands, face, clothing)

  1. Always neatly dressed and well-groomed, without assistance.
  2. Grooms self adequately, with occasional minor assistance (e.g., in shaving).
  3. Needs moderate and regular assistance or supervision in grooming.
  4. Needs total grooming care, but can remain well-groomed after help from others.
  5. Actively negates all efforts of others to maintain grooming.

E. Physical Ambulation

  1. Goes about grounds or city.
  2. Ambulates within residence or about one block distance.
  3. Ambulates with assistance of (check one):
     (a) wheelchair (1. gets in and out without help; 2. needs help in getting in and out); (b) railing; (c) cane; or (d) walker.
  4. Sits unsupported in chair or wheelchair, but cannot propel self without help.
  5. Bedridden more than half the time.

F. Bathing

  1. Bathes self (tub, shower, sponge bath) without help.
  2. Bathes self, with help in getting in and out of tub.
  3. Washes face and hands only, but cannot bathe rest of body.
  4. Does not wash self but is cooperative with those who bathe him.
  5. Does not try to wash self and resists efforts to keep him clean.

* Start by asking the patient to describe her/his ability to perform a given activity, e.g. feeding. Then ask specific questions as needed.

Reprinted with permission from Lawton MP: The functional assessment of elderly people. J Am Geriatr Soc 1971; 19(6):465–481.

SCALE FOR INSTRUMENTAL ACTIVITIES
OF DAILY LIVING (IADL)*

A. Ability to Use Telephone

   1. Operates telephone on own initiative: looks up and dials numbers, etc.
   2. Dials a few well-known numbers.
   3. Answers telephone but does not dial.
   4. Does not use telephone at all.

B. Shopping

   1. Takes care of all shopping needs independently.
   2. Shops independently for small purchases.
   3. Needs to be accompanied on any shopping trip.
   4. Completely unable to shop.

C. Food Preparation

   1. Plans, prepares and serves adequate meals independently.
   2. Prepares adequate meals if supplied with ingredients.
   3. Heats and serves prepared meals, or prepares meals but does not maintain adequate diet.
   4. Needs to have meals prepared and served.

D. Housekeeping

   1. Maintains house alone or with occasional assistance (e.g., domestic help for heavy work).
   2. Performs light daily tasks such as dishwashing and bedmaking.
   3. Performs light daily tasks but cannot maintain acceptable level of cleanliness.
   4. Needs help with all home maintenance tasks.
   5. Does not participate in any housekeeping tasks.

E. Laundry

   1. Does personal laundry completely.
   2. Launders small items; rinses socks, stockings, etc.
   3. All laundry must be done by others.

F. Mode of Transportation

   1. Travels independently on public transportation or drives own car.
   2. Arranges own travel via taxi but does not otherwise use public transportation.
   3. Travels on public transportation when assisted or accompanied by another.
   4. Travel limited to taxi or automobile, with assistance of another.
   5. Does not travel at all.

G. Responsibility for Own Medication

   1. Is responsible for taking medication in correct dosages at correct time.
   2. Takes responsibility if medication is prepared in advance in separate dosages.
   3. Is not capable of dispensing own medication.

H. Ability to Handle Finances

   1. Manages financial matters independently (budgets, writes checks, pays rent and bills, goes to bank); collects and keeps track of income.
   2. Manages day-to-day purchases but needs help with banking, major purchases, etc.
   3. Incapable of handling money.

* Start by asking the patient to describe his/her functioning in each category, then complement with specific questions as needed.

Reprinted with permission from Lawton MP: The functional assessment of elderly people. J Am Geriatr Soc 1971; 19(6):465–481.

SOCIAL COMPETENCE ACTIVITIES

Activities in the Home

Can you describe what your primary responsibilities have been in your home? Has this changed in recent weeks? If yes, in what ways?

e.g.: Who prepares the meals?
  – If the patient does, ask if his health has affected this activity.

Who does the shopping?
  – If the patient does, ask if his health has affected this activity.

Who does the laundry?
  – If the patient does, ask if his health has affected this activity.

Who cleans the house?
  – If the patient does, ask if his health has affected this activity.

Who does repairs around the house?
  – If the patient does, ask if his health has affected this activity.

Who does the yard work?
  – If the patient does, ask if his health has affected this activity.

Who runs errands?
  – If the patient does, ask if his health has affected this activity.

Work Questions

A. Do you work? That is, do you receive pay for the work you do? If yes:

(1) What kind of work are you presently doing?
(2) Are there some things at work you used to do that you aren't doing now?

B. If you don't work, did you stop working for pay because of illness? If yes:

(1) What kind of things do you do now that you think of as work (that is, things you are responsible for such as chores around the house, volunteer club duties)?
(2) Are there some things you used to do that you aren't doing now?

C. If you have never worked for pay or have not worked for pay for a considerable period of time unrelated to current illness:

(1) What kind of things have you done that you consider work (that is, things you are responsible for such as chores—yard work, repairs, cooking, cleaning, shopping—or volunteer work)?
(2) Are there some things you used to do that you aren't doing now?

Recreational and Social Activities

A. What kind of things do you do for recreation or just for fun? What about TV?

B. Has this changed in any way since your illness?

C. How much contact do you have with people not a part of your family, and where does this occur?

D. Do you keep in touch with your friends like you used to?

E. Are there things you'd like to do in the way of recreation or entertainment that you aren't doing right now?

F. What did you do (do you plan to do) on the most recent (upcoming) major holiday?

Adapted from Benoliel JQ, McCorkle R, Young K: Development of a Social Dependency Scale. Research in Nursing and Health 1980; 3:3–10.

APPENDIX B

INSTRUCTIONS FOR USE OF PREVENTION FLOW-SHEET

Susan C. Day and Todd Goldberg

The prevention flow-sheet is designed to help clinicians care for their older patients. The first page is the Health Maintenance Profile. It should be kept clearly visible on the front of the chart; this sheet contains information that is essential to the day to day care of patients (Problem List, Medication List, Immunization History and Health Status Review). The second page details a checklist of preventive care screening measures and is designed as a reminder system to provide a framework for periodic evaluation of the elderly patient as well as a way to record important results for quick review. Each is described in depth below. Both sheets, if placed prominently in the front of the patient's chart, should facilitate incorporating regular preventive care measures into routine patient care. Non-physician office personnel can help by entering basic demographic information and updating selected portions. An office nurse, particularly if trained in geriatrics, may be able to review current medications, collect basic information on functional status, and enter vital signs, and so forth.

A blank flow-sheet is accompanied by a model flow-sheet where the recommended screening intervals are included for easy reference. These recommendations are based on current knowledge of optimum screening intervals; as new information on screening in the elderly becomes available, these may change. In addition, these recommendations are targeted towards healthy, asymptomatic individuals. For any given individual, the screening program should be adjusted for that person's functional status, coexisting conditions and personal preferences.

HEALTH MAINTENANCE PROFILE

1. **Patient Identifying Information:** On each sheet, the patient's name, phone number and date of birth should be recorded for easy reference. Making note of a pharmacy number can also help facilitate medication renewals.

2. **Problem List:** The patient's currently active problems, as well as important inactive problems, can be recorded here along with the date that the problem was first noted.

3. **Medications:** The medication list should always be kept up to date. In order to facilitate accurate recording, there is space to designate the current dose and the date that the dose was started. Additional space is allotted beside each drug to allow for dose modification. There is also a column for "Comments," where important side effects, patient preferences regarding choice of drugs, etc., can be indicated.

240

4. **Immunizations:** The dates when the patient received the Pneumovax and tetanus-diphtheria immunizations should be noted. More space is allotted for the influenza (flu) vaccine, which may be given every year.

5. **Allergies:** All documented drug allergies should be recorded, along with a description of the specific reaction that occurred.

6. **Functional Status:** The key elements of the functional status examination are listed. The patient's baseline functional status may be briefly described, leaving space for notation of any important changes.

7. **Other Baseline Data:** Other key health habits and social information may be recorded here for quick reference.

PREVENTION CHECKLIST

1. **Comprehensive Evaluation:** Setting aside a formal session with a patient to perform a comprehensive history and physical may facilitate the regular performance of screening procedures. Recording the dates of recent complete examinations will help provide a reminder of when the next extended visit should be scheduled.

2. **Age:** Recording the patient's age may help provide a reference point for planning appropriate screening procedures for that individual.

3. **Review of Systems:** The review of systems for the elderly individual focuses on specific areas, such as sensory or mental status changes, bowel, or urinary symptoms, that have a high likelihood of being abnormal or are important to detect early. The checklist provides a reminder system for common symptoms in the elderly.

4. **Physical Examination:** Key aspects of the physical examination, emphasizing the cardiovascular examination and targeted areas for cancer screening, are listed. Adequate space for recording weight and BP is included.

5. **Diagnostic Tests:** Currently recommended screening tests are listed. A complete report of the findings may not be feasible in the limited space available; if test results are abnormal and require more lengthly discussion, this may be noted along with the date so that quick reference to a progress note can be made.

6. **Counselling Checklist:** Just as the areas that are important to focus on in the review of systems may change in the older individual, so may the areas of health maintenance that should be addressed by the practitioner. The patient's diet, vitamin use, exercise program, etc., should be discussed on a regular basis and note made on the flow-sheet of the dates of when such discussions occur.

7. **Other:** These spaces can be used to monitor areas of particular importance to a specific individual.

HEALTH MAINTENANCE PROFILE

Name: _____   Pharmacy No.: _____

Phone No.: _____   D.O.B. _____

Problem List (Date of Onset)		Medication	Dose	Date	Comment

Problem List (Date of Onset)

1. _____
2. _____
3. _____   *(Update*
4. _____   *each*
5. _____   *visit)*
6. _____
7. _____
8. _____
9. _____

Immunizations:

Pneumovax _____ Td _____

Flu _____

Allergies: *(Update each visit)*

Medication   Dose   Date   Comment

1. _____
2. _____   *(Update*
                    each
3. _____   *visit)*
4. _____
5. _____
6. _____
7. _____
8. _____
9. _____

HEALTH STATUS REVIEW

Functional Status   **Describe Baseline: Indicate Change**   **Other Baseline Data**

Functional Status	Describe Baseline: Indicate Change	Other Baseline Data
Dressing		
Feeding		Smoking
Continence	*(Review annually*	Alcohol
Bathing	*or after each*	
Toileting	*hospital discharge*	Exercise
Transfer	*or major illness)*	Living Situation
Telephone		Marital Status
Shopping		
Food Preparation		Driving
Laundry		Occupation
Mode of Transportation		
Responsibility for own meds		*(Review annually)*
Manages finances		

HEALTH MAINTENANCE PROFILE

Name: _____   **Pharmacy No.:** _____

Phone No.: _____   **D.O.B.** _____

Problem List (Date of Onset)	**Medication**	**Dose**	**Date**	**Comment**
1. _____	1.			_____
2. _____				_____
3. _____	2.			_____
4. _____	3.			_____
5. _____	4.			_____
6. _____				_____
7. _____	5.			_____
8. _____	6.			_____
9. _____	7.			_____
Immunizations:				_____
Pneumovax _____ Td _____	8.			_____
Flu _____				_____
Allergies:	9.			_____

HEALTH STATUS REVIEW

Functional Status	**Describe Baseline: Indicate Change**	**Other Baseline Data**
Dressing		
Feeding		Smoking
Continence		Alcohol
Bathing		
Toileting		Exercise
Transfer		Living Situation
Telephone		
Shopping		Marital Status
Food Preparation		Driving
Laundry		Occupation
Mode of Transportation		
Responsibility for own meds		
Manages finances		

PREVENTION CHECKLIST

Comprehensive Evaluation (Dates):								
Age at time of exam:								
ROS	Weight Change							
	Mental Status			*(Yearly)*				
	Hearing							
	Vision							
	Bowel							
	Urinary							
PHYSICAL EXAM	BP							
	Weight							
	Vision							
	Hearing			*(Yearly)*				
	Breast Exam							
	Pelvic							
	Prostate							
	Rectal							
	Gait/Balance							
DIAGNOSTIC TESTS	Cholesterol							
	Stool Occult Blood		*(Yearly)*					
	Audiogram		*(As indicated by a hearing screen)*					
	Mammogram		*(Yearly in the elderly until age 75)*					
	Sigmoidoscopy		*(Two exams, 1 year apart; if negative, every 3–5 years until age 75)*					
	Pap Smear		*(Three exams, 1 year apart; if negative, every 3 years until age 75)*					
COUNSELLING CHECKLIST	Diet							
	Vitamins							
	Exercise							
	Injury Prevention			*(Yearly)*				
	Community Resources							
	Medication Review							
OTHER								

PREVENTION CHECKLIST

Comprehensive Evaluation (Dates):								
Age at time of exam:								
ROS	Weight Change							
	Mental Status							
	Hearing							
	Vision							
	Bowel							
	Urinary							
PHYSICAL EXAM	BP							
	Weight							
	Vision							
	Hearing							
	Breast Exam							
	Pelvic							
	Prostate							
	Rectal							
	Gait/Balance							
DIAGNOSTIC TESTS	Cholesterol							
	Stool Occult Blood							
	Audiogram							
	Mammogram							
	Sigmoidoscopy							
	Pap Smear							
COUNSELLING CHECKLIST	Diet							
	Vitamins							
	Exercise							
	Injury Prevention							
	Community Resources							
	Medication Review							
OTHER								

INDEX

Entries in boldface type indicate complete chapters.

Abuse, definition of, 167-168
 elder, **167-181**
  diagnosis of, 175
  documentation of, 175
  emergency, 176-177
  evaluation of, 169-170
  functional assessment and, 170
  practice recommendations and,
   179-180
  prevention of, 169
  reporting laws and, 175
  risk assessment and, 170-172
  signs and symptoms of, 172-174
  support services and, 177-179
 management of, 175-179
 mental status and, 173
 patient history and, 172-173
 physical exam and, 173
 prevention of, 177-179
Abuser, high-risk, 171-172
Active life expectancy, concept of,
 199-200
Active neglect, 168
Activities of daily living, 143-148
 instrumental, scale for, 238
 scale for, 145
Adverse drug reactions, age-related
  changes and, 47-49
 cost of, 49-50
 obstacles to preventing, 50-52
 over-the-counter drugs and, 56-57
 prevention of, **47-62**
Aerobic exercise, 79
Alcohol, 96, 98-100
 drug interactions with, 100
 practice recommendations for, 104
Alcoholism, 96, 99-100
 elderly and, 4
Alternative living arrangements, 178
Alzheimer's dementia, 154, 161-163
 clinical diagnosis of, 162
 home care and, 211
AMA Resolution 112, 168
Angina, exercise prescription and, 78, 82

Angiotensin converting enzyme inhibitors,
 for hypertension, 70
Antidepressant drug treatment, 159-161
Assessment instruments, **215-239**

Balance and gait test, 233-235
Beck's Depression Inventory, 156,
 223-225
Benign prostatic hypertrophy, 186
Beta-adrenergic blockers, for hypertension,
 70
Bladder, physiology of, 184-187
Bladder record, 191-194
Blindness, agencies serving, 129
 See also Vision
Blood pressure, See Hypertension
Bone loss, screening for, 111-113
Bone mass, factors affecting, 109-110
 methods to assess, 113
Breast cancer, screening for, 29-31
Breast self-examination, 30-31
Burnout, caregiver, neglect and, 172
Burns, prevention of, 136

Calcium, and bone mass, 109-110
Calcium, dietary sources of, 117
Calcium channel blockers, 70
Calcium supplements, 117-118
 side-effects of, 117-118
Calcium therapy, for bone loss, 116-118
 older women and, 117
 perimenopausal women and, 116-117
 practice recommendations for,
  120-121
Caloric intake, recommended, 96
Cancer, elderly and, 4-5
 epidemiology of, 23-24
 screening for, **23-35**
  practice recommendations and, 34
  recommendations for, 27-33
  treatment and, 25
Cancer screening program, assessment
 of, 24-26
Captopril, for hypertension, 70

Cardiac risk, evaluation of, **63-74**, 76-77
Cardiovascular disease, elderly and, 4
    practice recommendations and, 72-73
Cardiovascular risk, reduction of, **63-74**
Cataracts, 127-128
Cervical cancer, screening for, 31-32
Cholesterol, 64-68
    diet therapy and, 67
    drug therapy and, 68
Chronic obstructive pulmonary disease,
    exercise and, 82-83
Cigarette smoking, 70-71, 100-103
    and bone loss, 110
    cost-benefit of cessation, 201
Cognitive impairment, 161-164
    and depression, 158-159
Colles' fracture, 107
Color perception, 130
Colorectal cancer, screening for, 27-29
Competence, screening and, 19
Compliance, screening and, 18-19
COPD, exercise and, 82-83
Coronary artery disease, **63-73**
    prevention of, 72
Cost, of adverse drug reactions, 49-50
    of immunization, 40-41
    prevention and, **197-207**
    See also individual chapters
Cost-benefit analysis, of prevention,
    200-202
Cost effectiveness, of prevention
    alternatives, 198-200
Creatinine clearance, changes of, with
    age, 47-48
Cyclic progesterone, 114

Delirium, 163-164
    vs. dementia, 164
Dementia, 154, 161-163
    assessment of, 154-156
    vs. delirium, 164
    medical illness and, 161-162
    organic, vs. of depression, 159
Dependence and injury, prevention of,
    125-139
Depressed mood, medical disorders
    causing, 157
    medications associated with, 158
Depression, assessment of, 154-156
    vs. depressed mood, 158-159
    elderly and, 3
    management of, 159-161

Depression (*Continued*)
    risk factors for, 155-156
    screening for, 157
    self-rating scale of, 220-221
Depression inventory, Beck's, 223-225
Diabetes, heart disease and, 71
Diet therapy, for serum cholesterol, 67
    See also Nutrition
Disease, cost of, 197-198
Diuretics, thiazide, for hypertension,
    69-70
Dosing schedule, optimizing, 52-53
Drug, ideal, characteristics of, 59
Drug-drug interactions, 47
    patterns of, 53-56
    summary tables of, 54-56
Drug prescriptions, number of, 51-53
Drug reactions, adverse, elderly and, 3
    prevention of, **47-62**
Drug regimen, individualization of, 58-59
    regular review of, 57-58
    simplifying, 52-53
Drugs, age-related changes and, 47-49
    cost of, 49
    and depressed mood, 158
    misuse of, 49
    monitoring of, 58-60
    over-the-counter, adverse reactions
        and, 56-57
    patient education and, 59
Drug therapy, for depression, 159-161
Drug therapy, for serum cholesterol, 68
Drug therapy, practice recommendations
    and, 60-61
Drug trials, elderly and, 50

Economic considerations of prevention in
    elderly, **197-207**
Educational needs,
    of clinicians, 6-7
Elder abuse, 5
Elderly, efficacy of prevention and, 1-5
    health behavior of, 5-6
Emphysema
    exercise and, 82-83
Enalapril, for hypertension, 70
Epidemiology, of cancer, 23-24
Estrogen, and bone mass, 109
Estrogen replacement therapy, 113-116
    contraindications for use of, 116
    effects of, 114
    effects of withdrawal of, 115

Estrogen replacement therapy (*continued*)
    older women and, 114-115
    perimenopause and, 113-114
    practice recommendations for, 120
    recommendations for use of, 115-116
Ethanol-drug interactions, 100
Ethical considerations, of screening, 18-19
Exercise, **75**
    adaptation of, for physical problems,
        81-83
    aerobic, 79
    benefits and risks, of 75-77
    bone density and, 118-119
    and bone mass, 110
    cardiac risk and, 76-77
    contraindications for, 83
    COPD and, 82-83
    elderly and, 3
    guidelines for assessment and
        prescription of, 79-81
    intermittent claudication and, 82
    low-intensity, 79
    motivations and, 83-84
    musculoskeletal problems and, 83
    practice recommendations and, 86
    programs for, 84
    target heart rate and, 82
    weight reduction and, 71
Exercise activities, benefits of (table),
    85
Exercise stress tests, 76-78

Falls,
    exercise and, 118-119
    prevention of, 118, 133-135
        hazards and, 135
    risk of, 110-111
Fiber, dietary, 90
Fish oil, for serum cholesterol, 68
Fitness, See Exercise
Fractures, osteoporotic, **107-123**
Function, elderly, 2-3
Functional assessment, 143
    cost-effectiveness of, 143
Functional deficits, **141-152**
    epidemiology of, 142-143
Functional incontinence, 187, 190
Functional status assessment, **141-152**
    barriers to, 148-150
    case study of, 149-150
    practice recommendations for,
        150-151

Functional status questionnaire, 143-148
Functional status scale, 236-239

Gait test, balance and, 233-235
Geriatric teams, **209-214**
Glaucoma, 128
    cost-benefit of prevention of, 204
Gout, heart disease and, 72
Grief and bereavement, 155

Haloperidol, 163
Hazards, and prevention of falls, 135
Health behavior, of the elderly, 5-6
Health maintenance profile, 240-243
Health promotion, clinicians and, 6-7
Hearing, loss of, 130-134
    assistive devices and, 132-134
    communication strategies and, 133
        devices for, 134
    environment and, 131-132
    primary care provider and, 131
Hearing aids, 132, 134
Heart disease, cholesterol and, 64-68
    clinical studies and, 63
    practice recommendations and, 72-73
    reduction of risk of, **63-74**
Hepatic metabolism, altered, drugs and, 49
Heterocyclic antidepressants, 159-161
High density lipoprotein, screening for, 66
Hip, fractures of, 107
Home care team, **209-214**
Home health care, **210-214**
    physician and, 212-213
    practice recommendations and, 213-214
Hypercholesterolemia, 64-68
Hyperlipoproteinemia, screening for, 66
Hypertension, 68-71
    cost-effectiveness evaluation of outcome
        and, 199-200
    elderly and, 4
    North Karelia Hypertension Program,
        199-200
    prevention of, cost-benefit of, 203
    treatment for, 69-70

Iatrogenic illness, drugs and, See Adverse
    drug reactions
Ideal body weight, 93
Immunization, **37-46**
    alternative sites for, 43
    benefits of, 39-40
    cost of, 40-41

Immunization *(Continued)*
    elderly and, 3
    patient attitudes and, 43-44
    physician attitudes and, 41-43
    practice recommendations and, 44-45
    promotion of, 43
Immunologic changes of aging, 39
Incontinence, urinary, **183-196**
    diagnosis of, 187-190
    flow diagram for, 188-189
    home care and, 211
    types of, 186-187
Individualization, of drug therapy, 58-59
Infection in the elderly, susceptibility to,
        38-39
    immunology and, 39
    institutionalization and, 39
Infectious diseases, immunization and, **37-46**
Influenza, epidemiology of, 37
Influenza vaccine, cost-benefit of, 201
    effectiveness of, 40
Informed consent, 19
Injuries, elderly and, 3
    practice recommendtions and, 137-138
    prevention of, 133-137
    sensory changes and, **125-139**
Institutionalization, infection and, 39
Instrumental activities of daily living, 143-148
    scale for, 146, 238
INSURE project, 205
Intermittent claudication, exercise and, 82

Kahn's 10-item Mental Status Questionnaire,
        157
Kegel's exercise, 190, 193

Lighting, vision and, 127, 129-130
Lipoprotein cholesterol, risk associated with,
        66-67
Liver, changes in, drugs and, 48-49
Low density lipoprotein, screening for, 66-67

Malnutrition, See Nutrition
Mammography, 29-30
MAST, 216-217
Medicare, costs and, 198
    home care and, 211
Medications, See Drugs
Menopause, and bone loss, 109-118
Mental function, **153-166**
Mental health, **153-166**

Mental states, mini-mental examination for,
        229-231
Mental status, screening for, 156-161
Mental status assessment, practice
        recommendations for, 164-165
Mental Status Questionnaire, 226-227
Mevinolin, for serum cholesterol, 68
Michigan Alcoholism Screening Test,
        216-217
Micturition, physiology of, 184-187
Mineral supplements, composition of,
        97-98
Mini-Mental State Examination, 157,
        229-231
Mobility, elderly and, 2-3
Monitoring, for drug therapy, 58-60
Monoamine oxidase inhibitors, 160
Mood, depressed, See Depressed mood
Motor vehicle accidents, prevention of,
        133-136
Multi-infarct dementia, 159, 162

Neglect, elder, **167-181**
        emergency, 176-177
        evaluation of, 169-170
        functional assessment and, 170
        practice recommendations and, 179-180
        risk assessment and, 170-172
        support services and, 177-179
    management of, 175-179
    resources for prevention of, 177-179
    signs and symptoms of, 172-174
    table of signs of, 174
Niacin, for serum cholesterol, 68
Nicotine withdrawal syndrome, 101
North Karelia Hypertension Program, 199-200
Nurse practitioners, 209-210
    screening and, 15-15
Nutrients, natural sources of, 93
Nutrition, **89-96**
    deficiencies of, signs and symptoms of,
        93
    elderly and, 4
    over-the-counter food supplements and,
        90-91
    practice recommendations for, 103
Nutritional assessment, questions for, 95
    Risk Index, 218-219

Obesity, 90, 96
    heart disease and, 71

Occult blood testing, fecal, 27-28
Occupational therapist, geriatric team and, 209-214
Osteoporosis, **107-123**
   definition of, 108
   elderly and, 5
   practice recommendations and, 119-121
   prevention of in women, 113-119
   risk factors for, 108-111
      table of, 110
   secondary, causes of, 110-111
   screening for, 111-113
      menopause and, 111-113
Overflow incontinence, 186-187, 190-191
Over-the-counter drugs, adverse interactions and, 56-57

Pap test, 31-32
Passive neglect, 168
Patient education, drug therapy and, 59-60
Pelvic examinations, annual, 32
Pharmacologic therapy, See Drugs
Pharmacotherapy, See Drug therapy
Physical abuse, 167
   self-maintenance scale, 145, 237
   therapist, geriatric team and, **209-214**
Physician, home care and, 212-213
Pneumococcal infections, epidemiology of, 37-38
   vaccine for, cost-benefit of, 201
      effectiveness of, 40
Postmenopausal women, osteoporosis and, 111-118
Prevention, of adverse drug reactions, **47-62**
   cost of, **197-207**
   cost-benefit of, 200-202
      discounting and, 202
   cost of alternatives of, 198-200
      of additional diseases, 204-205
      of additional pensions, 204-205
   for the elderly, **1-245**
      economic barriers to, 205-206
      economics of, **197-207**
      efficacy of, 1-5
   levels of, 14-15
   payers and, 202-204
   primary, 14
   secondary, 14
   tertiary, 14
Prevention Checklist, 241, 244-245
Prevention Flow-Sheet, 240-245

Preventive care, for the elderly, **1-9**
Preventive gerontology, concept of, xi
Primary prevention, 14
Productive aging, xi-xii
Prostate cancer, screening for, 32-33
Prostatic acid phosphatase measurement, for prostate cancer, 32-33
Protein binding, altered, drugs and, 48
Psychiatric consultation, 159

Quality-adjusted life years, 199
Quality of life, screening and, 13

RDAs, 94
Recommended daily dietary allowances, 94
Rectal examination, for prostate cancer, 32-33
Restricted activity, 2
Retirement, depression and, 155

Screening, for cancer, **23-35**
   criteria to justify, 13-15
      asymptomatic period, 14-15
      incidence, 14-15
      quality of life, 13
      tests, 14
      treatment availability, 13
   ethical considerations of, 18-19
   instruments, **215-239**
   patient factors affecting, 17-17
   physician factors affecting, 16-17
   program, evaluation of, 11-15
   practice recommendations and, 20
   principles of, 11-21
   recommendations, 12
      for specific cancers, 27-33
   test, characteristics of, 25-26
   value of, 15-16
SDAT, 161-163
Secondary prevention, 14
Self-help aids, 131-132, 137
Senile macular degeneration, 128
Sensory changes, **125-139**
   age-related, 126-133
   medications and, 138
   practice recommendations and, 137-138
Sensory loss, elderly and, 3
Sensory nerve hearing loss, 130-131
Sexual abuse, 167-168
Short Portable Mental Status Questionnaire, 226-227

Smell, age-related changes and, 132-133
Smoking, 100-103
    elderly and, 4
    nicotine withdrawal and, 101
    practice recommendtions for, 104
    treatment protocol for cessation of, 102
Social Competence Activities scale, 147,
        239
Sound perception, 130-132
Spouse, loss of, 155
Step testing, 77-78
Stress, caregiver, and neglect, 172
Stress incontinence, 186, 192-193

Taste, age-related changes and, 132-133
Team, interdisciplinary geriatric, 209-214
Tertiary prevention, 14
    functional status assessment and,
        141-152
Tetanus vaccine, 38
Tetracyclic antidepressants, 159-161
Thiazide diuretics, for hypertension, 69-70
Thioridazine, 163
Third-party payer, prevention and, 202-204
Tobacco, 100-103
Trazadone, 160
Treadmill tests, 78

Treatments, screening and, 13
Trycyclic antidepressants, 159-161
Triglyceride levels, screening for, 66

Urge incontinence, 186, 193-194
Urinary incontinence, 183-195
    elderly and, 5
    management of, 190-194
    practice recommendations and, 194
    summary table of, 192
Urination, physiology of, 184-187
Uterine cancer, screening for, 31-32

Vaccination, See also Immunization
    side effects of, 42
    status, 42-43
Vasodilators, for hypertension, 70
Violence, See Abuse, elder
Vision, changes in, 127-130
    low, agencies serving, 129
    primary care provider and, 128-130
Vitamin D, and calcium, 116-117
Vitamin toxicity, 90-92

Weight for height table, 93

Zung's Self-Rating Depressing Scale,
        156, 220-221